Cognitive-Behavioral Therapy in Groups

Cognitive-Behavioral Therapy in Groups

PETER J. BIELING

RANDI E. MCCABE

MARTIN M. ANTONY

THE GUILFORD PRESS
New York   London

© 2006 The Guilford Press
A Division of Guilford Publications, Inc.
72 Spring Street, New York, NY 10012
www.guilford.com

Printed in the United States of America

This book is printed on acid-free paper.

Last digit is print number: 9 8 7 6 5 4 3 2

Library of Congress Cataloging-in-Publication Data
Bieling, Peter J.
    Cognitive-behavioral therapy in groups / Peter J. Bieling, Randi E. McCabe, Martin
M. Antony.
      p. cm.
    Includes bibliographical references and index.
    ISBN-10: 1-59385-325-4 ISBN-13: 978-1-59385-325-9 (cloth : alk. paper)
    1. Cognitive therapy. 2. Group psychotherapy. I. McCabe, Randi E. II. Antony,
Martin M. III. Title.
    RC489.C63B54 2006
    616.89′142—dc22
                                                                    2006017072

For Audrey
—P. J. B.

For Liam
—R. E. M.

For Cynthia
—M. M. A.

About the Authors

Peter J. Bieling, PhD, is Associate Professor in the Department of Psychiatry and Behavioural Neurosciences at McMaster University and Director of Mood and Anxiety Services of St. Joseph's Healthcare, Hamilton, Ontario. Dr. Bieling completed his PhD in clinical psychology at the University of British Columbia and did his postdoctoral training at the Center for Cognitive Therapy, University of Pennsylvania, and the Beck Institute for Cognitive Therapy. He has authored many articles in the area of depression, particularly on the psychological factors associated with depression and vulnerability to depression. Dr. Bieling is also a Founding Fellow in the Academy of Cognitive Therapy and has written extensively about cognitive-behavioral therapy for depression. In addition to his research activities and academic work, he is an active therapist and teacher of cognitive-behavioral therapy and a consultant in private practice.

Randi E. McCabe, PhD, is Chair of the Clinical Behavioural Sciences Programme in the Faculty of Health Sciences, a postprofessional diploma program in psychotherapy training at McMaster University. She is Assistant Professor in the Department of Psychiatry and Behavioural Neurosciences at McMaster University and Associate Director of the Anxiety Treatment and Research Centre, a specialized anxiety clinic at St. Joseph's Healthcare in Hamilton, Ontario. Dr. McCabe has written numerous articles, book chapters, and conference presentations on anxiety, eating disorders, and cognitive-behavioral therapy. She has authored three books geared to consumers: *The Overcoming Bulimia Workbook, 10 Simple Solutions to Panic,* and *Overcoming Your Animal and Insect Phobias.* Dr. McCabe is actively involved in training other mental health professionals and has given many workshops on conducting cognitive-behavioral therapy and the treatment of anxiety disorders and eating disorders. She is on the editorial board of *The Clinical Psychologist* and also maintains a private practice where she focuses on eating disorders.

Martin M. Antony, PhD, is Professor in the Department of Psychology, Ryerson University, Toronto, and is Psychologist-in-Chief and Director of the Anxiety Treatment and Research Centre and the Psychology Residency Program at St. Joseph's Healthcare in Hamilton, Ontario. He received his PhD in clinical psychology from the University at Albany, State University of New York, and completed his predoctoral internship training at the University of Mississippi Medical Center in Jackson. Dr. Antony has published 20 books and more than 100 articles and book chapters in the areas of cognitive-behavioral therapy, obsessive–compulsive disorder, panic disorder, social phobia, and specific phobia. He has received career awards from the Society of Clinical Psychology (American Psychological Association), the Canadian Psychological Association, and the Anxiety Disorders Association, and is a Fellow of the American and Canadian Psychological Associations. He has also served on the Boards of Directors for the Society of Clinical Psychology and the Association for Behavioral and Cognitive Therapies, and as Program Chair for past conventions of the Association for Advancement of Behavior Therapy and the Anxiety Disorders Association of America. Dr. Antony is actively involved in clinical research in the area of anxiety disorders, teaching, and education, and he maintains a clinical practice.

Contributors

Arthur Freeman, EdD, Department of Psychology, Philadelphia College of Osteopathic Medicine, Philadelphia, Pennsylvania

Trinh An Nguyen, MS, Department of Psychology, Philadelphia College of Osteopathic Medicine, Philadelphia, Pennsylvania

David L. Penn, PhD, Department of Psychology, University of North Carolina, Chapel Hill, North Carolina

Amy E. Pinkham, MA, Department of Psychology, University of North Carolina, Chapel Hill, North Carolina

David L. Roberts, MA, Department of Psychology, University of North Carolina, Chapel Hill, North Carolina

Frederick Rotgers, PsyD, Department of Psychology, Philadelphia College of Osteopathic Medicine, Philadelphia, Pennsylvania

Jessica L. Stewart, PsyD, Old Rochester Regional School District, Mattapoisett, Massachusetts

Preface

Good ideas sometimes start over good food, and the seeds of this book were sown over lunch several years ago. At our usual spot, Bronzie's, the three of us one day were complaining about a problem we had in common. Each of us was in our own way responsible for running cognitive-behavioral therapy (CBT) groups in our clinics, including training students and junior therapists, and each of us was trying to get every drop of effectiveness that we could out of what we were doing. But each of us felt that we simply did not have all of the resources we needed. Like most, we had a collection of "how-to" protocols and manuals filled with bullet points of techniques that we were using, most with their origins in clinical trials, and we were following these as best we could. But we also noted that these protocols were often silent on issues that seemed to us as practical and important as the sequencing and execution of the cognitive and behavioral strategies they contained—questions like, How do you select people for group therapy? What kind of stance should a group leader take? What kind of leadership style works best? What should you do with a group member who dominates every week? What do you do if someone doesn't speak at all? Why do some groups seem to "gel," while others dwindle to almost no members? Why do some groups seem so rewarding to run, while others become a chore for therapists and maybe their members?

It occurred to us that we were asking questions that were hardly new, and that these were issues considered in another academic tradition—the group process literature. Surely, this work also had something to offer the dyed-in-the-wool CBT therapist? So the concepts percolated as we immersed ourselves in this literature, and gradually, carefully, we sifted through the theories (dense as they are) and tried to distill what we learned into real-world behavioral change in ourselves, in the supervision and advice we gave to trainees, and in our own attempts to optimize the way we were leading groups.

This work is the result of those years of experience and learning. Along the way we found a very receptive ear in Jim Nageotte at The Guilford Press, who encouraged us to formalize our thoughts and who immediately understood the gap we were trying to fill. The eventual result was this book.

In this volume, we try to answer the questions we posed. We attempt to bridge the gap between the typical CBT protocols to follow particular strategies and the real-world messiness that is inherent in translating these specific strategies in a group context. To do so, we illustrate the challenges in this translation with a formalized description of the interplay among group members as they think, feel, and experience together the powerful changes that occur during CBT. We also try to do justice to the complexities of being a group CBT leader and specify the set of skills that group leaders must know and practice if they are to be effective. Through this work, we have come to believe that considering processes in CBT groups is as basic as the mechanics of teaching thought disputation. Group CBT works best only when the interactional properties of the group modality are understood by group leaders and leveraged to maximize learning, change, and growth.

A book like this is not possible without a great team helping along the way. We gratefully acknowledge the organizational skills and editing of David Grant, who carefully went over each chapter. Our invited authors were wonderful not only in sharing their expertise in areas that were weaknesses for us, but also in supporting the overall mission of the book. Jim Nageotte provided terrific feedback, as did several peer reviewers who went well beyond critique to share some excellent ideas from their own perspectives. This feedback rounded out the book and provided key clinical and academic questions that help to close this volume. Finally, we want to thank Paul Basevitz, Susan Chang, Michele Laliberté, and Eli Swartz for their comments on particular chapters.

Contents

PART III. Comorbidity and Future Directions

PART I

General Principles and Practice of Cognitive-Behavioral Therapy Groups

Part I

CHAPTER 1

Cognitive-Behavioral Therapy Groups
POSSIBILITIES AND CHALLENGES

Cognitive-behavioral therapy (CBT) is an empirically validated form of psychotherapy that has been shown to be effective in over 350 outcome studies for myriad psychiatric disorders, ranging from depression to the anxiety disorders, and more recently to personality and psychotic disorders (Beck & Weishaar, 2000). Despite its relatively young age, both as a theory and treatment, the cognitive-behavioral approach has generated unparalleled volumes of research data. There is widespread support for both the therapy itself and many of its theoretical explanations for psychopathology (Bieling & Kuyken, 2003; Clark, Beck, & Alford, 1999).

Traditionally, CBT was described and practiced in an individual format. However, even the original, now classic text on treatment of depression by Beck, Rush, Shaw, and Emery (1979) described the use of a group format. The reasons for this exploration of a group approach then was simple and is as applicable now as in 1979: "More patients can be treated within a given period of time by trained professional therapists than can be treated individually" (Hollon & Shaw, 1979, p. 328). Some authors have found that in terms of therapists' time, groups offer as much as 50% greater efficiency when compared to individual treatment (N. Morrison, 2001). There may also be overall financial savings for the health care system when a group format is used (N. Morrison, 2001; Scott & Stradling, 1990). Efficiency may have been a factor when group CBT was first proposed in the late 1970s, but consideration of costs has since become paramount in health care. In some settings it is now all but impossible to deliver CBT in anything but a group approach due to limited funding.

Beyond the clinician efficiency argument, the efficacy of the group CBT approach has also been confirmed by carefully conducted research that started in the 1970s. For example, in the area of depression, small early studies by Hollon, Shaw, and other collaborators found that a CBT group was superior to several other treatments, but not as effective as individual CBT (Beck et al., 1979). Subsequent reviews and at least one meta-analysis since that time suggest a high level of efficacy, even to the point of equivalence between group and individual CBT for depression (Burlingame, MacKenzie, & Strauss, 2004; Robinson, Berman, & Neimeyer, 1990). In other clinical areas, for example, many different anxiety disorders, considerable evidence for the efficacy and effectiveness of a group approach has emerged (N. Morrison, 2001). The state of evidence for specific disorders is reviewed in the chapters that follow, but there is little doubt now that CBT groups are efficacious and effective.

Importantly, there is also a subset of clinical problems that lends itself to group work, and conceptually at least, would seem to be better treated using a group approach. Social phobia is a prime example, because the focal fear of other people, social evaluation, and concern about how one is perceived are readily tested in a group environment (Heimberg, Salzman, Holt, & Blendell, 1993). Group CBT for social phobia provides ample opportunities to practice exposures to a variety of social situations, to engage in role plays, and to provide different members with feedback about social interactions. Considerable data have since accumulated to support the efficacy of group CBT for social phobia.

The apparent success of the group approach in CBT based on efficacy and cost-effectiveness suggests that over time, more and more disorders are likely to be treated in this modality. Thus, it will be important to continue to refine and develop methods specifically designed for a group approach. Luckily, numerous CBT group protocols are now available in the literature, many based on carefully designed efficacy studies. A collection of approaches for specific disorders, including depression, panic, obesity, eating disorders, and work in specific populations, has also been published (e.g., White & Freeman, 2000). Thus, the literature on how to deliver group CBT continues to expand, with more and more resources becoming available.

Despite the success and availability of group approaches to a variety of disorders, the literature on group CBT contains a number of significant omissions. Because group protocols for CBT tend to be based on individual treatment strategies, it is understandable that such protocols tend to emphasize the adaptation of very specific teaching of principles and strategies of CBT techniques to a collection of individuals. However, this also results in too little attention paid to the simple fact that such strategies are being delivered to an interacting, evolving group. Some authors certainly have recognized that a group modality offers unique therapeutic opportunities. For example, CBT group approaches to depression and social phobia emphasize that patients may more readily recognize cognitive errors made by others than errors made by themselves, and that a group can produce many more examples of links between thoughts and feelings than would be possible in individual therapy (Hollon & Shaw, 1979; Heimberg et al., 1993). However, traditional CBT protocols for groups also imply that group CBT is similar to individual CBT, only the audience has grown from a single person to a handful. Few CBT group approaches meaningfully contemplate the ways in which group members interact with one another, and with the therapist(s). Moreover, when there are two therapists, they are likely to interact with one another, not just with group members. Finally, there is a sense in which "the group" interacts with each individual member throughout treatment. All of these interactions are more than incidental; they involve significant learning opportunities and exchange of information, and clearly involve an inherently "relational" component that is rarely addressed in traditional CBT protocols. The traditional CBT group approach by and large neither recognizes nor takes advantage of the fact that the group itself can create a milieu that either supports or undermines the overall goals of learning and using cognitive and behavioral strategies.

Training group therapists with extant protocols offers dozens of examples of important quandaries and dilemmas that evolve out of a group interactional context that have thus far been difficult to address with currently available treatment protocols. Learners (and some senior therapists!) of group CBT approaches find themselves asking questions such as the following:

- What do I do if one group member seems to not understand a point about evidence gathering but all the others do?
- What should I do if one group member gives nonconstructive, or even mean-spirited, feedback to another member?
- What can I do if the group as a whole seems to be doing less homework because a couple of members never do theirs?
- How can I involve a group member who never offers any examples?
- How can we stay on track when two of the people in group have a second disorder and keep talking about symptoms that no one else has?
- Should we offer an alternative approach to one group member who is clearly not doing well and not keeping up?

These questions, which clearly fall into the "troubleshooting" category, are rarely addressed in group CBT protocols. At an even more basic level, issues such as how best to use group discussion to illustrate the central point of a session or how to maximize the efficiency of reviewing or assigning homework are often not addressed in the CBT group literature.

These important issues can be addressed only by acknowledging that such groups are more than techniques delivered "simultaneously" to multiple clients. The group process issues must be also be considered and leveraged for success, but from the foundation that the principal mechanism of change is based on a cognitive-behavioral model. Indeed, a consideration of group process should not in any way conflict with or suggest a choice between expending time and effort on enhancing process versus focusing on teaching and implementing CBT strategies. Process and technique can and should ideally be symbiotic and rarely in direct competition. The focus of this volume is therefore, to a large extent, the integration of CBT strategies, and the understanding and enhancement of group process to aid in learning and understanding cognitive and behavioral strategies. We also offer specific protocols for disorders, as well as trouble shooting guides, integrating both techniques and the process of applying those techniques in real-world settings.

Interestingly, a similar pattern of evolution can be discerned in the literature on individual CBT in which the early work tended to focus on specific techniques and principles, followed over time by more and more emphasis on enhancing or optimizing the techniques by also considering the therapeutic alliance and interpersonal factors. In their well-known volume on interpersonal processes in CBT, Safran and Segal (1990) advocated for both a theoretical and practical integration of CBT techniques and the therapeutic relationship in which those techniques are communicated. This work added a number of dimensions to CBT, emphasizing the moment-to-moment experiential aspect of cognitive strategies for the patient, attunement of the therapist to the patient's interpersonal schema, as well as the affective, behavioral, and cognitive responses of the therapist to the patient. It is now common practice to emphasize, as the basis for productive CBT, that a strong collaborative therapeutic alliance and attention to both the internal and external reaction of the therapist to the patient are critical factors in individual CBT (Beck, 1995).

Similarly, our aim in this book is to integrate group process factors and CBT techniques. Just as Safran and Segal (1990) suggested that consideration of interpersonal factors in individual CBT should be construed as an evolution toward integration, we believe that considering group process factors in CBT represents the development of a more sophisticated and inclusive model of intervention. We believe that this integration can provide the answers to the several sample questions we posed earlier, and that focusing on such integration will help to set the stage for more clinical developments, research questions, and a richer understanding of the "effective ingredients" in group CBT.

THE GROUP PSYCHOTHERAPY LITERATURE

To begin this integration task, we first turn to the group psychotherapy literature, which has a long tradition of its own that predates CBT. The group psychotherapy movement, with its roots in psychodynamic models of pathology, focus on experiential (or encounter) groups, and historical antithesis to research, appears to be diametrically opposed to the scientist–practitioner mind-set of CBT. Moreover, data on the effectiveness of such generic groups are less clear, and not all aspects of group process can be readily investigated in the same manner as aspects of cognitive-behavioral models or their efficacy.

Stated most plainly, the well-proven techniques in a CBT group are seen as the intervention, and the group is simply the delivery system for those techniques. In the group psychotherapy literature, on the other hand, the group process itself is the intervention. Summarizing this perspective, Burlingame and colleagues (2004) write that in the traditional group approach, "high value is placed on interpersonal and interactional climate of the group, undergirded by the belief that the group is the vehicle of change and that member-to-member interaction is a primary mechanism of change" (p. 647). Writers from the group psychotherapy tradition focus not only on group process over techniques, but may also advocate for groups with heterogeneous diagnoses and an "open" format in which group membership changes as individuals enter and depart the group.

Certainly this process-based theoretical foundation is indeed a stark contrast to the CBT model and group approach. Pragmatically too, few CBT groups are run with an open format, and no empirically supported protocols suggest diagnostic heterogeneity as matter of course. Yet despite the readily apparent differences between these two clinical traditions, work on group process factors does offer many important insights that are useful for CBT. The group literature offers not only a carefully thought out, detailed perspective on the functioning of groups but also a more highly evolved set of strategies for troubleshooting when groups are not functioning optimally. In some cases, knowledge of group process can also be construed as atheoretical, based more on observation and inductive process than on a particular theory. For example, seminal writers such as Yalom attempt to distill from many different kinds of groups, ranging from large didactic groups to small and intense therapy, the effective ingredients that result in change processes in group members.

Indeed, perhaps the most comprehensive perspective in the group psychotherapy field has been offered by Irvin Yalom (1995) in *The Theory and Practice of Group Psychotherapy*. Yalom describes nine relevant therapeutic factors that groups offer, and how each of these can be fostered in the group environment to produce change. These factors are: (1) instillation of hope, (2) universality, (3) imparting information, (4) altruism, (5) the corrective capitulation of the primary family group and interpersonal learning, (6) development of socializing techniques, (7) imitative behavior, (8) group cohesion, and (9) catharsis. Each of these factors is seen to be important in a unique way and more or less present in almost any type of therapeutic group. Burlingame and colleagues (2004) offer a complementary theoretical model that extends this work, yet offers a very concise and specific model of groups that can be adapted to different modalities. These two complementary perspectives on group effectiveness and functioning are briefly described below, followed by an examination of how these factors are relevant to CBT delivered in groups, followed by the beginnings of an integration between CBT and the group factors literature.

Yalom's Group Factors

Yalom (1995) describes *instillation of hope* as a necessary ingredient in all psychotherapies, including group therapy. Yalom suggests that it is important for therapists to reinforce directly the potency of a group approach and to emphasize positive outcomes in members of other groups. Instillation of hope, including narratives of "overcoming" provided by members, appears to be an important component of many self-help groups, including Alcoholics Anonymous (Yalom, 1995).

Universality describes the discovery that others suffer from similar difficulties, often despite patients' conviction that their problems are unique and hence isolating. This factor is more unique to groups than instillation of hope, because it can often be difficult for patients in individual therapy to recognize that their disorder(s) have been experienced by others. Yalom (1995) describes the palpable relief that group members can experience when they, perhaps for the first time, recognize that they are not alone in their suffering.

According to Yalom, the *imparting of information* is a central feature of most groups. This can be further broken down into two specific categories of information, didactic instruction and direct advice. Didactic instruction can be in the form of psychoeducation about the nature of a particular diagnosis or problem, specification of a treatment plan, and a description of how a specific technique might alleviate suffering. At an implicit level, learning about the nature of interpersonal processes and the patient's own interpersonal impact can also occur (Yalom, 1995). The central source of change is seen to be provision of an explanation, a narrative to help the patient understand why and how problems came to exist. Direct advice from the therapist or a copatient may also provide new and helpful information for the patient. Yalom emphasizes the process of advice giving, rather than the content, as offering the most critical learning.

The interpersonal factor of *altruism* refers to the opportunity that group members are given to help one another in the group. If a group member benefits from advice given by another member, then both members benefit. The person receiving the advice obtains helpful information, whereas the person providing the advice benefits from helping another. Groups offer individuals who are often demoralized and marginalized many opportunities to provide others with help, whether by giving advice or offering support, empathy, or understanding. In this way, the group members learn that they can make valuable contributions and have much to offer. Yalom also describes altruism as a sort of antidote to the morbid self-preoccupation that often characterized distressed individuals (Yalom, 1995).

Groups, because they involve peers and "leaders," can also offer opportunities for *corrective recapitulation of the primary family group and interpersonal learning* (Yalom, 1995). Based on the work of attachment theorists such as John Bowlby, and Harry Stack Sullivan's emphasis on interpersonal relationships, the group is thought to constitute a *social microcosm*, a crucible in which the interpersonal patterns of each member will emerge and interact. This offers many opportunities, but in the case of particularly problematic interpersonal styles, can also cause significant strife between members and disrupt the group as a whole. Group leaders are important for helping to moderate rather than amplify these dysfunctional patterns. For example, excessive dependency may express itself as an unusually strong attachment to the group leaders and reliance on their advice and feedback. Similarly, individuals with early experiences of mistrust may have difficulty becoming meaningfully engaged with other group members. The corrective aspects of the experience are provided by both the group members and the leaders, who are able to observe objectively these interpersonal patterns in others. Rather than responding in a way that increases the dysfunction, the group should respond in a way that makes the individual aware of this pattern, so that his or her interpersonal functioning becomes more flexible and adaptive. The interpersonal learning is therefore thought to occur at a fully conscious level; individuals become aware of how they are constructing their interpersonal world and that they have the power to change it. Yalom also emphasizes affect and consequences of this learning. The more affect involved in this realization and behavior change, the more potent the experience (Yalom, 1995). Also, when patients attempt a behavior change and realize that the new behavior has better consequences than their former, more dysfunctional style, the new approach they have learned becomes part of an "adaptive spiral" (Yalom, 1995, p. 43) in which the new behavior gains strength both within and outside the group.

At a more basic interpersonal level, a group can offer *socializing techniques* that involve the development of more basic social skills, either implicitly or through direct exercises including role plays. Groups can give members opportunities to "try out" a variety of new skills or approaches and, unlike many real-world situations, receive direct feedback on the consequences of those actions.

Another area emphasized by Yalom from a traditional group perspective is *imitative behavior*. This factor is based directly on the work of social learning theorists, including Albert Bandura, who identified the process of vicarious or observational learning. In a therapy group, a group member can learn by observing other models of behavior, potentially including both the leaders and group members, from which he or she can gain important information about appropriate and effective interpersonal strategies.

Paralleling the importance of the therapeutic alliance in individual therapy, *group cohesiveness* is seen as a critical ingredient in the process and outcome of any group (Burlingame, Fuhriman, & Johnson, 2002; Yalom, 1995). Operationally, "cohesiveness" is defined as the attraction the members have for the group and for the other members. The ingredients of cohesiveness include acceptance, support, and trust. Similar to unconditional positive regard in individual therapy, the group ideally provides its members an environment in which they can disclose their most private emotions and thoughts, and know in advance that the group will understand and empathize. Yalom (1995) suggests that attendance and, in "open" groups, lower levels of turn-over are indicators of cohesion. Cohesion is typically described as an over-arching condition under which groups operate, and level of cohesion is seen to affect almost all other interpersonal aspects of group process.

Group cohesion has also been among the most studied aspects of group process, even though proponents of group approaches still lament the gap between clinical and research literatures in this area (Burlingame et al., 2004). Reviews of this cohesion research point to a number of discrete principles and practices to create a group with high levels of cohesion (Burlingame et al., 2002). These principles involve factors including pregroup preparation in which members are informed about group functions and roles, high levels of structure in early sessions, consideration of group membership to balance interpersonal and clinical factors, and leadership with a balance of control and expression of regard for all group members and their contributions. Clearly then, cohesion is itself a complex and dynamic grouping of factors, likened to a complex chemical reaction for which all conditions must be right (Burlingame et al., 2002).

Like cohesion, *catharsis* is a seen to be a critical variable in groups but one that defies simple categorization as a single type of event that occurs under specific conditions. Virtually any verbalization made by group members to the leader or to one another can involve an aspect of unburdening, sharing something that has not previously been articulated or even part of self-awareness. However, catharsis is also seen as necessary but not sufficient for a positive outcome: "No one ever obtains enduring benefit for ventilating feelings in an empty closet" (Yalom, 1995, p. 81). Equally important then is the response to the cathartic event, and obviously this could involve information or other kinds of feedback that fit the particular situation. Nonetheless, according to Yalom, a group that does not involve catharsis is unlikely to pro-vide the proper conditions for change.

Burlingame, MacKenzie, and Strauss Group Model

Burlingame, MacKenzie, and Strauss utilize a different framework that is informed on the one hand by Yalom's work and on the other hand by the developing literature on treatment outcome that supports the efficacy of a group approach in many disorders (Burlingame et al., 2004). The results of this dualistic approach are represented in Figure 1.1. With therapeutic out-come as the overarching "fact" to be explained, Burlingame and colleagues include a number of evident contributing factors. One of these is the "formal change theory," in other words, the treatment modality. In the case of CBT, this would correspond to a protocol or session plan describing the CBT princi-ples and techniques to be worked through. The modality occupies an impor-tant but by no means primary position in the Burlingame model. The second critical component in the model, the principles of small-group process, corre-

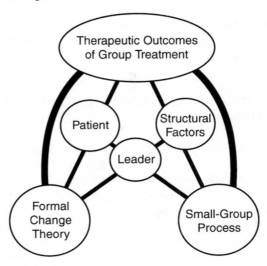

FIGURE 1.1. Forces that govern the therapeutic outcomes of group psychology. From Burlingame, MacKenzie, and Strauss (2004). Copyright 2004 by John Wiley & Sons, Inc. Reprinted by permission.

sponds in many ways with the processes described by Yalom, essentially the various interpersonal relationships that come into operation when a group of individuals gather in a "therapeutic" context.

The other three components are more specific but are seen to have a powerful and unique effect on outcome (Burlingame et al., 2004). One is the patient, in terms of not only his or her their specific disorder but also personal and interpersonal characteristics. Various factors, such as the individual's ability to be empathic to other group members, as well as a host of basic social skills, are believed to have a strong potential to interact with the specific treatment modality (Piper, 1994). Group structural factors make up another component that "explains" the positive impact of a group. This includes factors such as length and number of sessions, frequency of meeting times, group size, and the setting in which treatment takes place. Also considered here is the number of group therapists, and whether or not there exists a hierarchy of leadership.

The final component of the model is at the nexus of the other components (Burlingame et al., 2004). To a great extent, all aspects of group experience are seen to flow through a single source, the group leader(s). The model points out that the style and practice of leadership determine exactly how the formal change techniques are delivered in a group setting. Also, the leader helps to direct and redirect a host of group process variables throughout the moment-to-moment interactions for the duration of the group. The interpersonal approach taken by the leader and levels of warmth, openness, and empathy have been shown to predict cohesiveness and outcome, and are seen to parallel the importance of the therapeutic alliance in individual therapy (Burlingame et al., 2002).

APPLICABILITY OF TRADITIONAL GROUP FACTORS IN CBT GROUPS

We take the view that many of the factors we have described can be adapted or are readily evident within CBT groups, even though few writers have explicitly focused on both group process and CBT. Of course, there are also considerable points of divergence between the traditional group process literature and CBT models of intervention. Below we first consider the process factors as described by Yalom and how they can be related or adapted to a typical group CBT protocol. We then consider the Burlingame et al. model, which already includes a specific modality component, and discuss the implications of choosing CBT as a modality for various aspects of group structure, leadership, and selection of patients.

Yalom's Factors and CBT Groups

Usually as a first step, CBT protocols for specific disorders present participants with a model of their difficulties that emphasizes the possibility for change. In many clinics, information about the efficacy of CBT is also described either in written literature or in early discussions with therapists. From a group perspective, this process is consistent with both *instillation of hope* and *imparting didactic information*. Participants are provided with a model of their difficulties, one that both explains their condition and offers a systematic way to relieve their suffering. Traditionally in CBT, psychoeducation is intertwined with change strategies; for example, explanations of a biopsychosocial model of depression emphasize that changing one system, thought content, can change affect, behavior, and physiology (Greenberger & Padesky, 1995). Within a group context, the possibilities for positive change offered within the group should be consistently emphasized. Instillation of hope can also be enhanced through discussion of case examples, for example, describing other people who have overcome similar problems using the same type of interventions.

Another aspect of group process that likely plays a significant role in CBT is *universality*. The gathering together of individuals with specific disorders is often the first time one sufferer has ever met, let alone gotten to know, another sufferer. This is especially true for those disorders that are less common, for example, obsessive–compulsive or personality disorders. Similarly, some individuals, given the nature of their difficulties, are reluctant to discuss their inner experiences with others except in this new group circumstance. Individuals with social phobia often feel isolated in this manner not only because, like many people with psychiatric disorders, they perceive their problem to be unique, but also because they are the least likely to share their experiences or talk with others in everyday social situations. In the initial phases of CBT group work, individuals often openly express their surprise that other individuals, at this time and this place, have the same problems and have chosen to work on those problems in the group. *Universality* can also be enhanced when group members describe their own difficulties and some background about themselves. After a round of introductions and some autobiographical information, group member often express incredulity that individuals with such different backgrounds could suffer from the same kinds of problems. Such recognition, and the sense of belonging this experience of other group members provides, appears to be very useful in setting the stage for the introduction of more specific CBT strategies and helps to create a milieu that supports cohesion in subsequent sessions.

Once the group begins to focus on specific CBT strategies, for example, thought monitoring and examination of evidence for thoughts, other group factors come into play and can be used to support learning and change. A group can offer many opportunities for its members to express *altruism* whenever a new strategy is introduced. In the case of evidence gathering, therapists typically demonstrate the Socratic approach using one group member's example. Therapists ask questions about both the facts that support a particular thought and evidence that does not support that thought. Group members could and should be encouraged to participate in this questioning process, and this sets the stage for altruism. By asking such evidence-gathering questions of one another, group members can help each other obtain new information or see the events and thoughts in their lives in different ways. The group member whose example is being discussed clearly benefits from these multiple perspectives, but the group members asking these helpful questions also will feel that they are making valuable contributions to one another. Also, by seeing the beneficial impact of asking questions of others, the group members are more likely to ask themselves similar, useful questions. Moreover, it is not uncommon for therapists to discover that the best questions about a thought record examined in the group come from other group members. This important process of group members contributing to the Socratic dialogue needs to be encouraged early on in sessions, for both the altruistic benefit it offers and the diversity of questioning strategies for automatic thoughts that result from broad group participation.

As a CBT group progresses through the discussion of various behavioral strategies, *socializing techniques* and *imitative behavior* become more and more important. A group may offer many opportunities for group members to practice new behaviors with one another. The most obvious application of these is with interpersonal behavior, for example, in practicing to be assertive or to engage in a social interaction that previously engendered anxiety. More broadly, most CBT groups would discuss experiments and action plans within areas that a group member may need to explore in more detail. As in contributing to Socratic dialogue, group members should be encouraged to offer input into developing more adaptive behavioral approaches to their problems. Moreover, if one group member is able to stop a self-defeating behavior, reduce reliance on a dysfunctional compensation strategy, or engage in an anxiety-reducing exposure, other group members have access to a model that has succeeded. When handled optimally, such examples of positive change can engender more hope and purpose in other group members. Encouraging group members to be pleased about one another's successes and to discover how such successes help others to make progress is an important task for therapists to consider. Finally, because the completion of homework tasks is so critical in CBT, therapists need to focus on socializing the group, as a whole, toward the importance and benefit of working on homework. Completion of homework by members offers many opportunities to reinforce the importance of this therapy task, thereby supporting the desire of the other members to imitate homework completion.

As in Yalom's analysis, group *cohesion* in CBT is a factor that combines a sense of trust in and support from other group members. As described earlier, the creation of cohesion is itself a complex "chemical" process; the addition of the specific CBT approach is yet another variable to be considered in that mix. Cohesion has traditionally been seen to occur around the group, but it could be extended to encompass the CBT approach itself. Group members and therapists who share a sense of enthusiasm for the active change strategies of CBT are likely to reinforce each other. However, group cohesion is clearly a varying and variable product and process of CBT groups. When cohesion is high, it is not uncommon for members of CBT groups to exchange phone numbers with one another, to offer each other support around the tasks of treatment. Sometimes groups will continue to meet even after the therapy has ended. This is a clear indicator of attraction of group members to the group, and it is important also to consider the "attraction" to a CBT model. If group members choose to meet or speak outside of group time, therapists may wish to consider to what extent such contact can encourage use of cognitive and behavioral strategies, and reinforce principles taught in treatment. Also important, the trust and support aspects of cohesion set the stage for important self-disclosures. In almost any specific category of disorder, an individual may have "secrets" or cognitive–emotional material that they have rarely, if ever, disclosed to anyone else, let alone to a group. All other things being equal, the higher the level of cohesion, the more likely group members will regularly disclose important affective and cognitive content. The presence of cohesion also increases the probability that highly private revelations will be well received, even if such disclosures have the potential to be upsetting to others. When group members have an affinity and unconditional regard for one another, they are more likely to accept one another throughout the therapy process.

Cohesion can also be low, and this tends to be a particular problem when there is an associated lack of progress toward important clinical goals. There are examples of CBT groups that "fall apart" when a significant number of members drop out. Just as in groups with high cohesion, the reasons for a lack of cohesion are complex and may be difficult to alter, especially if group members are in direct conflict with one another. Putting into place carefully considered measures to increase cohesion, for example, the composition of group members, choice of leaders and leadership style, and preparation of members for the group, will reduce the likelihood that the group will disband prematurely. Cohesion clearly is not static. A group that seems cohesive in early sessions may become less so if progress for some or all members becomes difficult, or if group members have a negative interaction in some way. Troubleshooting and "midcourse" corrections are often necessary to stay on track and in step with the treatment protocol.

Two other group factors described by Yalom may be less relevant to CBT, largely because these factors are, at a theoretical level, antithetical to CBT models and therapeutic strategies. First, *catharsis* alone is unlikely to be seen by most CBT practitioners as useful. Certainly disclosure of private and troubling affect, cognition, and behavior is critical to CBT. However, this disclosure is usually seen only as a first step toward modification of these problems, not an end in itself. Thus, a CBT group should create a forum in which individuals are comfortable and encouraged to reveal private information, even if catharsis is not the ultimate goal of such revelations.

The second group factor that may be less relevant in CBT is *corrective recapitulation of the primary family group*. Because CBT focuses largely on the "here and now" and does not view most problems as rooted in problematic attachment experiences, CBT group protocols are unlikely to focus on this area. Traditional group psychotherapy is more likely to involve a "working through" of early developmental experiences, focusing on recollections of parenting and members' expressing affect and discussing these experiences with one another. However, there are two less direct ways in which CBT groups do relate to early learning, if not recapitulation. First, CBT strategies concerning core beliefs are likely to involve an examination of the origins of such beliefs. This is done to aid understanding of how such beliefs were learned rather than to create a reexperiencing or interpretation of such experiences. Nonetheless, a CBT group should foster an environment in which early experiences can be shared and discussed when needed. Second, just as beliefs about the meaning of situations are uncovered in CBT, these same strategies often result in the discovery of problematic or self-defeating beliefs about other people. Those "interpersonal" beliefs or schemas are likely to be brought to the group experience, as to other relationships in the individual's life, and are often brought to bear in interactions with group members and therapists. For example, a depressed patient who has difficulty trusting others may experience difficulties in trusting fellow group members and the therapists. Not only should this belief itself be targeted in treatment, but it also has the potential to undermine learning from the therapy experience, because the individual doubts whether others are genuinely motivated to help him or her. As a result, the patient may withhold information, not express doubts, or not be motivated to follow up on strategies he or she has learned. Clearly, creating an environment in which such beliefs can be shared and then "tested" through experiments with other group members would be very useful for someone with mistrust beliefs.

Importantly, not all group CBT treatments are likely to deal with interpersonal beliefs or core beliefs in this manner. For example, in some anxiety conditions, such as panic disorder, there may be little focus on interpersonal relationships by design of the protocol. However, in groups for depression, social phobia, and certainly personality disorders, beliefs about others are an important focus of the treatment. A supportive and trusting therapeutic milieu will help participants to share their beliefs about others. How the group receives and responds to these beliefs is an important and very real source of learning for participants. In that sense, a CBT group is indeed an important "micro" social environment that can go a considerable distance toward correcting interpersonal distortions.

The Burlingame et al. Model

The approach advocated by Burlingame and his colleagues adds three factors not considered explicitly by Yalom: the structure of the group context, patient characteristics, and leadership. Each of these areas is certainly touched on by group writers, but the Burlingame model separates these factors into discrete entities since they have been targets of research and conceivably can be linked to outcome in specific ways (Burlingame et al., 2004).

Structure of the group context is typically specified in most CBT protocols, though not necessarily with an explicit rationale. Many common themes emerge across protocols. First, most CBT groups are closed; that is, there is no regular provision for people to join or depart from a group in progress. There are important reasons for this choice, mainly that CBT is a set of skills that should be taught and learned in a linear manner. This choice makes plain that a CBT group emphasizes content of the modality over process. Frequency of meetings is another near-constant factor; most CBT groups meet once per week for between 1 and 2 hours. Again, this choice likely reflects the notion that learning can only take place when intervals between sessions are relatively small, and that optimal learning cannot occur when the duration of any one session exceeds 60–120 minutes. One potentially compelling area of clinical and research interest involving structure is provision of booster groups (Burlingame et al., 2004). Once the acute phase of treatment has ended, it may be desirable to provide occasional booster groups to support wellness, or stated differently, to help the patient avert relapse.*

---

*Emerging studies suggest that maintenance individual psychotherapy promotes stability and prevents relapse in depression (Jarrett et al., 2001; Lenze et al., 2002). Whether this is also the case in the group approach would be important to discover.

The second factor in the Burlingame model considered here is patient characteristics and individual differences. Certainly these do come into play in CBT groups, most obviously based on the primary Axis I diagnosis of the patient. Extant and efficacious protocols for CBT are largely built for a single diagnostic category, and in many cases, efficacy of these approaches is established in individuals with a single Axis I disorder. However, in real-world applications of such protocols, it is likely that significant Axis I and, possibly, Axis II comorbidity and heterogeneity may occur. This may be the case even in settings where patients are selected for a group based on their *primary* diagnosis. These adaptations to a true "effectiveness" context have implications for not only the CBT protocol being used but also the group process. Particular types of diagnoses, especially on Axis II, will have important implications for each individual's predominant interpersonal style, ability to have insight into that impact, and ability to be empathic to others. Also, patients with multiple Axis I disorders will present a different set of complaints, symptoms, affects, and thoughts compared to patients with a single Axis I disorder. Group therapists therefore need to consider the level of flexibility in their protocol and the impact of working with any single individual's unique set of symptoms and functional impairments. A large degree of diagnostic heterogeneity can overwhelm almost any protocol, forcing therapists to invoke such a variety of techniques that group therapy begins to resemble individual CBT with 10 diverse people at once! Clearly this is not ideal from a technique or process perspective; thus, we consider many of these questions explicitly in this volume.

Beyond Axis I and II disorders lies the issue of an individual's "suitability" for CBT. Safran and Segal (1990) pioneered an approach to suitability for CBT in individual therapy that consisted of an interview to determine the level of fit between client and the treatment modality. The 10 specific dimensions considered consisted of a number of broader factors, including abilities to describe affect, emotion, and cognition, compatibility with the rationale of CBT, a desire to engage in an active treatment, and the ability to form therapeutic relationships. The scores on this instrument have shown moderate correlations with both client and therapist ratings of success in treatment (Safran & Segal, 1990). It may be important to consider whether similar factors are useful in a group context, and potentially to add several dimensions of group process; that is, how will this particular person interact with other group members, and what interpersonal impact will he or she bring to the group experience?

Another issue regarding patient-related characteristics concerns patient motivation or potential to change in CBT group. Preparation of a patient for CBT has certainly been considered in individual treatment and may also be considered for group treatment. In individual CBT, emerging "preparatory" approaches have been based on the transtheoretical model of change and motivational interviewing (Rowa, Bieling, & Segal, 2005). Also, the traditional group approach emphasizes the importance of informing group members about the functioning of the group, and their roles and responsibilities, but whether such preparation is necessary or useful in a more didactic group has not been well considered up to this point.

Finally, the Burlingame model places leadership at the nexus of the different group factors. In the area of leadership and leadership style, few CBT group protocols make explicit recommendations despite leadership's presumed importance in the group's experience. In the absence of that recommendation, it tends to be assumed that the interpersonal "style" of a group leader would be very similar to the approach taken in individual CBT. The prerequisites would therefore include empathy, an emphasis on collaborative empiricism, and the ability to foster guided discovery through Socratic dialogue (Beck, 1995). However, beyond these basic requirements, we postulate that leaders of CBT groups also need additional skills that arise from the unique features of the group context. Some have likened the role of the CBT group therapist to that of an orchestra conductor or film director, a person who helps control the action but is clearly not a part of the production (White, 2000). Indeed, group leaders need to be sensitive to a host of group factors, balancing attention to in-session process and affect in each member on the one hand with the need to cover the necessary material in the time available on the other. Thus, there will be times when leaders must make difficult decisions about both process and techniques. Group leaders need to consider connections between patients' experiences with one another, and especially those group interactions that foster learning. In a sense, the best leadership style is one that allows technique to be enveloped in a healthy group process, or allows process to make the techniques feel "live" through the groups' examples.

In many ways, leaders of CBT groups face challenges above and beyond those faced by leaders of more traditional group psychotherapy. Whereas the latter can devote all of their energy toward emphasizing and deepening process, CBT therapists must balance their attention to group relationships with the need to teach certain principles and associated techniques. This requires many difficult decisions throughout the group experience, and often leads to necessary compromises. Thus, there is little doubt that leadership style is an important variable in conducting a CBT group.

DEFINING "PROCESS" FOR CBT GROUPS

One of the clearest challenges that arise from any attempt to integrate the traditional group approaches with CBT is the distinction between group process and techniques. As described earlier, the notion of "process" dominates the approaches of Yalom and other group theorists. However, despite the importance of this concept in group approaches, it often lacks an operational definition; there is a tendency for the general notion of process to be attached to almost every group event. This tendency muddles and confuses the extent to which certain theoretical frames underlie "process." On the one hand, for example, didactic education seems more like a technique anchored in theories of learning than a process. On the other hand, recapitulation of the primary family group relies heavily on a psychodynamic formulation of psychopathology, and it too is often construed as an aspect of "process." This lack of clarity may account for the difficulty with advancing a systematic research agenda for group theories that others have observed (Burlingame et al., 2004).

For our purposes, we distinguish between "process" and "technique" within a CBT group. The latter refers to the commonly understood learning tools and strategies by which patients are educated about their disorder, or are taught to examine their behaviors, thoughts, and feelings, and any strategy designed to change this cognitive-behavioral system. We define "process" as the interpersonal interactions among group members, and between group members and group leaders, and lay out a specific description of these factors in Chapter 2.

PROBLEMS IN CBT GROUPS

Thus far, we have focused on critical group factors and the role these factors can play in the process and learning that occurs in CBT. CBT group therapists also readily acknowledge that every group they treat is different, and that there are clear differences in how "well" groups function. This complex judgment can be based on lack of progress on outcome variables, a low rate of homework completion or, as described earlier, lack of cohesion. Some groups overcome such obstacles; homework completion is targeted with problem-solving strategies by therapists and compliance increases, or group members, with the aid of the therapists, resolve a disagreement and find common ground. When difficulties in a group occur, group factors, rather than the CBT model of intervention, are often responsible. When a group is deemed to be not going well by therapists (or members), this should trigger an examination of what factors are in play. This identification process also points to potential solutions, again, likely related to group process rather than CBT techniques per se.

Aside from specific process variables, CBT groups can function poorly due to the other factors considered here: patient factors, structure, and leadership. Perhaps the mix of patient characteristics in a particular group has impaired the ability of members to make connections with one another. In some instances, a single group member who stands apart from others on some dimension can impede the formation of cohesion in the other members. Structure factors can also impede learning of CBT skills. For example, in groups that reach a certain size (i.e., $n > 12$), leaders quickly run into difficult decisions about involving each group member and being able to "cover" the material in the protocol. Such groups risk becoming underinvolving for their members and more didactic than experiential. Finally, group leaders may have to reexamine their approach when a group is not going well. Is the leadership style too rigid or not focused enough? Is time being effectively managed to cover material and explore group members' examples? All of these factors may need to be considered when running a CBT group, perhaps more so when the group members seem to be struggling or making no forward progress.

CONCLUSIONS

Understanding and working with group process variables can have two significant advantages. First, facilitating these factors may enhance outcome and set the stage for more change, greater levels of intra- and interpersonal learning, and a sense of lasting benefit for group members. We would argue that bringing these models of group process to the CBT context would significantly enrich a clinician's understanding of how to work effectively and optimally in a group setting. Second, awareness and attendance to such factors may help to resolve problems that inevitably arise in a group context. Optimal CBT groups involve a carefully constructed protocol that includes the critical information and exercises to support specific cognitive and behavioral techniques. But these techniques should also be embedded in a comprehensive understanding of group process factors that, in every possible sense, are constantly interacting with the delivery of techniques to influence the overall experience of the group for its members.

The rest of this book is devoted to a further, detailed exploration of these ideas. Rooted in a CBT model, we consider process, patient factors, structure, and leadership style, both generically and for specific disorders. In the remaining chapters of Part I we describe the generic techniques, interventions, and process factors that are likely common to nearly all CBT groups. Chapter 2 more explicitly explores group processes in CBT, focusing on how to marshal these process variables to enhance the group members' experiences, learning, and changes to symptoms and functioning. Chapter 3 provides an overview of specific cognitive strategies for educating patients about the importance of different levels of cognition and the consequences of cognitive processes for affect and behavior. Chapter 4 shifts the focus to behavioral strategies and how these are best communicated and illustrated in a group context. These chapters serve as foundations for the integration of techniques with the process variables introduced here. Chapter 5 focuses on issues that are not always described in specific protocols but are critical for setting the stage for a successful group. In Chapter 6 we describe common pitfalls and obstacles to running successful groups and strategies to resolve these common problems. These issues include ways to structure and lead CBT groups, and we present a number of methods for determining what type of group to conduct and possible leadership configurations.

In Part II we present protocols and methods for treating specific disorders in CBT groups, focusing on both techniques and group processes unique to that type of group. The treatments for disorders described here represent the most common types of difficulties treated with CBT, as well as disorders for which some amount of efficacy data exists. Included in Chapters 7–15, respectively, are panic disorder and agoraphobia, obsessive–compulsive disorder, social phobia, depression, bipolar disorder, eating disorders, substance abuse, personality disorder, and schizophrenia. Unlike the chapters on techniques that are common across a number of disorders, the chapters in Part II focus on techniques and interventions that are unique to a specific disorder. In addition these chapters consider the group process factors that are most critical for that specific disorder, offering troubleshooting and suggestions for optimizing outcomes.

Part III focuses on two additional areas that need to be considered in CBT group work. Co-occurrence of Axis I disorders is the norm in most tertiary care or specialized clinics. Unfortunately, extant protocols for CBT groups rarely take comorbidity into account. Chapter 16 describes the impact of comorbidity on both the application of CBT techniques and group process. Finally, Chapter 17 describes some of the unresolved issues in the clinical and research literature on Group CBT and offers some directions for future work.

CHAPTER 2

Group Process in CBT
USING GROUP DYNAMICS PRODUCTIVELY

Group process has been well described and has a substantial evidence base; for example, a PsycINFO search from 1872 to 2003 reveals 2,102 sources for the term "group process." Yet few sources on CBT groups consider these factors explicitly; combining the seach term "group process" with CBT returned just three papers. Other writers have lamented this lack of information as well. More than 20 years ago, Rose, Tolman, and Tallant (1985) published a study in the *Behavior Therapist* highlighting the role that group process may play in CBT outcome studies. Not surprisingly, they found that there was a lack of attention given group process and its potential role in confounding treatment outcome. Some 20 years later, in this volume, we are attempting to examine group process explicitly from a cognitive-behavioral framework. To this end, we began a search for an operational definition of "group process." The general concept has been approached in a number of areas, including sociology, social psychology, and social work, which makes our search challenging. With respect to clinical psychology, the main source for describing group process has been Irvin Yalom's classic work *The Theory and Practice of Group Psychotherapy*, originally published in 1970 and most recently revised in 1995 for the fourth edition.

Some writers have made a distinction between "process" groups and "structured" groups. "Process groups" focus on the here-and-now group interaction, with the view that the group functions as a vehicle of change driven by group member interaction; "structured" groups, of which cognitive-behavioral groups are a prime example, focus on predetermined session activities consistent with specific therapeutic strategies (Burlingame et al., 2004).

According to this conceptualization, CBT groups, as a form of structured group, are distinct from process groups; thus, it is not a surprise that process factors have been neglected in studies done within a cognitive-behavioral framework.

Others would argue that where there is a group, there is process, regardless of the type of group. According to this view, unique features associated with a group format are theoretically or empirically associated with patient outcome. Moreover, these "process" factors have an influence on group members, over and above the influence of a specific theoretical approach to treatment (Burlingame et al., 2004).

One way that group process may play a role in CBT groups is through facilitation of self-disclosure. As Rose et al. (1985) noted, self-disclosure is necessary for the group to gain access to covert cognitive processes that represent potential treatment targets. In addition, feedback from the group, as well as the therapists, plays a role in helping to shift distorted cognition and reinforce more realistic appraisals. Thus, group process is likely to have a significant impact on CBT group outcome.

Consider the following example. William completed a 12-session group for panic disorder with agoraphobia at a specialized anxiety clinic. Upon completion of treatment, his panic attacks were reduced; however, he still experienced significant agoraphobic avoidance and anticipatory anxiety. His family physician referred him to a different anxiety clinic a year later, when William took a leave of absence from work because of his anxiety symptoms. During the assessment at the new anxiety clinic, William was asked about his previous treatment experience and what components he found helpful or not helpful. William reported that he was not able to benefit from the group, because he was never able to disclose his true fears. He indicated that everyone in his group was worried about passing out, vomiting, or having a heart attack. His concern was about losing control of his bowels and soiling himself. He stated that he was so embarrassed about the nature of his fears that he was never able to disclose them in either the initial assessment or the group. Not until the therapist assessed him a second time and reviewed a list of common fears of people with panic was William able to share his concerns. It is clear in this case that his lack of disclosure in the group prevented the therapists from addressing William's core fears. In addition, his lack of disclosure stemmed in part from process factors within the group. Most likely, William lacked a strong sense of belonging, trust that this "novel" fear would be properly acknowledged by others, and encouragement from group leaders, who failed to recognize the extent to which William was withholding such critical information. These issues are rooted far more in process than in technique.

Although the empirical evidence examining process factors and treatment outcome in CBT is scant, available data indicate that group process factors in CBT groups are recognized by patients as important to the therapeutic experience (Glass & Arnkoff, 2000). Furthermore, these factors are predictive of patient improvement (Castonguay, Pincus, Agras, & Hines, 1998).

WHAT IS GROUP PROCESS?

As we surveyed the literature, it was a challenge to find a precise definition of "group process," because most studies discuss "process" issues and "process" variables, without reference to a specific articulation of what group "process" is. When we polled our clinical colleagues, a definition was just as elusive, and responses such as "Group process includes those factors unique to the group setting that influence group functioning and treatment outcome" were the norm. What are those "factors"? According to A. P. Beck and Lewis (2000), "group psychotherapy process" is the study of the entire group as a system, including changes in the development of the group, interactions between the group members and the therapist (subsystem), interactions among group members (subsystem), interactions between therapist and cotherapist (subsystem), and the interactions of these subsystems with each other and how they are influenced by the group as a whole. This definition of group process is broad and encompassing, yet does not provide us with an operational definition of specific factors consistent with a cognitive-behavioral approach.

Yalom (1995) defined process as the "here-and-now" interactions between group members, the therapist, and the group itself. This process is limited unless there is an "illumination of process" whereby group members reflect on the here-and-now experience that has just occurred. The therapist's role is twofold: to facilitate both here-and-now experience and reflection on that experience (e.g., what information the experience tells us about the relationship of a group member to other group members, the therapist, the group as a whole, and the task of the group). This view, based on an interactional psychotherapy approach, lends itself to process-oriented groups. However, this view has applicability for conceptualizing group process within a CBT model as well.

UNDERSTANDING GROUP PROCESS
WITHIN A CBT MODEL

In 1994, Satterfield presented a hybrid model of conducting cognitive therapy "through a group rather than simply in a group setting" (p. 185). This model integrated group dynamics within a CBT group approach, focusing on how the power of the group could enhance the efficacy of cognitive therapy. Satterfield's hybrid model focused on three group process variables: group cohesion, group developmental stages, and isomorphism (simultaneous interaction on different levels: individual, dyad, subgroups, and the group as a whole).

Our conceptualization of group process within a CBT framework takes a different approach from the hybrid model of Satterfield (1994) and is based on Burlingame and colleagues' (2004) conceptualization of group treatment. Based on this perspective, therapeutic outcome in a CBT group is determined by both the formal CBT strategies and the small-group process present in the group context. The group leader plays a pivotal role in determining whether the treatment proceeds essentially as individual therapy within a group setting or from the perspective of enhancing the CBT by recognizing and building on group process factors.

There are definitions of group process that specify the critical "factors" more precisely. For example, Burlingame et al. (2004) describe "group process" as the theoretical mechanisms of change operative within the group, including group development, therapeutic factors, degree and timing of group structure, and interpersonal feedback. Within this model, therapist factors (e.g., leader characteristics, attention to group process), patient factors (e.g., interpersonal skills, empathy), and structural factors (e.g., length, frequency, setting) are proposed to interact with group process to influence treatment outcome.

DEFINING GROUP PROCESS WITHIN A CBT FRAMEWORK

Becoming even more precise, we put forth a definition of "group process" that aims to operationalize the variables involved. Group process is the set of factors that arise from conducting therapy within a group setting. Factors that we considered in our definition of process in CBT groups include the following:

- The effects of group members' symptoms on one another.
- The effects of group members' personality styles on one another.
- The effects of improvement/worsening in one group member on the others.
- The ways in which group members interact with one another.
- The therapeutic relationship between the therapist and group (e.g., whether they like and trust one another).
- The therapeutic relationship among group members (e.g., whether they like and trust one another).
- The therapeutic relationship between cotherapists (if cotherapist is present).
- The effects of dropout and absenteeism on the group.
- The effect of individual variables on the group:
  - patient expectations
  - patient satisfaction with treatment
  - patient variables that predict outcome
  - patient suitability for group treatment
- Group mechanisms of change:
  - inspiration
  - inclusion

- group learning
- shifting self-focus
- group cohesiveness
- emotional processing in the group setting.

These factors interact with delivery of the specific cognitive-behavioral intervention to influence treatment outcome. These may not be exhaustive, as with other taxonomies of process factors; we have attempted to distill clinical experience in leading CBT groups, and previous influences including the work of Yalom and Burlingame, reviewed in Chapter 1.

USING GROUP PROCESS IN CBT GROUP TREATMENT

According to Yalom (1995), group therapy is associated with specific mechanisms of change that are unique to a group format. These mechanisms of change also represent group process factors. Yalom referred to these interdependent, overlapping constructs as the "therapeutic factors" unique to the group. In Chapter 1, we adapted Yalom's factors to a CBT setting and found that some concepts were highly relevant, whereas others would have little relevance in a CBT-based intervention. In this section, we extend our discussion of process in CBT by proposing a new taxonomy of process factors that reflects this earlier work but proceeds from CBT precepts. Our emphasis here is to consider group process variables that may be utilized with specific interventions to enhance the delivery and impact of CBT. We define each aspect of CBT process, followed by appropriate examples and sample dialogues that illustrate this factor in action.

Optimism

Positive expectations and associated feelings of hopefulness toward recovery are related to better therapeutic outcome. Although this therapeutic factor is not unique to group CBT, the sources of inspiration in the group therapy setting are different. In addition to information provided by the therapist, clients receive information from other group members and observe others getting better over time. In addition, the group serves to enhance motivation to recover by providing an atmosphere that supports behavior change. CBT strategies for maximizing positive expectations for recovery and enhancing motivation occur throughout the course of treatment. During the assessment and inception phase, therapists provide information about the effectiveness of the group approach (from actual group data or the research literature). CBT therapists can rely on the substantial empirical base for the effectiveness of the therapeutic strategies to engender an optimistic attitude and positive expectations regarding therapy outcome. During treatment therapists are able to provide positive reinforcement for practicing strategies, attending group, and tackling problems in a direct way. Therapists can also encourage group members to provide positive feedback to fellow group members, as well as call attention to improvements and progress (e.g., use the exposure hierarchy as a way of highlighting a group member's progress) and have the group reflect on that progress. Over time, more and more of this positive feedback is typically provided from one group member to another based on modeling done by therapists in the initial phases of treatment. For example:

THERAPIST: Let's go around and hear what each group member has planned for exposure practice this week. Also, let us know where your exposure practice ranks in terms of your exposure hierarchy and ratings.

TONY: I am planning to drive to the city. It is number 3 on my list. My anxiety rating is 70 and my avoidance rating is 85.

THERAPIST: Looking back to just before you started group, what were your ratings like?

TONY: My anxiety rating was 95 and my avoidance was 100. That has come down a lot. Before I started this group, I would never have driven to the city.

THERAPIST: What do people think about the progress Tony has made?

POLLY: I think it is wonderful. I can see that group members have already made changes and it has only been four sessions. It makes me more hopeful that this treatment will work for me too.

In this example, the therapist has used exposure hierarchy ratings to highlight Tony's progress, both for him and for other group members.

Inclusion

In the group setting, patients realize that they are not in isolation with their problem; rather, group members have been included in the group for the very fact that they have a shared problem. The CBT therapist can promote a group member's feelings of inclusion by drawing links between the patient's symptoms and experiences, and promoting dialogue among group members on their feelings about having a specific disorder and their attempts to overcome it. For example:

THERAPIST: Now that we have gone around and heard from group members about their symptoms and experiences, we can see that although each person has a unique experience, there are certain similarities that you all share. What do people think or feel about what they have heard?

RON: I feel a great sense of relief. I have been struggling with this anxiety for so long, and I always thought I was alone in this.

KATIE: I have to say I feel like you are all actors, because what you have said is so much exactly like what I have been living with, it is hard to believe that you haven't been planted here to say exactly what I have been experiencing.

GROUP: (*Silence.*)

THERAPIST: What about for others?

POLLY: It is nice to feel that I am not alone in this, but I do worry that hearing about other people's anxiety might make mine worse.

THERAPIST: I am glad you shared that, Polly. Although people may find that their anxiety does increase as we start to work on it directly in therapy, our data tell us that it is exceptionally rare for us to have a group member actually get worse. You have raised a normal concern that is good for us to talk about.

In this example, we can see that checking group members' thoughts and feelings in the here and now is important for not only helping them build a sense that they are not alone but also in giving each group member an opportunity to process doubts that may have interfered with his or her therapeutic progress.

Group-Based Learning

Learning through the group can happen through a number of pathways, including didactic means by the therapist, advice and feedback received from other group members, and observational learning of both the therapists and group members. Psychoeducation is a cornerstone of CBT, but so is experiential, problem-based learning. In the group setting, the CBT therapist should present material in an interactive way that encourages active participation by group members. If a whiteboard is used to present models or information, the CBT therapist should use Socratic questioning to help group members discover new information or provide examples to individualize the model to their own unique experiences. In terms of advice and feedback from other group members, the CBT therapist can facilitate provision of feedback and advice so that it is given in a helpful way, ideally through guided discovery between group members. CBT therapists can encourage modeling behavior in the group setting through therapist- and group member–assisted exposure, role plays, and sharing of strategies and approaches to problem solving among group members. For example:

KATIE: I didn't do very well this week. I was able to go to the grocery store, but I wasn't able to go alone. I took my daughter with me. I got very anxious in the store but was able to stay there until my anxiety came down. I am kind of disappointed that I wasn't able to do it by myself.

THERAPIST: What do people think about how Katie did this week?

RON: Even though you took your daughter with you, it is still a major accomplishment that you went and stayed.

POLLY: I agree, even though you felt anxious, you stayed. It seems like you are focusing on the negative—what you wanted to do but couldn't—and not on what you actually did.

THERAPIST: Katie, what do you think about what people are saying?

KATIE: It is helpful to have that perspective; it's true that I need to focus on what I did do. I was focusing on the negatives, and that really brings my confidence down. I feel better about what I was able to do this week.

In this example, the therapist uses the group to provide feedback, giving Katie a different perspective. As a result, Katie has learned to evaluate her progress in a more evenhanded fashion. Using the group in this way is a more powerful way to learn, because the group provides the key ingredients of the "lesson," which is likely to be more meaningful and persuasive than if the therapist alone had emphasized that same point.

Shifting Self-Focus

The benefit of being able to help other group members is an important aspect of the group experience. In addition, the group provides an atmosphere that shifts focus from the self to focus on other group members and on the group itself. CBT therapists can promote this shift by facilitating group members in providing support, giving reassurance, and sharing strategies with the group. In a sense, support provided to others reflects back, benefiting each individual. For example:

TONY: I found that I was so stressed at work this week I felt too anxious to do the exposures I had planned. I was worried that if I did them, I would really have a bad week.

THERAPIST: Do others find that you are worried about doing exposures when you're already stressed or not feeling well and if so, how do you manage?

POLLY: I can totally relate. I just tell myself that whether I do the exposure or not, I am going to feel anxious. At least if I do it, then I know that I will feel much better afterward.

TONY: That is true. I did feel even worse that I didn't do the homework I had planned, and I felt anxious anyway.

RON: Tony, is there a way that you can cut back on your stress at work so that you have more time to work on your exposures? I know, for me, I need to save some energy for doing the homework, so I've rearranged some other things until after the group.

TONY: You're right. I probably need to do the same thing.

In this example, we not only see that Tony benefits from the input of group members but also that the group members are able to derive a sense of effectiveness from being able to help a fellow group member.

Modification of Maladaptive Relational Patterns

The group provides a corrective social learning experience for maladaptive interpersonal patterns that have developed through early experiences. As Yalom (1995) noted, the group represents a social microcosm, in that group members interact with each other the way they would interact with others in the external world. Thus, group provides an excellent opportunity for interpersonal learning. Although a focus on socializing techniques and skills is an explicit component of CBT treatment for social phobia, it is also an implicit component of any group. The CBT therapist can facilitate awareness of interpersonal patterns and the effect that a group member's style may have on other group members. By focusing on current interactions among group members and cotherapists, interpersonal patterns can be identified. The therapist can then elicit feedback, modify maladaptive appraisals, and encourage different ways of behaving that may be more adaptive or in line with personal goals and values. Interpersonal learning may also occur through other group process factors, including group education and altruism. In addition, the group leader may utilize specific CBT techniques (e.g., exposure, role play, identification of maladaptive appraisals and core beliefs) to facilitate corrective experience within the group setting.

Group Cohesiveness

According to Yalom (1995), group cohesiveness in group therapy is the equivalent of the therapeutic alliance in individual therapy. "Group cohesiveness" may be defined as the conditions that hold group members within the group (e.g., feelings of comfort and belonging, valuing the group, and unconditional acceptance by other group members; Bloch & Crouch, 1985). Promoting group cohesion is an important task for the group therapist. In comparison to noncohesive groups, cohesive groups are more likely to have increased participation, increased acceptance of group members, increased self-disclosure, increased sense of security for group members, increased openness by group members, and less susceptibility to disruption (e.g., dropout, deviation from group norms; Yalom, 1995).

The CBT group therapist can use a number of strategies to increase cohesiveness:

- Increase homogeneity of the group in pregroup selection.
- Encourage consistent attendance.
- Provide a safe environment for self-disclosure, largely through modeling of acceptance, empathy, and helpful feedback.

- Promote sharing of information.
- Make connections between two or more group members' experiences.
- Attend to group process in the here and now.

Emotional Processing in the Group Setting

The group setting promotes open expression and processing of emotion. By balancing the agenda of each group session with processing thoughts and feelings among the group members in the here and now, the CBT group therapist can promote expression and processing of feelings in a way that is in line with the goals of the group. In addition, processing in the here and now may help to elicit important automatic thoughts, assumptions, beliefs, and behaviors that become a target for intervention. In the example that follows, the therapist is introducing the concept of cognitive distortions when she notices that a group member is doodling on a paper in front of him and appears disengaged. The other group members appear interested and attentive. It may be that some members of the group have also noticed the disengaged member. Instead of continuing with discussion of cognitive distortions in the group, the therapist shifts to the here and now to process what is happening.

THERAPIST: Before we go on to talk about examples each of you may have, I just want to check in with the group. Tony, I noticed that you seem distracted. Can you tell us what is going on for you?

TONY: Nothing.

THERAPIST: Oh. How does what we were covering fit for you?

TONY: Well, I am just feeling like it doesn't fit. I'm discouraged because I don't think this therapy will help me. It seems like a lot of work, and I don't see how it can ever make this anxiety go away.

THERAPIST: Does anyone else ever feel discouraged about overcoming their anxiety?

POLLY: (*Nods her head.*)

KATIE: Yes, I sometimes feel that way too.

THERAPIST: What do you do to stay hopeful, Katie?

KATIE: I just try to keep an open mind. I mean, what do I have to lose by trying this treatment? If I don't try, then how will I ever get rid of this anxiety?

THERAPIST: Tony, what is it like for you to know that other people also feel discouraged sometimes?

TONY: Well, I guess it makes me feel more normal. Maybe I can give this a try. Katie's right. I really don't have anything to lose, because my life has already been ruined by this anxiety.

In this example, the therapist has shifted from introducing a CBT concept to processing a group member's feelings about the treatment in the here and now. By attending to the emotional climate of the group, and strong emotions in one group member, the therapist has not only refocused and validated that one individual but has also opened this line of inquiry for the entire group and made it a subject that can be shared and addressed. In addition, left unattended, the disengaged group member was at risk of believing that he was not getting sufficient understanding or support from the group. As a result of this intervention, group cohesion has likely increased; group members have been invited to support one another and have also learned that their therapist is responsive to their emotional state and not just solely interested in teaching strategies. The therapist was also able to elicit the discouraged group member's automatic thoughts about treatment ("Treatment will not work") as well as his beliefs about the future ("This anxiety will never go away"). She has now accessed "live" material that can be used to illustrate the concepts she was introducing in the session as part of her agenda (cognitive distortions).

In this section, we have attempted to capture the major factors representing mechanisms of change unique to group therapy from a CBT perspective. These are summarized and operationally defined in Table 2.1. Whether we have been overinclusive or underinclusive in our attempt is an empirical question, and one that we hope will be a focus of future inquiry. In any case, the purpose and goals of the group will determine the therapeutic factors that may be a focus of attention. In any single group there may be certain factors at the forefront. It is up to the CBT group therapist to identify those factors that are operating and to then work with these processes in parallel with the CBT-specific group agenda.

ATTENDING TO GROUP PROCESS WITHIN A CBT STRUCTURE

It is helpful to think of these same group process factors within the technique-specific structure of CBT group therapy sessions. The structure of these sessions often includes the following components: homework review, presentation of new information, practicing skills (e.g., examples, role play, exposure), and planning homework for the week.

Homework Review

Homework review is an important part of each CBT group therapy session in which group members relate their experience practicing the skills or strategies that they learned from the previous session. This is an opportunity to reinforce CBT principles, provide encouragement and positive feedback, and problem-solve obstacles or challenges that may have gotten in the way.

TABLE 2.1. Group Process Factors: Mechanisms of Change from a CBT Perspective

Process factor	Description	Therapeutic strategy
Optimism	The group provides an atmosphere that promotes an optimistic, hopeful outlook on overcoming the problem, as well as motivational activation.	• Provide data on effectiveness of approach. • Provide positive reinforcement of group participation. • Facilitate group members to provide positive reinforcement of other group members. • Highlight improvement and progress. • Use group members' experience to promote positive expectations. • Utilize the group to promote cognitive shifts in expectations.
Inclusion	The group raises awareness of a shared problem and provides a sense of belonging and reduced isolation.	• Link group members' symptoms and experiences. • Promote dialogue among the group members about having the specific problem and attempts toward recovery.
Group learning	The group provides an opportunity for learning on a number of levels.	• Provide psychoeducation in an interactive manner. • Use Socratic technique to help group members to discover new information. • Facilitate provision of feedback and advice from other group members. • Use group to provide a range of perspectives and appraisals. • Utilize therapist- and group member–assisted exposure and role plays.
Shifting self-focus	The group promotes helping of other group members, shifting emphasis from the individual to the group.	• Facilitate group members to provide support, share information and strategies, and give reassurance.
Modification of maladaptive relational patterns	The group provides a corrective learning experience for maladaptive interpersonal interactions.	• Facilitate awareness of interpersonal patterns and the effect one has on other group members. • Focus on current interactions in the group. • Elicit feedback. • Modify maladaptive appraisals. • Encourage alternative ways of behaving. • Utilize specific CBT techniques to facilitate corrective experience: exposure, role play, identification of appraisals and core beliefs.

(continued)

TABLE 2.1. *(continued)*

Process factor	Description	Therapeutic strategy
Group cohesiveness	The attractiveness of a group to its members facilitates cognitive and behavioral change.	• Encourage consistent attendance and commitment to group. • Promote a safe environment for self-disclosure. • Promote sharing of information. • Make connections among group members' experiences, thoughts, and feelings. • Attend to other group process factors in the here and now.
Emotional processing in the group setting	The group provides a place for open expression and working through of emotions, thoughts, and behaviors, allowing for the identification of therapeutic targets for intervention.	• Encourage expression of feelings in real time. • Examine feelings associated with specific thoughts and courses of action. • Encourage processing among the group members.

In CBT group therapy where there is an inattention to group process, the homework review looks like individual therapy moving along a circle as each group member reviews his or her week and how the homework went. Often, this can take up to 5 or 10 minutes per group member, with the therapist and cotherapist asking questions of each person. If one were to look around the group during such an instance, one would likely see that some of the other group members have "zoned out," are doodling on a paper, looking out the window, or generally appear "disengaged" from what is going on within the group. Such an approach casts an explicit and implicit spotlight on one group member, literally excluding all the others. Consider the two examples that follow:

Lack of Attention to Group Process

THERAPIST: Who would like to tell us how their week went with the homework?

GROUP: (*Silence.*)

THERAPIST: Katie, would you like to fill us in on how things went for you?

KATIE: Sure, I guess. This week went pretty good. I found that I tried to stay in some situations that usually I wouldn't, so that I could experience some anxiety.

THERAPIST: That's great! Can you tell us about one of those situations?

KATIE: Well, I went to the grocery store, and when I got anxious I stayed where I was and kept going down the aisle even though I felt like bolting. I took a basket instead of a cart, so I was feeling really nervous, because usually I feel less anxious with a cart.

THERAPIST: Why is that?

KATIE: Well, if I have the cart, then I feel safer, like if I get nervous I will have something to hold on to.

COTHERAPIST: That is really good Katie. It sounds like you really challenged yourself, so that you could experience some anxiety. Who would like to go next?

Attention to Group Process

THERAPIST: Who would like to tell us how their week went with the homework?

GROUP: (*Silence.*)

THERAPIST: Katie, would you like to fill us in on how things went for you?

KATIE: Sure, I guess. This week went pretty good. I found that I tried to stay in some situations that usually I wouldn't, so that I could experience some anxiety.

THERAPIST: (*Nods head.*)

KATIE: Well, I went to the grocery store, and when I got anxious I stayed where I was and kept going down the aisle even though I felt like bolting. I took a basket instead of a cart, so I was feeling really nervous, because usually I feel less anxious with a cart.

THERAPIST: That's great! Did anyone else find that they had to challenge themselves a bit so that they experienced some anxiety?

RON: Yes, I let my wife drive when we went out, which triggered quite a bit of anxiety, as I usually like to be in control and be in charge of driving.

THERAPIST: That's excellent. Polly, I saw that you were also nodding your head.

POLLY: I had a very similar experience to Katie. I went to a store by myself. Usually I take my children, which makes me less anxious.

COTHERAPIST: That is interesting, Polly. It sounds like both you and Katie practiced eliminating a safety behavior so that you would experience some anxiety. Katie, what happened when you were at the store without your cart?

KATIE: Well, I did get quite anxious, because I had nothing to hold onto if I felt lightheaded. I kept going down the aisle even though I felt like bolting.

THERAPIST: That is really great. Who would like to go next?

With either of these approaches, the therapist reviews homework and how the week went. In the first approach, the therapist's style is efficient and gets the job done. However, the lack of attention to group process fails to marshal the power inherent in the group. In the first example, group members are likely to learn that when one group member is talking, they are not a part of the interaction and therefore do not have to pay a lot of attention, and above all, that they have nothing to learn from a discussion between a group therapist and another member of the group. In the second approach, the therapist builds group cohesion by having the group members relate their experiences to each other, and highlights similarities. This keeps the other group members engaged and interested. These participants are likely to learn, over time, that homework review is relevant for the entire group, that they can learn from similarities and differences between themselves and others, even when they are not being questioned directly themselves.

Presenting New Information

Often, a portion of the group session is focused on the presentation of new information, whether this is psychoeducational in nature or laying the groundwork for learning a new strategy or skill. In CBT group therapy where there is a lack of attention to group process, this portion of the session often resembles what takes place in a classroom. In that scenario, the therapist and cotherapist are the teachers working on a blackboard and the group members are the students. Typically, the therapists actively present the new information and the group members absorb it passively. In contrast, when there is a focus on group process, the therapist and cotherapist present new information in a more interactive style whereby material is solicited from the group and then processed within the group. Consider the following two examples:

Lack of Attention to Group Process

THERAPIST: Today we are going to talk about our thoughts and how they can be distorted. People with anxiety tend to distort their thoughts by overestimating the probability of a bad thing happening and underestimating their ability to cope. They also tend to think that these scary outcomes will be much worse than they realistically are. This first type of distortion is called probability overestimation. The second type of distortion is called catastrophization. Does that make sense to people?

GROUP: (*Members are nodding their heads.*)

THERAPIST: Okay, does anyone have any questions or thoughts about these two types of distortions?

GROUP: (*Silence.*)

THERAPIST: Okay, why don't we all look at your homework and see if any of your thoughts would be good examples of probability overestimation or catastrophization.

Attention to Group Process

THERAPIST: Okay, today we are going to talk about our thoughts and how they can be distorted. When you think about the word "distortion," what do you think it means?

TONY: It means that it is shifted from the truth.

THERAPIST: Exactly, we all see things in our own way, which is often a distortion from the way things really are. Can anybody think of an example of this?

POLLY: In my family, my brother always thinks that he does all the work around the house but really he doesn't. His thoughts are obviously distorted! (*Group members laugh.*)

COTHERAPIST: That is a great example! Now let's think about when you all are feeling anxious. How are your thoughts distorted?

RON: I tend to be focusing on the "what ifs"—like what if I have a heart attack? What if this numbness down my arm is a sign that I am going to die? Maybe I should go to the hospital.

THERAPIST: And why are those thought distortions, Ron?

RON: Because I always have them but nothing ever happens.

COTHERAPIST: That is a nice example. So it sounds like, based on your own experience, you have felt these physical sensations many times but nothing bad has ever happened. However, every time you have them, you focus not on what is realistically likely but rather on the potential danger.

RON: Exactly.

THERAPIST: Do other people find that they tend to do that as well?

GROUP: (*Members nod.*)

THERAPIST: Okay, we actually have names for the types of anxiety distortions that people with anxiety tend to make. The first one is called probability overestimation. Who wants to guess what that is?

POLLY: Well, that sounds like what Ron was describing. Overestimating the chances of a bad thing happening. I do that when I think I am going to pass out every time I am anxious, even though I never have.

THERAPIST: Exactly. That is a good example too. The second type of distortion that anxious people tend to make is catastrophization. Who can guess what that is?

KATIE: Well, I guess it is like it sounds. Thinking that something is a catastrophe.

COTHERAPIST: Exactly. And what does that mean?

KATIE: Well, thinking it is worse than it really is?

THERAPIST: Can anyone think of an example for this?

TONY: Yeah. I think that when I am anxious, people will notice and it will be awful.

THERAPIST: Right. When you are anxious, it feels really horrible and people may notice. But is it really a big deal if people notice?

TONY: Not when I really think about it. In fact, even though I worry about people noticing, I am not even sure if people really can tell when I am anxious.

By focusing on group process and presenting the new material in a more interactive manner in the second example, the group is more engaged and participative in the process of learning the information rather than absorbing it passively. Both approaches have the therapist asking at least some Socratic questions, but in the second example the questions are much simpler and phrased in an open-ended manner, so that many more people are likely to contribute. The therapists also carefully build the information from multiple perspectives, doing a much better job of guided discovery. In the second example, the therapists are far more likely to hold the attention of the group members and have group members looking for opportunities to contribute to the dialogue.

Practicing Skills/Exposure

After group members practice new skills, exposures, or role plays in the group, it is important to process the experience with the group as a whole before moving on in the session. Therapists should focus on members' thoughts and feelings about the experience and try to make connections between group members' experiences. This helps build group cohesion and also provides important feedback. Consider the following example, which took place in a therapy session after the group returned from doing exposures at a shopping mall:

THERAPIST: How do people feel about how the exposures went?

TONY: I feel good about it. Although I was anxious taking the bus on the way down, I felt less anxious on the way back.

THERAPIST: That is great. (*Looks around at the group.*)

RON: I had a different experience. Although I was anxious about going to the mall, when I got there I wasn't really anxious at all. My anticipatory anxiety was much worse than the actual situation.

COTHERAPIST: That is interesting. Did other people find that?

POLLY: Yes, although I was really anxious when we were walking around the mall, it wasn't as bad as I thought it would be before we got there.

THERAPIST: What about for you, Katie?

KATIE: Well, I am not doing as well as everyone else. I felt anxious the whole time.

THERAPIST: What do other people think about Katie not doing as well as everyone else?

TONY: Katie, you did a good job just even going. It was really hard for me too, when I did this for the first time a couple of weeks ago. We are all at different stages. I think it will go better for you next time.

COTHERAPIST: That brings up a great point. Often in the group people tend to compare themselves to how others are doing. It is important to remember that everyone is starting at a different place and will be working at a different pace.

In this example, it is clear that if the activities were not discussed in the group, Katie would have gone home feeling that she was not progressing as well as everyone else. This could also make her vulnerable to dropping out. In addition, having a group member tell Katie that she was doing a good job is much more powerful then if the therapist had told her. Processing CBT exercises in the group context enables other group members to provide feedback, help one another, and learn from each other's experiences.

Planning Homework

Homework can also be planned with attention to group process. Instead of having each member go around and plan his or her homework with the therapist, group members can be involved to help think of potential homework practices and problem-solve potential obstacles. This helps keep the group engaged in the process and uses the group to its potential. It also serves to increase motivation of group members when they return to group the following week, because they know that the other group members are interested in how things went.

Therapeutic Strategies Within Session and Across Treatment

The previous examples reveal a number of interventions and strategies that the group therapist can use to conduct CBT effectively, while also paying attention to and using group process. Other issues of process that need to be attended to in a CBT group to maximize the potency of the group experience include the following:

- Achieving a balance between group members and therapists in terms of "air time."
- Ensuring that each group member receives a similar amount of attention from the group.
- Achieving a balance between focusing on the individual, particularly during guided discovery, and taking issues back to the group for general feedback.
- Managing group members that miss sessions and processing the effect this may have on the group.
- Addressing the fact of "dropouts" in a group and the effect this has on sense of cohesion.
- Balancing interaction between cotherapists and supporting one another's interventions.
- Balancing working on specific skills/agendas and group members' thoughts/feelings in the here and now.
- Processing progress in the group (how members feel about being in the group, particularly at the start of treatment, how treatment is going, etc.).
- Allowing group members to provide feedback or answer questions posed to the therapist.
- Using Socratic questioning and interactive methods to present new information and elicit relevant material from group members.

STAGES OF GROUP DEVELOPMENT

All groups are believed to develop over time in distinct phases: preparation, initial stage, transition stage, working stage, and final stage (Corey, Corey, Callanan, & Russell, 2004). In the preparation phase, group leaders meet with members individually to screen for their appropriateness for the group treatment options, review the goals of treatment, provide education on how group treatment works, reduce apprehension about participating in group therapy, and discuss the importance of confidentiality. Although Corey and colleagues discuss the stages of group evolution in reference to an intensive, short-term residential group therapy session (20 hours over 3 days), the stages they describe may also be useful for examining the unfolding of a CBT group. In fact, Corey (2000) discusses behavioral group therapy and rational-emotive behavior therapy from a group development perspective in terms of six stages as illustrated in Table 2.2. Although it remains an empirical question whether CBT groups go through different stages, it has been our clinical experience that the group does evolve over time in repeatable and predictable sequences. In the next section we review each of the stages of group evolution from a CBT context, along with specific interventions and strategies that the therapist may use to facilitate group process.

TABLE 2.2. Stages of Group Development and Therapist Tasks

Stage	Development	Therapist tasks
1	Pregroup issues: Formation of the group	• Plan group. • Recruitment. • Screening. • Pregroup meeting. • Preparation of group members.
2	Initial stage: Orientation and exploration	• Set structure of group. • Explore expectations. • Define goals. • Build group cohesion (trust). • Manage initial anxiety of group members.
3	Transition stage: Dealing with resistance	• Help members work on concerns that brought them to group. • Manage resistance, anxiety, and conflict.
4	Working stage: Cohesion and productivity	• Transition to allow group members a more active role. • Provide feedback and reinforcement. • Facilitate interaction. • Be aware of therapeutic factors of group process and manage these factors accordingly to produce behavior change. • Support motivation for change. • Process current here-and-now patterns in the group at appropriate times. • Encourage translation of increased understanding to action.
5	Final stage: Consolidation and termination	• Reinforce changes. • Process experience in group. • Provide further resources as appropriate. • Support continued work on treatment goals. • Discuss incorporation of skills learned in group to situations of daily life. • Develop continued goals. • Set foundation for utilizing group experience (knowledge and skills) when necessary.
6	Postgroup issues: Follow-up and evaluation	• Hold follow-up group to check in on progress. • Identify obstacles and process issues. • Provide further resources if needed. • Evaluate outcome of group. • Schedule individual follow-up, if desired.

Note. Data from Corey (2000).

Initial Stage

Pregroup individual meetings are recommended to educate prospective members about the group and group process before it begins. This is also a final opportunity for the group leaders to screen prospective members to ensure their appropriateness for the group. In the initial stage, the identity of the group is formed. Norms are established and members develop an understanding of the group experience. Members get acquainted, trust is developed, and initial resistance may occur. The latter term is important to define before moving on.

The concept of resistance is rooted in psychoanalytic theory, yet we can operationalize resistance from a cognitive-behavioral framework (Leahy, 2001). Resistance is the interruption of therapeutic progress (e.g., noncompliance) due to factors related to the patient (e.g., lack of understanding of the therapeutic rationale, lack of readiness for action-oriented treatment, lack of commitment to treatment), the therapist (failure to develop strong therapeutic alliance, lack of clarification around the rationale for a specific therapeutic strategy, focus on the wrong problem), or the therapeutic strategy (inappropriate treatment strategy for patient). Strategies for working with resistance in the group setting are covered in depth in Chapter 6.

In the initial stage, the main tasks of the group leaders are to build cohesiveness (develop trust within the group), impart group structure, and establish treatment targets or goals (Corey, 2000).

Specific strategies for attending to and managing group process during this phase include the following:

- Ensuring that the therapist and cotherapist are spaced appropriately in the group.
- Going through introductions (e.g., have group members go around and say their name and something about themselves, such as a hobby, a pet, or a favorite place to travel). An ice-breaker exercise may also be useful (e.g., have group members pair off in dyads and share something about themselves, then report back on the group member they have met when the group resumes).
- Encouraging group members to participate spontaneously, without calling on them by name or going around in a circle.
- Reviewing the norms of group (e.g., expectations for participation, attendance, missed sessions, homework requirements, confidentiality).
- Discussing group members' reactions, thoughts, and feelings about being in the group.
- Normalizing anxiety or apprehension that members may feel about being in a group.
- Encouraging interaction among group members.
- Making associations between group members' symptoms to encourage group cohesiveness.

- Asking other group members if they can relate to a particular group member's experience to promote group cohesion.
- Encouraging group members to go at their own pace.
- Transition from being directive to allowing group members to become more active in the group.

Transition Stage

In the transition stage, often just a few sessions into a CBT group, group members have become more comfortable in the group and conflict may arise as group members voice concerns about the group leaders, other group members, or the therapy and techniques. Group members may become more aware of their thoughts, feelings, and behaviors, as well as their symptoms. They may express concern that their symptoms have worsened since the group started or wonder whether the group leaders can help them if they themselves have not experienced the problem the group is focused on. Group members may not be ready to engage in treatment actively, or they may be apprehensive or ambivalent.

Working Stage

In the working stage, the group actively works on material in the group and between sessions. These middle sessions also feature the bulk of the techniques. During this phase it is important to continue to encourage feedback, particularly support and positive reinforcement between group members for changes and progress. Group leaders also need to encourage sharing of difficulties and obstacles group members are encountering, as well as unresolved issues. Homework should be planned collaboratively, ideally with feedback from the group around what types of work or exercises would be most useful for the group as a whole. It is also important to remind group members that time is passing, so that they are prepared for termination and gain motivation to practice the CBT skills they are developing outside of the group.

Final Stage

In the final stage of the group, members are considering how they will proceed once the group has ended. As in individual therapy, it is important to allow time for discussion of termination issues, including thoughts and feelings about the group ending. A formal "good-bye" exercise or closing can be included. There should also be time devoted to a review of what members have gained from the group (where they were, where they are now, and where they are going), what obstacles they have overcome, and what goals they will continue to work on. Sharing the "effective ingredients" of the group for each group member will be important for relapse prevention and maintenance of CBT skills.

POTENTIAL PROBLEMS

A number of problems may arise in conducting group therapy. These problems interfere not only with the CBT agenda but also with group process and the therapeutic efficacy of the group intervention. Problems that arise may include the following:

- Problems with group process (e.g., formation of subgroups or emergence of a nontherapeutic group culture).
- Problems in leadership (e.g., leadership style or skills).
- Problems with individual group members' personality styles or expectations (e.g., lack of disclosure, passivity, hopelessness).

These problems may be addressed by managing group process, as well as using specific CBT interventions (examining beliefs about the group, the role of each group member in the group, etc.). A more elaborate examination of the potential problems and challenges that arise in group treatment is conducted in Chapter 6.

RESEARCH DIRECTIONS

The empirical literature on group CBT effectiveness continues to grow, with an emphasis on the question of symptom change. As Greenberg noted in the A. P. Beck and Lewis (2000) text on the process of group psychotherapy, "In studying change, the majority of psychotherapy researchers have tended to focus on the easier question 'Has change occurred?' and have left the much more difficult question 'How does change occur?' to those of heartier souls" (p. xiii). This is certainly true of the empirical literature on CBT group effectiveness. Given that group process factors likely do play a role in outcome, there is a need for future research on CBT group effectiveness to study these factors and their relation to outcome. Greene (2000) draws attention to this issue as follows: "It is ironic that the most empirically studied group therapy modality [CBT] ignores the group qua group as a potential therapeutic agent" (p. 24). To study group process factors operating within a CBT group, we must first understand these factors from a CBT perspective. This chapter represents a first step in that direction. It is our hope that our discussion of group process within a CBT framework may stimulate much needed research on the role these factors play within CBT group therapy.

CHAPTER 3

Cognitive Strategies in CBT Groups

This chapter describes some of the most frequently used cognitive therapy techniques and how they can be adapted and applied to a group setting. In addition to presenting these techniques, the definition of CBT group process is considered and its various aspects (described in Chapter 2) are conveyed in sample dialogues and attached descriptions of each strategy. One obvious challenge in presenting these strategies is that there likely exists no absolute or correct way to determine how many cognitive techniques are essential in CBT and how to classify the different strategies. Previous authors describing CBT have opted for different presentations, some using a relatively delimited number of domains (Beck, 1995) and others using a "compendium" approach featuring dozens and dozens of very specific strategies (Leahy, 2003; McMullin, 2000). An additional consideration is that cognitive strategies will be presented differently depending on the disorder being treated. Indeed, in Part II we describe specific protocols for different disorders and examine techniques that are unique to each disorder. We emphasize here the relatively more broad cognitive strategies that are likely to be present in nearly all protocols and provide examples of dialogue to illustrate these that might occur in groups with a variety of different diagnoses.

The areas of technique we describe are intended not only to be fundamental but also to be building blocks for more varied and specific offshoots, analogies, or Socratic dialogue. Familiarity with the areas described here should be prerequisite prior to use of disorder-specific protocols. Moreover, there are instances in which CBT might be administered in a heterogeneous group with multiple disorders. The areas we describe would likely be useful in almost all diagnostic categories.

We have grouped the techniques into four broad categories: (1) connection between thoughts, situational triggers, and the elicitation of negative affect, including depression and anxiety; (2) use of evidence gathering and thought distortions to become more objective about one's thoughts; (3) use of experiments; and (4) exploration of underlying beliefs and assumptions. Throughout, we also focus on the three fundamental concepts of cognitive therapy that underlie each of these domains: collaborative empiricism, Socratic dialogue, and guided discovery (A. Beck & Weishaar, 2000). The group modality alters each of these fundamental precepts of cognitive techniques in very specific ways. We next define each of these terms, taking into account group process factors.

Collaborative empiricism is achieved when therapist and patient join forces to investigate thoughts and experiences in a manner that is reminiscent of the scientific method. This requires developing hypotheses about thoughts and testing these through logical analysis and collection of factual evidence. Importantly, this partnership helps to demystify the process of change since the techniques for change are shared openly and step-by-step (A. Beck & Weishaar, 2000). Of course, in a group, the essential elements of this definition are left intact; however, the relationship must necessarily expand to include interactions between therapists and group members, and interactions among group members. In a sense, group members become therapists for one another, asking questions rather than providing direct advice or feedback. The role of therapist also becomes more complex because collaborative empiricism needs to be cultivated not only between therapist and patient but also between patients. This requires direct modeling and feedback about the need to ask questions and more subtle forms of socialization. Therapists also need to reflect on that process through summaries and reiteration of the process, namely, collaborative empiricism, by which the group has assisted its members with examining their thoughts. This is useful for ensuring generalization of the empirical approach when group members are applying the approach, by themselves, between sessions.

Socratic dialogue, a series of interconnected questions that lead to a more logical, objective conclusion about one's inner experiences, is also a common theme for all cognitive techniques (Beck & Young, 1985). In fact, asking open-ended and open-minded questions is probably one of the most critical and distinguishing features of CBT. Four basic steps in this questioning process have been described: (1) characterizing the problem specifically and accurately; (2) identifying the associated thoughts, beliefs, and interpretations; (3) understanding the meanings of the thoughts for the patient; and (4) assessing the consequences of thoughts and their basis in evidence (Beck & Weishaar, 2000). Although the questions in a Socratic dialogue should neither lead nor trap the patient into agreeing with the therapist's view (which is, of course, inevitably biased), the questions are intended to stimulate consideration of alternative perspectives and uncover information that was not previously considered.

In individual therapy, the clinician has the task of asking questions that will help to illuminate new information and new perspectives. Cognitive therapists can quickly become adept at formulating questions, anticipating possible answers, and even considering the question that might follow the one currently being asked, or at least considering possible answers and where these might lead. However, this process becomes much more complex in a group. Multiple individuals, including cotherapists and other patients, will be asking questions of the patient whose example is being considered. Thus, therapists must not only keep up with the questioning strategy they are using, but they must also process, in an "online" manner, where questions asked by others will lead the discussion. Therapists must also evaluate the usefulness, or therapeutic value, of questions group members ask of one another. Although this seems like a difficult, even impossible task, in practice it is important to consider that many lines of questioning, even in individual therapy, can come to an unproductive end. Multiple lines of questioning must very often be used to discover useful information, and unless an example runs well over the allotted time, there is no harm in using multiple types of questioning or starting over using a new questioning approach. Nonetheless, an important component of the therapist's work is to teach group members to ask useful and therapeutic questions of one another, in addition to being ready to ask themselves useful questions. This is a process that readily develops over time. In early sessions, therapists are more likely to be asking most of the questions, while group members observe and learn strategies. Over time, more and more of the questioning strategies can be left to the group, with occasional "course corrections" from therapists. For therapists, this can also be illuminating and surprising, because group members very often ask highly useful questions that the therapists may not have considered. This only reinforces the value and power of Socratic dialogue and the importance of multiple perspectives inherent in a group of individuals.

The final underlying factor common to many cognitive techniques is *guided discovery*. Here, the therapist helps to illuminate meaning of thoughts and problems in logic, or helps to create situations from which the patient learns new information and different ways of thinking, acting, and feeling. In a group setting, guided discovery takes on the additional dimension that there are multiple possible guides in addition to the therapist. Although therapists undoubtedly retain a considerable portion of authority and lead the group through exercises and examples, the group significantly influences that process. For example, if a therapist wishes to help a group member to create an experiment to test the validity of a thought, the therapist might suggest a basic approach, with group members making additional suggestions or modifications. The advantage of having the group help to guide discovery is that this often makes the process more creative. However, therapists as leaders must retain the option of not heeding group suggestions that are not helpful or valid for the specific example being considered. Group members often make helpful suggestions, but this is not universal, and at times the input of the group may impede guided discovery. Such difficulties are considered explicitly in Chapter 6, which offers a guide to troubleshooting both process and technique factors.

The three change strategies in cognitive therapy—collaborative empiricism, Socratic dialogue, and guided discovery—are evident in each of the four technique content areas we describe next. We recognize that our presentation of those four stages of cognitive therapy technique is somewhat arbitrary and caution therapists that we do not intend for these techniques always to be presented exactly as described here. Instead, we would ask therapists to regard collaborative empiricism, Socratic dialogue, and guided discovery as a set of philosophical principles or values. Keeping these principles of the intervention in view, therapists can construct an infinite number of specific techniques that might be suited to a particular group in a specific instance.

COGNITIVE TECHNIQUES I: CONNECTING THOUGHTS TO SITUATIONS AND AFFECT

Eliciting automatic thoughts and educating patients about the connections between this "inner dialogue" and their affective reactions to events are often the first areas examined by the group. In some instances, group members will have had an opportunity to record events that changed their mood or other symptoms and to have made an initial attempt to record what they recall thinking or saying to themselves. Other times, group members may be asked to recall a recent situation that elicited strong negative feelings, anxiety, or other symptoms they are seeking to change.

In either case, group members are sensitized to the idea of "shifts" in their emotional state, and will be encouraged to take the opportunity to record what was happening at that time, and what they were feeling and thinking. This may seem straightforward, and it is in many instances; however, some group members have considerable difficulty identifying mood shifts or articulating their thoughts. There are other ways to elicit thoughts, initially by asking questions about what was happening in the person's mind, or by providing generic examples that might parallel the patient's experience. Another alternative is to have the person imagine the situation as if it were happening again; this allows group members who have some initial difficulties with the process to remember their thoughts.

This process, the recording of thoughts, is usually done on something that resembles the daily record of dysfunctional thoughts (DRDT). Many different and specific forms of this record exist, usually customized for the specific disorder of interest. However, almost all forms will have columns to represent the situation encountered, the emotion or symptoms, and the recorded thoughts. In the example to follow, group members would have been asked to attempt to complete only those three columns of the record, so as to sensitize them to the idea of recording their thoughts. This can take some practice; some group members will find the idea of writing down their internal, often negative dialogue to be somewhat unusual and even acutely uncomfortable. Even those group members who have no difficulty with this recording are unlikely straight away to record those thoughts that contain the most emotional content, which we would term the "hot" thought (Greenberger & Padesky, 1995). Through further questioning and dialogue, the group helps each member refine the ability to record thoughts and become more and more aware of which thought is "hot" and of central importance to his or her experience.

The example that follows, while obviously involving a specific circumstance, could well occur in almost any kind of group setting, especially where depression and anxiety are prominent features. The example also lends itself to exploration with the other techniques we describe here and is thus carried forward in the rest of the chapter. The setting is a review of homework in which the group member has, for the first time, recorded an incident that was upsetting. Also of importance, therapists need to be aware that an initial discussion of negative thoughts can be an area of considerable sensitivity to each group member. More than likely, patients will be sharing information about their thoughts that they have never communicated to anyone, much a less a group of people they have only recently started to know. The therapist illustrating this technique has the following goals, and the dialogue reflects each of these:

1. Help the patient connect the event with a certain set of thoughts that have important consequences for affect.
2. Lay the groundwork for "shaping" the group's thought records so that all members becomes more likely to record the "hot" thoughts they are experiencing.
3. Model questions one can ask oneself (or others) to specify thoughts and their connections to events and emotions.
4. Emphasize the importance of understanding one's thoughts as an initial step to change emotional responses.
5. Maintain positive group processes, particularly inclusion, cohesiveness, and emotional processing, so that group members experience the group as a welcoming, supportive environment in which to share and explore their private thoughts and affect.

THERAPIST: Now that we have had a chance to put the first part of Ron's example on the white board, let's explore it a bit more. So, to make sure we're all on the same page, the situation was this: Your friend called you to ask if you'd help him fix his garage door; you went over and it was pretty daunting. You guys worked on it for a while, then your friend had to go to work, but you stayed there and tried to fix it until just after midnight. The emotions you experienced then, and since, are sadness and anxiety, and you've been feeling tense. Does that seem right so far?

RON: Yeah, that's pretty much it.

THERAPIST: Okay, and the thoughts you wrote down are "This thing is a mess; it's so old"; "I wish I had the right tools for this"; and "I can't believe I can't fix this." That sounds like it must have been kind of frustrating. Do other people feel like they understand Ron's experience?

POLLY: I think so. I know I get frustrated when things are broken and I can't fix them.

KATIE: Me too, Ron. I think it was good of you to stay even after he left. That must not have been a fun way to spend your whole evening.

THERAPIST: Okay, let's remember that for now, the thing we want to do is to focus on thoughts; later on we'll focus on what to do with those thoughts. Ron, were there any other thoughts you had that you might not have recorded?

RON: I'm not sure. I guess it's interesting what Katie said. My friend thought it was weird that I wanted to stay; he told me to go home, too. But I just felt like I had to get that done.

THERAPIST: I wonder if that's important. Why would you say you "had" to get it done? What are the thoughts about having to get it done?

RON: Well, I guess when someone asks for your help, it's up to you, and they're relying on you. If you can't do it, you've let them down. And I'm pretty good at fixing stuff like this. I should have been able to do it.

THERAPIST: Were you thinking these things then?

RON: Sure. That's true.

THERAPIST: So let's write that down. "It's up to me"; "I should have been able to do it"; and "If I can't do it, I'm letting him down." Those sound like other thoughts you were having then. (*Writes thought on board.*)

KATIE: But you did a lot for your friend already; that doesn't seem fair.

POLLY: He's lucky to have you as a friend. I don't have many friends that would help me out that way.

(*Silence.*)

THERAPIST: So Ron, that's some interesting feedback, I think, but for now let's focus again on thoughts you did have. Remember that, for all of us, the first step is to understand our thoughts. Later on we'll explore the thoughts in detail.

RON: Okay.

THERAPIST: Now that we've listed this new thought, look at them again and tell me which one was the most upsetting to you.

(*Pause.*)

RON: I guess it's the idea that I'm letting him down. I felt like I couldn't leave until it was done, and that was really weighing on me.

THERAPIST: That's a difficult thought, so we call that thought the "hot thought." (*Circles the thought.*) It's the one that results in the strongest emotions, and often it's the thought that drives a lot of other thoughts. Do other people think that if they were in the situation Ron was in and had the thought Ron had—that they were letting someone down—they'd also feel sad or unhappy?

POLLY: Definitely, that's hard for me, too. You know, like when I know someone is disappointed with me.

KATIE: I can see that, but I still think what Ron did was pretty helpful.

THERAPIST: Those are good points everyone. The main thing for now is to begin talking more about which thoughts we have that are the most troubling, contain the most emotion, or really drive how we feel and act. Hot thoughts are those thoughts that would make anyone having them feel a strong negative emotion. Let's look at someone else's example next.

In this example, the therapist first summarizes the information, but the first significant impetus for the interventions to follow is the therapist's belief that not all the most relevant thoughts have been recorded yet. The therapist engages the group, then asks Ron directly whether there were any other thoughts going on that were not recorded. Indeed, perhaps based on a cue offered by another group member, Ron describes a completely new but seemingly important theme: his perception of what his friend would think, and a strong imperative to to not disappoint his friend. Group members subsequently offer some supportive feedback that, in a sense, questions the need for the thought or its validity. These statements are not necessarily related to the point of the example, exploring Ron's hot thoughts. However, they have the advantage of contributing to process factors, including group cohesion, inclusion, and shifting self-focus. In essence Ron learns (and so do other group member through modeling) that the group is receptive to and supportive of discussing these thoughts, and the group members learn that they have something important to contribute in helping one another. Once Ron agrees on what the hot thought is, the therapist checks to see whether the group relates to this particular experience and the thought attached to it, as well as making a more general psychoeducative point about what a hot thought is.

Subsequent examples would be used in an attempt to work with each group member to locate a hot thought. This could take an entire session, and the homework would involve members completing a DRDT and identifying, on their own, the hot thought by asking themselves which thought was most troubling or upsetting.

COGNITIVE TECHNIQUES II: USE OF EVIDENCE GATHERING AND THOUGHT DISTORTIONS

Once group members are able to identify their painful "automatic thoughts," the group can begin to focus on reexamining these negative conclusions. Employing a Socratic approach, the group members learn to question their thoughts and take a more wide-ranging, objective view of the facts involved in a situation that they found emotionally distressing. This dialogue typically consists of many informational questions and then synthesizing questions that help patients to integrate the new information in a way that differs from their original conclusion (the hot thought). Critical questions in this process typically involve having persons think about their experience from another perspective, considering factors that they did not at first consider, and pointing out any logical leaps that might not be warranted by the actual facts. It is important to emphasize that evidence gathering and examination for distortion do not represent "positive thinking," nor should questions to be used to trap patients or invalidate their thoughts. Instead, the questions enable patients to look at the situation objectively and nondefensively.

The most common way to determine whether a negative thought might be distorted is by eliciting the "evidence" for and against the negative thought. First, all the facts—not interpretations or suggestions, but the objective facts that support the negative conclusion—need to be listed. Next, group members learn to ask questions that identify factual information that is not consistent with the original conclusion. The kinds of questions therapists ask vary according to the situation. Broadly defined, questions that gather evidence against the automatic thought are usually (1) ascertaining all the situational parameters related to a negative thought, especially those outside of the patient's control or responsibility; (2) asking patients to shift perspective on the situation by having them perceive the situation "through" another person; and (3) having patients focus on information that is incomplete or unsubstantiated. Once a more complete picture of the situation emerges, patients are asked to formulate a "balanced" thought that takes into account all of the evidence from the questioning process. This process usually helps to illuminate the kinds of cognitive errors, or distortions, patients made when they did not take into account all of the information. Typically, the group takes an example from one of its members, and both therapists and group members are encouraged to participate in asking questions of the person supplying the example. In addition, therapists summarize and highlight questioning strategies that will be useful beyond the context of the current example, so that group members consider such questions for their own thoughts.

Systematic errors in cognitive processing, or *cognitive distortions* (Beck et al., 1979), are often the basis for negative thoughts. Various lists of cognitive distortions exist, and different distortions are seen in different kinds of disorders. Most generally, cognitive distortions include the following:

- *Arbitrary inference*: Drawing a specific conclusion without supporting evidence or even in the face of contradictory evidence. An example of this is a harried worker, who cannot accomplish all of his or her tasks one day, thinking, "I'm a horrible employee."
- *Selective abstraction*: Conceptualizing a situation on the basis of a detail taken out of context, ignoring other information. An example is

the person who takes one piece of negative feedback from an evaluation with 10 pieces of positive feedback and becomes sad and hopeless.

- *Overgeneralization*: Abstracting a general rule from one or a few isolated incidents and applying it too broadly and to unrelated situations. After having difficulty with an unruly child in a class, a teacher concluded, "All of these children are ill-mannered."
- *Magnification and minimization*: Seeing something as far more or less significant than it actually is. After a woman on a date unintentionally mentioned that her former boyfriend had left her, she thought, "Now I've done it. He knows there's something wrong with me."
- *Personalization*: Attributing external events to oneself without evidence supporting a causal connection. At a party, a woman overheard someone saying that there weren't enough interesting people at the gathering, and she thought, "I know he's talking about me."
- *Dichotomous thinking or black-and-white thinking*: Categorizing experiences in one of two extremes; for example, as complete success or total failure. A woman who was cooking a family dinner felt that one of her dishes had not turned out perfectly, and she thought, "The entire dinner is ruined."
- *Mind Reading*: This error occurs when someone believes he or she knows what another person is thinking, without any direct evidence. A woman's friend did not return her call about plans for the weekend, and the woman thought, "She's fed up with my depression and doesn't want to be around me."

Teaching group members about these distortions in conjunction with evidence gathering is extremely useful, because once these concepts are understood, patients can quickly tackle their own cognitive errors. Once patients have identified their "usual" cognitive errors, they are able to correct their thinking more efficiently.

Use of these cognitive strategies in group follows the usual pattern for presenting techniques. Therapists provide a brief but careful didactic overview, in this case describing both the need to gather evidence around one's thoughts and possible distortions. Next, an example is provided by one of the group members. The therapist initially walks through the example, taking a leadership role in the process as the group learns the technique. Gradually, and over the course of further examples, the group leaders take on a less directive role, potentially helping the group to initiate questions, and correcting the course of questions only as needed. Eventually, each group member will have multiple opportunities both to ask questions of others and to have his or her particular example examined by the group.

The sample dialogue that follows, for the sake of efficiency, carries on the DRDT described earlier in which Ron's automatic thought was "It's up to me; if I can't do it I'm letting him down," in response to not having been able to repair a friend's garage door. This dialogue takes place in a subsequent session, where the aim is to gather evidence for that thought and identify any cognitive distortions that might be taking place. The goals of the therapist here are as follows:

1. Uncover evidence around the hot thought that is useful for Ron to consider.
2. Model and shape asking of Socratic questions by the group, as opposed to direct advice giving or offering reinterpretation or rationalizations.
3. Help group members to see how such questions can apply to their own thoughts.
4. Work with Ron and the group to identify whether a cognitive distortion has taken place.
5. Illustrate the usefulness for all group members of identifying cognitive distortions.
6. Continue to foster positive group process, particularly inclusion, group learning, and shifting self-focus.

The dialogue begins after the therapists have explained the evidence-gathering process and the distortion concepts using a "textbook" example to illustrate these didactic points.

THERAPIST: So let's take this thought—"It's up to me, if I can't do it I'm letting him down"—in the situation that Ron has told us about, trying for several hours to fix his friend's garage door and not being able to do that. Now we'd like to try out the evidence-gathering approach we've just talked about. The first step here then is to ask yourself, Ron, what evidence you have that supports your conclusion that you let your friend down. Remember the evidence has to be a fact, not an interpretation or an opinion.

(*Silence.*)

RON: Well, he did say he needed to get this fixed to get the car in and out, and since I couldn't fix it, he would have had to call somebody and pay for a repair.

THERAPIST: Okay, that is some information that we can write down. If other people have a question about this situation, one that might help Ron with the evidence collecting, feel free to ask it.

KATIE: Ron, did your friend say something to make you think he was disappointed?

RON: No, but he told me before I started that he was at his wits' end with that thing, and that if we couldn't repair it that night, he would call someone to fix it . . . and he said he didn't want to pay for that.

KATIE: I just think that your friend would have no right to blame you or hold you responsible.

THERAPIST: Let's hang on to that for just a minute. I just want to remind us all that for now we should be thinking about questions to ask Ron to help gather evidence, not trying to reach a conclusion yet. I understand what you're getting at, Katie, but let's think of that as a question for Ron.

KATIE: Okay. I guess the question in my mind is that it doesn't seem like his friend said anything directly about being disappointed in Ron. Is that right? (*Looks to Ron.*)

RON: No, he didn't. The last thing he said to me was that I should go home and not worry about it. He'd take care of it in the morning, and he was thankful that I tried.

THERAPIST: So that's a fact that I think belongs in the "evidence against" column. What do you guys think, and what do you think, Ron?

RON: Yeah, it's true. He didn't say he was disappointed in me.

POLLY: I just want to say that I think that is definitely evidence. I can see that his friend would want to have the door fixed, and none of us would want to pay for it, but I can't imagine blaming my friend after he tried to help me.

THERAPIST: I see what you are saying, Polly. Can you turn that into a question you could ask Ron?

POLLY: Umm . . . I guess what I would ask is, has this friend ever blamed you for something like this in the past? Do you think he's a good friend and appreciates you, and does he normally get mad at you for things? I'm not sure I'm being clear.

THERAPIST: That's a good start. Polly, are you asking whether there is a history of this friend blaming Ron or being disappointed?

POLLY: Yeah.

RON: Not at all. We do favors back and forth all the time. . . . I'm sure next week I'll ask him to come over and help me with my eaves trough or something.

THERAPIST: My question would be, has there ever been a time when your friend was helping you and the job was tough or didn't go well?

(*Silence.*)

RON: One time (*Smiling.*) I had a tree taken down, and he and I tried to pull the stump out. That was a fiasco; we had no idea what we were dealing with. Eventually a guy came with a backhoe and ripped it out. It was a huge job.

KATIE: So when the two of you couldn't do it yourselves, were you disappointed with him?

RON: No. The job was way too much for two guys. Unless we'd had some dynamite!

THERAPIST: So is it possible that, in this situation, what we've discovered is that the garage door needs to be fixed by a professional?

RON: Yeah, or replaced because it is ancient.

THERAPIST: So the evidence says that we have no fact that points directly to your friend actually being disappointed with you, even if he's frustrated by the door being broken. What we do know is he said "thank you" for your help, we know you've had a long history of helping each other, and when the two of you couldn't remove the stump, you weren't disappointed in him, and that perhaps this problem needs a professional fix.

RON: When I hear it like that, the whole thing looks pretty different.

THERAPIST: That's great. So what we all learn from this is that we can take a situation that we think we know all about, then step back and ask each other questions that put it into a different light. As we go along, it's important to remember that we can ask these questions of ourselves too, and whenever we feel a very strong emotion about a situation, we should be asking ourselves these types of questions about evidence.

In the evidence-gathering portion of this example, the therapist asks the first question and elicits what evidence Ron has for his automatic thought. As the dialogue suggests, group members tend to jump in quickly, typically pointing out possible evidence against, or even alternative interpretations, rather than asking questions to weigh that evidence. Such statements are certainly supportive, increasing inclusion and cohesion, and need to be welcomed by therapists, while at the same time being honed to maximize group learning. Where possible, the therapist consistently aims to create a Socratic dialogue, turning an observation into a question that can be directed to Ron. Note also that the therapist asks a question that leads to an answer from Ron and a related "follow-up" question from another group member that is even more helpful. This is an example of the therapist seeding a questioning strategy, and it is not unusual for other group members to pick up that theme. Finally, the therapist summarizes what has occurred and redirects group members to question their own thoughts, and in this way maximizes group learning from the example.

To complete this technique, the following dialogue focuses on the application of a thought distortion to this situation:

THERAPIST: Now let's see if we can look again at the list of thought distortions we handed out earlier. And let's look at Ron's example for which we just gathered all that evidence. Ron, when you look at that evidence and the list of distortions, do you think that any of those apply here?

(Silence.)

RON: Umm, I'm not sure. The way I'm seeing it now, I guess I jumped to a conclusion that wasn't warranted.

THERAPIST: Okay, anybody else see something on that list that fits the situation, and how it fits the situation?

POLLY: It seems to me that this would be "mind reading," because Ron made an assumption about what his friend was thinking about him and what happened. Am I right?

THERAPIST: There may be no perfect answer, but I think that what you and Ron are saying about this is situation is similar. What do others think?

KATIE: I think it was mind reading.

RON: Me too. You know it wasn't like this was about fixing that door; it's what he was thinking about me. The more I think about it, the more mind reading seems like the one that fits.

THERAPIST: Okay, that's the important part. Remember that the distortion list might help you figure out if you've made a kind of error in your thinking, and it might help you to catch yourself more quickly.

KATIE: Boy, do I relate to that one. I think I'm mind reading all of the time, especially with my husband.

THERAPIST: Sometimes discussing these distortions will help you realize that you do them quite a bit, so it's good that you've noticed that, Katie. Let's talk about when that happens for you in more detail next.

This dialogue would be typical of a group trying to apply the thought distortion list for the first time. Ron has some amount of uncertainty, and other group members make suggestions that help to illustrate the "correct" answer. Group learning is in evidence as the group members move toward a consensus. Also notable is that with little prompting, this discussion triggers another group member to contribute a potentially useful example.

COGNITIVE TECHNIQUES III: EXPERIMENTS

Aside from identifying a distortion and useful evidence, a DRDT may also point to a lack of information or leave the individual with unanswered questions about the meaning of a situation. In such instances, patients are encouraged to conduct an *experiment*, essentially a plan to gather the information they need to reach a conclusion about the accuracy of a negative thought. The experiment in cognitive therapy embodies collaborative empiricism and asking questions in an open-minded manner. Many experiments involve some form of returning to the situation and gathering more information, but the essence of any experiment is to form a hypothesis about a thought and a way to test that hypothesis. For example, in the situation described in the group dialogue, where a group member has been "mind reading," the group member could be encouraged to check his or her conclusions with the other person involved in the situation.

The key to a powerful experiment is to create two hypotheses that are credible and important, and that can be proven by facts to be either true or false. In individual treatment, often the patient's hypothesis is related to his or her automatic thought—that is, a negative conclusion about a situation. The therapist, at least initially, typically offers an alternative hypothesis that represents a more balanced, evenhanded view of the situation. Therapist and patient then work together to develop a simple methodology to "test" each of their ideas. Before any exploration is carried out, discussion should take place about what information is likely to emerge and what that information will mean to each person's hypotheses. Both the therapist and the patient are likely to have an attachment to their hypotheses, but both commit to allowing the evidence that emerges to influence their view.

In a group setting, the hypotheses and methods of the experiment are influenced in a more complex way by the entire group. However, group members can also contribute novel and useful suggestions for testing ideas. In the sample dialogue, the therapist focuses on the following objectives:

1. Clarification of the patient's hypothesis and an alternative, balanced hypothesis.
2. Development of a method for testing those ideas that is compelling for not only the patient but also for other group members.
3. Maximization of learning by reminding group members about how they can use experiments themselves.
4. Focus on group factors, including cohesion and shifting self-focus.

Prior to this dialogue, the therapist(s) would have presented the concept of an experiment didactically and with a preplanned, simple example. For the sake of simplicity, the dialogue focuses on the situation Ron encountered with his friend:

THERAPIST: So, Ron, going back to that situation with your friend and fixing his garage door, it seems you weren't sure what to conclude. Your initial automatic thought was that your friend was disappointed in you, and we couldn't find a lot of direct evidence for that. At the same time, that was just how it felt to you. I'm wondering if we can use that as an example for creating an experiment like we've just talked about.

RON: Sure.

THERAPIST: Okay, let's see what we can do with that, and hopefully, if we all put our heads together, we can come up with something. As we described, we start with hypotheses, and it seems that your hypothesis, from your hot thought, is "He's disappointed with me." The next step would be the alternative hypothesis. Any ideas?

POLLY: I think he was probably grateful to you.

KATIE: Me too, even if he was frustrated with the door.

THERAPIST: Okay, that seems like it's related to the evidence. Ron, are you okay with the alternative hypothesis—"He's not disappointed, he's grateful"?

RON: Well, I don't believe that, but that's what other people seem to think.

THERAPIST: That's okay, so long as we come up with a way to distinguish between these two hypotheses; in other words, we need to come up with a way to test out which of these two opposing ideas is true. Any ideas?

KATIE: I think you could ask him. Call him up and ask what he thought of you helping him the other night maybe?

RON: What if he doesn't mention anything about how he felt about what I did?

THERAPIST: Hmm, I think that asking him is a good start, but I can also see that what you need to know might not come up.

POLLY: Why not ask him directly whether he was disappointed in you?

THERAPIST: That would get to the heart of it.

RON: I can ask him. That's probably the only way it will come up.

THERAPIST: All right, so based on your hypothesis, he'd answer that he was disappointed in you. The alternative hypothesis predicts that he will say he was grateful to you.

RON: I guess that's true, but even if he says "thank you" and all that, how will I know for sure he's not upset, like if he didn't want to tell me how he really felt about it?

THERAPIST: That's really important, Ron, and useful for all of us. It might seem like asking your friend is a good way to find this out, but it is only useful if you think that is the best way to get the information. Whenever any of us does an experiment, we want it to really get at all the kinds of information we need. So, in this case, how else could we determine whether he is disappointed?

POLLY: If he was upset with you, maybe he'd be less likely to help you with something.

KATIE: Like that old saying, action speaks louder than words. Sometimes I think people can say things that are nice, but it means a lot more when they actually do something about it.

THERAPIST: So maybe another way would be to ask him to help you with something, and see whether he says he's not disappointed *and* he's willing to help you with something.

RON: That would be good to know.

POLLY: I'm not sure if it applies, but if this was me, the most important thing is that whatever happened doesn't affect the relationship.

RON: That's true for me, too. I think that speaking to him about it and seeing whether he's willing to help me out next time is important.

THERAPIST: All right, so that's the experiment, then. Step 1 is to ask him whether he is upset or disappointed with you after working on the garage door, and Step 2 is to ask him to help you with something. His response to those two questions will tell us something important and let you know if your initial thoughts were accurate. Any experiment needs to have predictions made in advance, so that we all understand what it means to get one kind of answer or another. Do other people feel like this experiment makes sense when you are wondering whether you might have been mind reading?

POLLY: Sure, there's a way to really check out what the other person was thinking, and the way to do that is to ask.

KATIE: And to see whether people's actions match their words. I'd like to know that even more than what they say.

This example dialogue illustrates a simple experiment, following up with someone else to check a "mind-reading" observation. This being a first attempt at designing an experiment, the therapist takes the lead in generating hypotheses and suggesting possible modifications to make the experiment more conclusive. Ron finds the first approach, asking his friend, to be useful but not conclusive. This leads to further consideration, by the group, of adding a second kind of test. Here, collaborative empiricism really comes to the fore, with group members making additional suggestions based on their own intuitions and experiences. Finally, the therapist includes other group members in the wrap-up, since this kind of cognitive distortion and experimental method is likely to be useful for a number of the group's members.

COGNITIVE TECHNIQUES IV:
EXPLORING UNDERLYING BELIEFS
AND ASSUMPTIONS

For most patients, problematic situations and thoughts occur repeatedly, and certain "cognitive themes" emerge over the course of many thought records. Such themes are indicative of patients' more deeply held beliefs about themselves, others, and the world. These beliefs, which are thought to be rooted in early life events and learning, are variously called core beliefs or schemas (Beck, 1995; Clark et al., 1999). The process of understanding early learning and how it leads to patients' beliefs and current problems is a more fluid and open-ended process compared to the DRDT. However, helping patients to understand their underlying beliefs helps them to change the factors that give rise to many of their troubling automatic thoughts and provides alternatives to self-defeating coping strategies.

Conditional Assumptions

One of the most common strategies for identifying beliefs is the downward arrow (Greenberger & Padesky, 1995). This approach begins with an automatic thought, and rather than disputing that thought with evidence gathering, patients are encouraged to deepen their level of affect and explore the thought with questions, such as "What it would it mean if this thought was true?" This typically leads to the emergence of an underlying conditional assumption, a level of cognition that typically takes the form of "if . . . then" statements. These "rules" often specify a circumstance and an emotional consequence that is dysfunctional. For example, a patient whose thought records reflect concern, time after time, with letting others down might have the belief, "If I cannot please everyone around me, it is awful."

Largely, these rules exist at a level of awareness such that the patient has rarely been able to reflect on them. In these instances, it is often the therapist who picks up on a kind of "emotional rule" that seems to reoccur in the patient's difficulties. A number of situations may share some features and cause similar emotional responses. Often, this means that similar rules are in operation across these situations. The therapist might initially verbalize this rule, then a collaborative effort can be made to modify the specific wording of the conditional assumption. Other times, patients may be aware of their conditional beliefs and are able to state "the rules" that seem to govern their emotional and behavioral responses to situations.

Another useful conceptual issue is the distinction between "positive assumptions" and "negative assumptions." A positive assumption is an "if . . . then" statement in which the outcome, the "then," is positively valenced from the patient's perspective. In other words, a positive assumption is a case where the patient, if he or she satisfies some condition, can gain a positive outcome. The difficulty with these beliefs is that the condition is often rigidly defined and difficult to maintain. For example, a patient may have the belief, "If I do everything right all the time at my job, I will be all right." A negative assumption is also an "if . . . then" statement, but in this case the outcome is negatively valenced from the patient's perspective. In some instances, negative assumptions can be seen as the "flip side" of positive assumptions. In the previous example, a negative assumption version might be, "If I make a mistake at my job, I will be a failure." Here the precedent (a mistake) leads to a negative consequence (sense of failure).

In a group setting, it is useful first to present the concept of conditional assumptions or emotional rules didactically and provide examples similar to those presented above. Usually, examination of beliefs will occur after many group sessions, by which time group members are highly cohesive and also have considerable knowledge of one another's difficulties. Thus, group process plays a very important role in uncovering beliefs, since group members have some understanding of one another's typical ways of emotional responding to situations. In the sample dialogue that follows, the therapist utilizes the downward arrow method to uncover a conditional assumption that underlies the example with Ron. The therapist's goals in this dialogue are as follows:

1. Explore the emotional rule underlying the particular automatic thought.
2. Illustrate the "if . . . then" nature of this and most such assumptions.
3. Discuss the negative emotional consequences of the assumption and the need to modify this.
4. Focus on emotional processing, group learning, and modifying maladaptive relational patterns, particularly when conditional assumptions are interpersonal.

THERAPIST: So, if we were to try the downward arrow with your example, Ron, we start with the automatic thought "It's up to me. If I can't do it I'm letting him down." We know we could gather evidence for this thought, but in this case, we are going to assume that it is true and just ask another question: What does that thought mean? What if it's true?

RON: It's like it's all on my shoulders, a burden for me.

THERAPIST: You feel responsible for fixing it and so not disappointing him.

RON: Yeah, and that's just the way I am. Whenever people ask me to help, it's like I can't say no.

THERAPIST: Okay, we're really getting there. Remember, we are looking for a kind of rule that you have for yourself.

KATIE: To me, Ron, it sounds like you take on all this responsibility when it isn't yours to begin with.

RON: I know. That goes way back, too. I guess it is that when people ask me to help, I have to help them or I feel terrible, guilty.

THERAPIST: Getting these rules down for the first time is not easy; it's a process that we work on. But in this case, it sounds like the rule is something like "I must always help other people, and if I don't I'm a bad person."

RON: That's what it feels like. As I said, I think that kind of rule has been with me for a long time.

THERAPIST: Okay, let's go with this for now and just explore it a bit more. If that's the rule you have, what is the problem with it? What do others think?

POLLY: It's like the examples you showed us earlier—it's pretty extreme.

KATIE: Like it's too much of a good thing. It's nice to help people when you can, but what if you can't for some reason? As long as you try, that's the important thing.

RON: Well, I know this leads to a lot of guilt.

POLLY: I think it could also lead to people taking advantage of your generosity.

RON: Maybe it could.

THERAPIST: Okay, let's summarize a bit. It seems like we have identified a negative assumption that if you don't help everyone all the time, you are a bad person. What it means for you is that whenever you don't or can't help someone, you feel guilty and down on yourself. Sometimes, when we first see these kinds of rules, we don't always recognize that they might be problematic. Other people, in this case Katie and Polly, are saying that they see this rule as too rigid and maybe needs to be changed. What do you think, Ron?

RON: I'd like to talk about it more. I know I get really caught up in that idea, even now.

In this dialogue, the therapist helps to "shape" Ron's answers to the downward arrow questions given that this is a first attempt by the group to discuss beliefs. Group members offer some supportive statements that are also potentially useful in modifying the patient's assumptions, since the group members represent an important source of corrective information for Ron. Also typical is that fellow group members perceive the rigidity in Ron's conditional assumptions even while he is ambivalent.

Associated with conditional assumptions or rules are compensatory or coping strategies. The ultimate goal of these coping strategies is directly related to a conditional assumption. These strategies can logically be defined as the behavior a person selects in order to ensure that (1) the positive assumptions are made true, and (2) the negative assumptions are made false. Thus, pragmatically, this means that patients are motivated to engage in any behavior that will satisfy their assumptions in an attempt to regulate affect. For example, with Ron's belief about needing always to help others, he may overextend himself and sacrifice to considerable lengths to provide help to anyone who asks. In most cases, the key consideration is to determine what behaviors are associated with conditional assumptions, then to specify what these behaviors are intended to do.

The following sample dialogue carries on the discussion to explore Ron's compensatory strategies and whether they are adaptive:

THERAPIST: So this belief about needing to help others obviously has some emotional consequences, and like most beliefs, it probably also leads to some behaviors, because these kinds of beliefs usually motivate people to act in certain ways. In your case, Ron, maybe we can start by having you tell us about "helping" situations.

RON: Well, the thing is, I spend a lot of time on those, whether it's my family or friends. Even when my kids ask for help with their homework—how much is enough? I find myself explaining things or even doing them; it's exhausting sometimes.

THERAPIST: Maybe we can call this "overhelping" for now. What are the consequences of that?

POLLY: Ron, I think it's great that you care that much about your kids to help them like that, and I know that this isn't about being a parent, but I find that with homework, my kids really have to learn it themselves. If I'm doing it for them, I'm not doing them any favors. Do you see what I mean?

RON: I do know. My wife says that too. (*Pauses, wipes his eyes.*) I'm really worn down by that, and a part of me knows I shouldn't be doing their math for them.

KATIE: Ron, I think you're a very good person for helping all those people, but look what it's doing to you.

RON: It's frustrating, like I'm swimming upstream.

THERAPIST: Unfortunately, that's the kind of consequence that often comes out of the combination of a conditional assumption and the coping strategy for it. The conditional assumption is often hard to live up to, and trying to keep up with it can have some pretty rough consequences, often with more bad consequences than good.

POLLY: Are you saying that it is bad to help people? That it isn't worth it?

THERAPIST: Good question. It might seem that way. Helping people when you can is admirable, but at what cost?

POLLY: Like helping people can be too much of a good thing?

KATIE: You can't help people if you're depressed and exhausted.

THERAPIST: That's the general approach. Any behavior can become problematic when it is too rigid or people overdo it. Often those behaviors have more bad than good consequences that we can explore with a list of pros and cons, and that can help us make decisions about trying alternative behaviors.

Again, the example illustrates a number of positive group factors, and both corrective and supportive information offered by group members. Notably, there is sufficient cohesion and comfort for one group member to provide feedback about parenting, providing her own information and supportively questioning a fellow group member at the same time. The next step in working with conditional assumptions and coping strategies is alternative beliefs and reducing reliance on coping strategies. More balanced and less rigid beliefs often emerge in the Socratic dialogue, though initially, more therapist direction may be required. The next sample dialogue focuses on the following:

1. Identifying an alternative conditional assumption that is more functional.
2. Examining the consequences of the new conditional assumption for behavior.
3. Facilitate group learning and emotional processing.

THERAPIST: So, Ron, we've seen that your belief might lead to a number of problems, and you've been thinking it's too rigid. What do you think is an alternative belief that you can live with?

RON: I still feel it's important to help people, although I'm seeing that I can try, but I can't determine how everything turns out.

THERAPIST: That's a great start. Remember that the alternative belief probably isn't the opposite of your current belief, because that could be rigid in the opposite direction. It's more something in the middle.

POLLY: So, in a way, part of the belief stays the same—like about helping people.

THERAPIST: It can. The key is it's flexible and doesn't lead to problematic consequences.

RON: So I should help people when I can but not overwhelm myself.

KATIE: That's kind of what I think we should all do.

THERAPIST: Most balanced beliefs are pretty reasonable. Maybe we could write, "I help people as much as is reasonable, but I'm not responsible for everyone." What kinds of behaviors would be related to that? Would that lead to any negative consequences?

RON: I'd still help people when I could, but not blame myself if it didn't work out.

THERAPIST: That makes sense. Anything else?

POLLY: I think that belief might help Ron to not overextend himself?

RON: If I believed what was on the board, it would for sure.

THERAPIST: That's great. Remember that getting used to these new beliefs will take some time, and at first this will seem very new. The trick is to try these ideas out and measure how well they work by how you are feeling.

This dialogue illustrates the variable and often less structured process that comes along with a focus on conditional beliefs and compensatory strategies. Nonetheless, collaborative empiricism, Socratic dialogue, and guided discovery are in evidence, as are a number of group factors that allow this example, and the experience of this belief, to be a shared experience among all group members.

Core Beliefs

The deepest form of cognition that most groups focus on is core beliefs. These represent extreme, one-sided views of self, other, and the world that give rise both to the conditional assumptions and coping strategies described earlier. Core beliefs are believed to primitive, extreme views formed as a result of early experiences (Clark, Beck, et al., 1999). Content for these beliefs varies for each individual, but it is important to emphasize that core beliefs are ways of understanding the world and tend to be "rational" in those circumstances under which they form. The most important precursor to identifying core beliefs is to explain these concepts in therapy. Patients are encouraged to see their automatic thoughts as outgrowths of something deeper and that more profoundly affects their interpretations of events over time. The rationale, early learning, should also be provided, because it is important for patients to understand that their negative core beliefs are not accidental or random, but rather are understandable outcomes of their experiences. Core beliefs often take the form of absolute statements, such as "I'm a failure," "I am unlovable," or "I am in constant danger." Patients usually experience considerable affect when exposed to their core beliefs; they can often become tearful, sad, or very anxious. This is usually a sign that a highly salient type of processing has been tapped.

Many of the techniques used for changing automatic thoughts (e.g., examining distortions, evidence gathering) can be applied to working with deeper levels of cognition, although changing beliefs takes longer and requires more effort than altering a negative automatic thought. In addition to these techniques, three other processes help to change core beliefs, all of which are facilitated by the group and group processes. First, patients need to have some narrative concerning the development of these beliefs. Second, patients need to view these experiences more objectively and sympathetically, acknowledging that they learned something negative and potentially damaging. Third, it is important to engender hope that these kinds of beliefs can be "relearned" with the help of the group experience. Once patients have acknowledged the need to change core beliefs, they can be encouraged to create an alternative core belief, just as they worked on an alternative thought to their automatic thought and alternative conditional assumptions. Once the alternative belief is identified, patients are encouraged to gather evidence for the old core belief and the more adaptive alternative core belief. This encourages patients to see their subsequent experiences through a new filter and assess which of the two beliefs is a better fit to their current reality.

As with other cognitive techniques, the therapist first provides an overview of the rationale for working on core beliefs and examples to illustrate the point. Next, the therapist selects a suitable example, keeping in mind the high level of affect that can sometimes accompany this discussion. The sample dialogue demonstrates some of the necessary fluidity in discussions about core beliefs; evident in the discussion are aspects of psychoeducation, affective processing, review of historical information, and application of cognitive change strategies. To keep the dialogue concise, the starting point is when Ron identifies a potential core belief, "I'm inadequate," through his homework. The goals of the intervention are as follows:

1. Identifying a core belief and its historical context.
2. Identifying a potential alternative belief.
3. Developing strategies for strengthening that alternative core belief.
4. Facilitating group learning and emotional processing.

THERAPIST: Ron, you've written down that you think your core belief is "I'm inadequate."

RON: Yeah. That's not what I think, it's what I feel.

THERAPIST: Okay, can we use this as an example? I think this will be very useful for you and the group.

RON: Sure.

THERAPIST: Going back to last week's discussion, remember that a core belief is usually a pretty extreme belief we have that comes from early on, and that these beliefs really drive lots of other "rules" we have for ourselves and the automatic thoughts that pop into our minds. Now in this case, Ron, do you have a sense of where that core belief comes from?

RON: I think so. As I've talked about a bit here, my parents were pretty tough on me. They expected a lot, nothing was ever good enough, no way to make them happy . . . . (*Stops, looks pained.*)

THERAPIST: Ron, that sounds like it's a difficult thing to remember, but I think it's important. What do people think would happen to a kid in Ron's situation, where parents really expected a lot, maybe for the kid to be perfect?

KATIE: I just want to say to Ron that I think he's a good person.

RON: Thank you. It's hard for me to believe that.

KATIE: Well, I think it's true, but what I also wanted to say is that I think we are all products of how we grew up and what we heard.

POLLY: I agree. Ron you seem like a person who really helps and takes care of others.

THERAPIST: So, there are two things I'm hearing that I just want to point out. One is that it sounds like people are saying that growing up with really high standards might lead anyone to develop some negative beliefs. The second thing is that what things are like today, for example, how we have come to know Ron, is not at all similar to his beliefs about himself. Do people agree with that? And what are you reactions to that, Ron?

RON: That makes sense to me. I kind of felt like this thing that pushes me to do all those helping things also sometimes make me feel terrible.

THERAPIST: That's really important for everyone to look at. Core beliefs often really push us to have other beliefs about things that are important, those "if . . . then" conditional beliefs we have.

RON: I've been working on that, and it's better. Like I'm judging myself less on those things.

THERAPIST: Great. For those conditional beliefs, remember how we developed an alternative belief for you to try out. We have to do the same kind of thing for core beliefs, so come up with a core belief that you think is more realistic, more fair, and more helpful for you in your life today. Any thoughts about that?

RON: I was thinking about that while doing the homework; I'm not sure I have an answer.

POLLY: The more fair way, I think, is to say that you are adequate. That seems true to me.

KATIE: I think so, too.

THERAPIST: Ron, does that seem close?

RON: Yeah, it would be something like that, I'd think.

THERAPIST: Okay, we can revisit that later, but for now, let's say that the alternative core belief would be "I'm adequate." At first that might seem like a strange thing to say to yourself. That will be true for many of you when we talk more about alternative core beliefs. Moving toward a new core belief might seem strange at first, but it is a process that takes time. After a while, that belief will become stronger.

KATIE: That makes sense to me. When we first talked about this, I kept thinking about how hard it is to change habits, you know, things you've done since you were a kid, or just things that have been that way for a long time.

THERAPIST: That's true. What it takes to do this is to slowly work on collecting evidence that supports your new belief. Kind of like we've done with thoughts and other beliefs, it's important to notice when something good is happening that supports the new belief. In this case, we should consider a positive events log, a place for Ron to collect information that supports the idea that he is adequate.

POLLY: How long does that take?

THERAPIST: It might take several weeks, maybe even month. Another thing we can do with core beliefs is put them on a continuum, so let's write "I'm inadequate" here on the board at one end, and on the other end write up the alternative, "I'm adequate," then make a line between them. Let's imagine making an "X" somewhere along this line to represent Ron's sense of where he is right now in terms of believing either of these two ends of the spectrum, and down here at the "Inadequate" end is 0 and at the "adequate" end is 100. Ron, where would you put yourself on that line today?

RON: I'd say about 15, closer to inadequate.

THERAPIST: Okay, so the idea would be to move this "X" along by gathering more information. Maybe through the homework and our discussion you've already chipped away at the "indaquate" belief, at least to the point where you are having some doubt that it's right.

RON: For sure. It's something I want to work on.

The example illustrates the importance of combining group process with therapist direction. Group members make useful suggestions, and this is counterbalanced with carefully directed questions from the therapist to shape the group interaction further to cover two distinct strategies for changing core beliefs: the positive events log and continuum approach (Greenberger & Padesky, 1995).

CONCLUSIONS

Cognitive techniques used in groups are anchored in a cognitive model of psychopathology, and the principles of all cognitive interventions including collaborative empiricism, guided discovery, and Socratic dialogue. Specific interventions are constructed from these component pieces; indeed, the presentation of skills and techniques in this chapter does not in any sense exhaust possible strategies therapists might adapt or innovate in specific applications. Rather, this chapter provides an overview of the most critical components and some sample approaches to creating cognitive change. The essence of cognitive intervention in group is to keep the traditional CBT principles in mind, and at the same time considering process factors. An ideal cognitive intervention in a group mixes teaching of technique with the activation of process factors that deepen and enrich the learning and change experiences for all group members.

CHAPTER 4

Behavioral Strategies in CBT Groups

This chapter reviews the use of behavioral strategies in group treatment. Although the primary emphasis is on exposure-based strategies (e.g., situational exposure, role-play and simulated exposure, imaginal exposure, symptom exposure), the chapter also includes sections on behavioral self-monitoring, social skills training, and problem solving. Behavioral activation for depression, which is covered extensively in Chapter 10, it is not covered in this chapter. Nor are relaxation training (see Bernstein, Borkovec, & Hazlett-Stevens, 2000) and emerging behavioral treatments, such as acceptance and commitment therapy and mindfulness-based meditation (see Hayes, Follette, & Linehan, 2004). Additional discussion of these approaches is available elsewhere (e.g., Antony & Roemer, 2003). Although this chapter provides some general description for each strategy discussed, the emphasis is on how these methods can best be presented and implemented in a group format.

ADVANTAGES AND CHALLENGES IN DELIVERING BEHAVIORAL TREATMENTS IN GROUPS

Overall, there is considerable evidence supporting the use of behavioral treatments in groups. A number of studies and meta-analytic reviews have reviewed the relative effectiveness of group and individual treatments for particular disorders (see Part II of this book). Both appear to be effective, with little consistent evidence to suggest that either individual or group therapy is more effective. However, comparative studies have often ignored variables other than efficacy, such as the cost of treatment, rates of treatment refusal and dropout, and treatment satisfaction. In addition, little is known about predictors of who is likely to benefit most from group versus individual treatment. Despite the lack of empirical research on the relative costs and benefits of delivering behavioral treatments in a group format, clinically, group treatment seems to have a number of strengths and liabilities relative to individual therapy.

Advantages of Administering Behavioral Treatments in Groups

Some of the advantages of delivering behavioral treatments in groups are similar to the advantages for any group treatment. For example, because they take less therapist time per client, groups often provide an opportunity for behavioral therapy to be offered at a lower cost compared to individual treatment. In addition, group treatments allow for behavioral practices that would be difficult to arrange in the context of individual treatment. For example, exposure exercises for social phobia require opportunities for social interaction, and a group format provides such opportunities readily.

Groups also allow clients to get a wider range of feedback on their performance during social skills training. In a group, there are more "heads" in the room for the purpose of brainstorming solutions to one another's problems. Often, group members suggest homework practices for one another that had not occurred to either the therapist or to any particular client. Groups also provide opportunity for shared learning. Clients can model nonfearful behavior for one another and also learn from one another's experiences. For example, listening to a discussion about another group member's exposure homework can help other members to think differently about how they might plan their own homework for the coming week.

Group treatment also provides peer support that may not be present in individual treatment. Being part of a group reminds clients that they are not alone in their struggle; they often value the support and inspiration they get from other members in the group. Although support from the therapist is important, support from others who share a particular problem is a unique feature of group treatment. Hearing from another group member that his or her fear eventually decreased as a result of exposure may be more credible than a similar message coming from a therapist.

It is not unusual for group members to push one another to try more challenging exposures, or to catch one another relying on subtle avoidance strategies. Group treatment may foster a sense of responsibility among clients to not let one another down (a form of peer pressure). It also helps to reduce the "therapist versus client" dynamic that sometimes arises during individual therapy with a client who is noncompliant. Finally, conducting behavioral practices in groups can also be a lot of fun compared to individual treatment.

Challenges in Administering Behavioral Treatments in Groups

As with some of the advantages of group behavioral treatment discussed earlier, several of the main disadvantages of administering behavioral therapy in groups are challenges that are likely to arise in any group treatment. For example, group treatment is usually more challenging to schedule than individual treatment. It can be difficult to find a time that is convenient for all members, and it is sometimes difficult for individuals to catch up following a missed session, which may lead some clients to drop out. Therefore, we recommend that, whenever possible, therapists try to meet with clients who have missed a session for at least a few minutes before the next meeting to fill them in on what they missed.

Compared to individual treatment, group treatment provides less time per client for reviewing homework, dealing with compliance issues, practicing in-session exposures, and setting up homework practices for the week following each session. In addition, although group treatment is less expensive than individual therapy, overall, it may be more time consuming for clients (typically, group sessions last 2 hours, whereas individual sessions are often shorter). Finally, just as some behavioral practices (e.g., exposures involving social interaction) are easier to do in groups, others (e.g., driving) are easier to practice in the context of individual therapy.

For groups in which clients differ in their levels of motivation, comprehension, or symptom profiles, it may be necessary to "pitch" the group for the "average" member. As a result, clients with poor motivation, difficulty comprehending the material in the group, or unusual symptom presentations may not get as much out of the group as they might from individual therapy. Such clients may benefit from a few individual sessions in addition to the group. In addition, some participants may be reluctant or embarrassed to bring up issues (e.g., symptoms having to do with sexuality, past experiences that they regret) in front of group members that they might have brought up in individual therapy. Finally, just as positive experiences among some group members can be a source of inspiration to others, negative experiences among group members (e.g., a bad exposure experience) can affect other group members negatively.

EXPOSURE-BASED STRATEGIES

Exposure is perhaps the most established strategy for combating fear. It is a key component of treatment for each of the anxiety disorders and is often used when treating other disorders in which fear and avoidance are important features (e.g., eating disorders, body dysmorphic disorder, hypochondriasis). In this section, we discuss general methods for implementing exposure-based treatments in a group format. Strategies for integrating exposure into the treatment of particular conditions are also discussed throughout various chapters in Part II of this book. A more detailed discussion of exposure may be found in a recent book by Rosqvist (2005).

Types of Exposure

In Vivo Exposure

In vivo exposure involves confronting a feared object or situation directly (i.e., in reality, as opposed to in imagination). Examples include practicing driving to overcome a fear of driving, attending parties, meetings, and other social gatherings to combat social anxiety disorder, and eating "forbidden" foods to combat a fear of gaining weight in anorexia nervosa. When an individual is fearful of a particular object, situation, or activity, *in vivo* exposure is typically the most effective exposure approach. Studies comparing *in vivo* exposure to imaginal exposure for situational fears have generally found situational exposure to be the most effective (e.g., Emmelkamp & Wessels, 1975).

Conducting situational exposures in groups can be a challenge, particularly when group members fear different types of objects and situations. In fact, when treating groups, it is not uncommon for group time to be spent reviewing homework and planning future exposures, and to have the actual *in vivo* exposure practices occur between group meetings. In these cases, it may be useful to suggest that clients work with a supportive family member or friend during exposure practice, if they need extra support or coaching.

Although exposure practices between group sessions are important, conducting exposures during group time can be a valuable experience. We recommend trying to do some exposures in group, if possible. One way to accomplish this is to break a group up into smaller groups that comprise individuals with similar concerns who can practice exposure together for part of the group session. If the group has multiple therapists, each therapist can take responsibility for coaching several group members during their exposure practices. If group practices are impractical (e.g., in the case of driving fears), some group members can practice exposures individually during group time. For example, in a group with obsessive–compulsive disorder, three participants could work on contamination exposures, while several others work on imaginal exposures to frightening words (see the section below on imaginal exposure), and one client works on leaving rooms without checking for possessions that may have been left behind. In a group focused on overcoming agoraphobia, several members could practice being at a mall, while others practice standing in line at a supermarket or driving alone on the highway. Before splitting up the group for exposures, it is often helpful to begin the session together to review homework and plan the practices, then meet as a group again after the practices are completed to discuss the outcome and assign new homework. In a 2-hour group session, that should leave up to an hour for the exposure practices. Longer meetings (e.g., 2½ hours) may be necessary, in some cases, to accommodate in-session exposures.

Simulated Exposures and Behavioral Role Plays

Simulated exposures are a form of *in vivo* exposure in which an individual practices confronting a situation that approximates the actual feared situation but is not quite the real thing. Examples include role-playing a job interview, with the therapist or another group member playing the part of the employer, or practicing a presentation, with group members playing the part of the audience. Exposures to stimuli in photos, videotapes, or three-dimensional computer simulations (i.e., virtual reality) may also be considered examples of simulated exposures, and are used most often for treating certain types of specific phobias (e.g., phobias of blood, needles, spiders, snakes, and some other animals), primarily on an individual basis (see Antony & McCabe, 2005; Antony & Watling, 2006). Simulated exposures or role plays are useful when (1) the client initially finds it too difficult to practice exposures in the actual situation, or (2) when it is inconvenient or impractical to practice exposure in the actual situation.

Simulated exposures are often used for in-session exposure practices during group treatment for social anxiety disorder (Heimberg & Becker, 2002). Practices typically involve having group members role-play various social or performance-related scenarios. Some practices may involve the entire group (e.g., having group members role-play engaging in casual small talk at a party). Other practices may involve breaking the group up into smaller groups, so that members can practice exposures that are relevant to them. For example, two group members might be role-playing a job interview, while several others practice eating in front of one another.

A possible disadvantage of role playing in front of other group members is that the role-play situation may be quite different from the real-life situation that is being simulated. In real life, conversations tend to occur in isolation, whereas a role-played conversation in group therapy may have the added component of an audience. Clients may feel pressure to make a good impression on not only the person they are talking to but also the audience. Also, clients may well "minimize" a positive performance and good feedback because it occurred in the protected setting of a therapy group. Nonetheless, an observant CBT therapist could point out that a group situation, with an audience, may actually be more pressure than the same "real-world" situation without several potential critics looking on.

Imaginal Exposure

Imaginal exposure involves exposing oneself to feared stimuli in imagination. This form of exposure was initially introduced as a component of systematic desensitization, one of the first exposure-based treatments to be studied systematically (Wolpe, 1958). As mentioned earlier, *in vivo* exposure is generally preferred to imaginal exposure, particularly when treating situational fears. However, there are a number of situations in which imaginal exposure may be appropriate. First, imaginal exposure is appropriate if an individual is afraid of his or her thoughts, images, or urges. For example, a client with obsessive–compulsive disorder who fears thoughts and images having to do with Satan might be encouraged to practice thinking about, writing about, and talking about images that trigger the fear (Rowa, Antony, & Swinson, in press). Similarly, imaginal exposure is commonly used for treating people with posttraumatic stress disorder who are fearful of traumatic memories following a sexual assault or other trauma (Foa & Rothbaum, 1998).

In some cases, imaginal exposure may also be useful for fears of external objects or situations. For example, if a client refuses to practice *in vivo* exposure due to extreme fear, imaginal exposure may be a good initial step before trying *in vivo* exposures. Also, imaginal exposure may be useful when regular *in vivo* exposure practices are impractical or when a feared situation is impossible to create on a regular basis (e.g., if a client is anxious about his or her upcoming wedding, a situation that is difficult to simulate).

Imaginal exposure may involve (1) having a client describe a feared memory or image out loud (e.g., Foa & Rothbaum, 1998), (2) having the therapist read a description of a feared image or scenario to a client (e.g., Craske, 1999), or (3) having a client silently bring a feared image to mind. Regardless, the process of imaginal exposure is very much a private experience. Different clients will typically need to work on different images, and for many clients in the group (i.e., those who are not afraid of their thoughts, images, or urges), imaginal exposure may not even be relevant. At our center, we typically do not practice imaginal exposure in groups. If imaginal exposure is warranted for one or more group members, therapists spend some group time describing the procedures and may demonstrate the process with one or more clients. However, clients are expected to do most of their imaginal exposure practices for homework, between group sessions.

Symptom Exposure

Symptom exposure (also referred to as "interoceptive exposure") involves practicing exercises designed to induce various feared symptoms and sensations, until the sensations are no longer frightening. In the same way that clients who fear situations are encouraged to expose themselves to the feared situation, and clients who fear their thoughts or memories are encouraged to bring them on using imaginal exposure, clients who are frightened of the physical symptoms associated with their anxiety or panic may be encouraged purposely to trigger the symptoms, initially in a safe setting (e.g., at home or in a therapist's office), and eventually in the context of feared situations.

Although well over a dozen exercises have been used to induce feared symptoms, some of the most effective of these include (1) breathing through a small straw for 3 minutes (to trigger smothering sensations), (2) hyper-ventilating for 60 seconds (to trigger breathlessness, dizziness, racing heart, and other symptoms), and (3) spinning in a chair for a minute (to trigger dizzi-ness) (Antony, Ledley, Liss, & Swinson, 2006). Symptom exposure is often a component of evidence-based treatments for panic disorder (e.g., Barlow, Gorman, Shear, & Woods, 2000). In addition, it is sometimes useful clinically to include symptom exposure to deal with fear of particular sensations in other anxiety disorders. For example, someone with social anxiety disorder who fears sweating while engaged in public speaking might be encouraged to wear warm clothing during a presentation. Additional details on how to implement symptom exposure strategies are described elsewhere (Antony & Swinson, 2000a).

Symptom exposure is usually quite easy to implement in a group setting, particularly when treating panic disorder, which by definition is associated with anxiety over experiencing physical sensations. Typically, all group mem-bers initially try each symptom induction exercise at the same time and record in diaries any symptoms they experience, as well as the intensity of their fear and the extent to which the experience was similar to their naturally occurring panic attacks. After each exercise, members also share their experiences with the other group members. Once clients have identified the exercises that are most relevant to them (i.e., the ones that produce similar symptoms to those experienced during typical panic attacks), they are encouraged to repeat the relevant exercises six or seven times, until their anxiety has decreased. This is repeated twice per day, until the exercises no longer trigger fear. Practices typ-ically occur during group sessions, as well as for homework.

Developing an Exposure Hierarchy

An exposure hierarchy is a list of situations that an individual fears and/or avoids, rank-ordered with the most frightening items at the top, easier items at the bottom, and moderately difficult items in the middle. Sample hierarchies are reprinted in Chapters 6, 7, and 8 of this book. Generally, exposure hierar-chies include 10–15 items. Hierarchy items should be as detailed and descrip-tive as possible, specifying the variables that impact upon an individual's fear in each situation on the list. For example, "riding a bus alone at rush hour, sit-ting away from the door" is a much more descriptive item than simply "riding a bus."

In individual therapy, items are typically generated collaboratively, with the therapist and client each proposing possible items based on their discus-sions about feared situations, as well as the client's responses to items on standard questionnaires, such as the Mobility Inventory for Agoraphobia (Chambless, Caputo, Jasin, Gracely, & Williams, 1985) or the Yale–Brown Obsessive Compulsive Scale (Goodman et al., 1989a, 1989b). After an initial list is generated, the therapist and client refine the items, ensuring that they are sufficiently detailed to describe situations relevant to the client's goals, that they are practical to assign for exposure practices, and that they cover a range of difficulty levels and a range of situations representative of those feared by the client.

Once the item list is finalized, the client rates his or her fear level (using a 0- to 100-point scale, where 0 = *no fear* and 100 = *maximum fear*) and the extent to which he or she would be inclined to avoid the situation, using a 0- to 100-point scale (0 = *never avoids*; 100 = *always avoids*). Alternatively, because fear and avoidance ratings tend to be very highly correlated, a single fear/avoidance rating can be generated for each item. The final step is to reorder the list, putting the items with the highest fear ratings at the top and those with the lowest ratings at the bottom.

At our center, we typically develop the hierarchy during an individual session with each client, before a group begins. An advantage is that this approach ensures that each client has a carefully constructed hierarchy and the therapist has had a chance to have some individual time with each client before the group starts. Also, the individual meetings provide each client an opportunity to address any last minute concerns or questions about the group.

It is also possible to develop the hierarchies during one of the group sessions. This can be done in one of two ways: (1) to provide detailed instructions (both verbally and in writing) during the group session, or (2) to request that clients develop their hierarchies for homework before the next session. Sending clients home with several sample hierarchies will facilitate the process. Feedback can then be provided to each client at the next group session. Alternatively, clients can actually develop their hierarchy in the group session. While clients work on their hierarchies, the therapists can move around the room, answering questions and providing feedback.

Introducing Exposure to the Group

The following dialogue illustrates how exposure can be introduced to a group, including strategies for dealing with doubts about whether exposure is likely to work.

THERAPIST: Can anyone think of a situation or object that was once frightening to you, but that no longer bothers you? Maybe a childhood fear of the dark, or a fear of diving into the pool for the first time?

RICK: I know I was afraid of dogs as a child, because I remember being terrified when my parents brought home a new puppy.

JENNIFER: I remember having to sleep with the light on when I was a kid. I was afraid of being alone in the dark.

THERAPIST: Anyone else?

NADINE: I don't remember having any childhood fears, but I definitely was much more afraid of driving a couple of years ago than I am now. In fact, driving isn't really a problem anymore, except on highways.

THERAPIST: How did you get over your driving fear?

NADINE: My husband had been driving me to work every day for several years. When his work schedule changed and he could no longer drive me, I had no choice but to drive myself to work. It was very difficult at first, but it gradually got easier.

JENNIFER: I don't know how my fear of the dark went away. It just seemed to get better. I think at some point my dad wouldn't let me have my light on any more.

THERAPIST: How about you, Rick? How did you get over your fear of dogs?

RICK: It just went away. I think it got easier after being around the new puppy for a while.

THERAPIST: All three of you accidentally stumbled upon what is perhaps the most important principle underlying all effective treatments for fear and phobias. One of the most effective strategies for overcoming any fear is repeated exposure to the situation. At least three of you have experienced the effects of exposure in the past: your fears of dogs, the dark, and driving. When we apply the principles of exposure to the situations that you fear now, you will again notice a reduction in your fear. The more exposure you do, the more quickly you will overcome your fear.

GITA: I've tried exposure in the past. About a month ago, I pushed myself to go to a concert. I completely panicked. Now, I'm even more scared than I was before I forced myself to go to that concert!

THERAPIST: That's not an unusual experience. Not all exposure is helpful. For example, if you were afraid of snakes, it wouldn't help you if I were to pull out a snake and throw it at you. That kind of exposure would probably make a snake phobia worse. Rick, based on your experience in overcoming your dog phobia, how do you think someone might overcome their fear of snakes through exposure?

RICK: Well, I think the exposure would have to be slow and gentle. No surprises.

THERAPIST: Absolutely. In everyday life, exposures are often unpredictable, and out of the person's control. They're also extremely brief, because the person often escapes if he or she feels panicky, and they are usually too infrequent. In contrast, the recipe for effective exposure requires that practices be predictable, under the person's control (so you know you can end the practice if you need to), prolonged (ideally lasting until your fear has come down), and frequent. Exposures that are too spaced out are less likely to make a difference in the long run. Here is a handout listing these guidelines, as well as several others that will help to ensure that you get the most out of your exposures. Let's take some time to go through each item on the handout. (*Therapist distributes handout.*)

Guidelines for Effective Exposure

The following guidelines should be considered when helping group members to plan exposure practices. We recommend reviewing them with the group when exposure is first introduced, and reminding clients about these principles from time to time over the course of treatment.

Predictability and Perceived Control

Predictable exposures have been shown to lead to better outcomes than unpredictable exposures (Lopatka, 1989). To the extent possible, it is important to ensure that clients know what to expect during an exposure practice. For practices that are inherently unpredictable (e.g., when driving, it is impossible to know exactly what the other cars on the road will do at any given moment), it may be useful for the client to anticipate possible scenarios and to think through how he or she might deal with each scenario in advance of the exposure.

Studies on the effects of controllability (i.e., the extent to which the client has control over the rate of exposure and the ability to end the exposure, if necessary) have yielded mixed findings, with some showing that control by the client leads to better outcomes and others finding no differences (for a review, see Antony & Swinson, 2000a). In light of these findings, as well as other studies suggesting that a lack of perceived control contributes to anxiety problems (Barlow, 2002), it is generally recommended that clients never be forced to do anything that they have not agreed to do. Exposure is believed to work best when clients have a sense of control over the process.

Spacing of Exposure Practices

Exposure sessions spaced closely together (e.g., daily) have been found to work better than exposure sessions that are more spaced out (e.g., weekly) (Foa, Jameson, Turner, & Payne, 1980). Furthermore, spreading out the last few sessions of exposure may lead to even better long-term outcomes (Tsao & Craske, 2000), though other studies have found no advantage in expanding the space between later sessions (Lang & Craske, 2000). Given that CBT groups typically only meet once per week, the best way to ensure frequent exposures is to encourage clients to practice between sessions, though it should be noted that research on the relationship between homework compliance and outcome following CBT for anxiety disorders has been mixed (Schmidt & Woolaway-Bickel, 2000; Woods, Chambless, & Steketee, 2002).

Duration of Exposure Practices

Stern and Marks (1973) showed that a single exposure session lasting 2 hours leads to more fear reduction than four 30-minute exposures occurring over the course of an afternoon. Ideally, exposures should last long enough for an individual's fear to decrease to at least a moderate level. It is generally recommended that clients plan to stay in situations until they feel comfortable. If an exposure is inherently brief (e.g., a social anxiety exposure that involves asking someone for directions), the practice should be repeated again and again, until the individual's anxiety has decreased. In group treatment, it may be difficult to set up in-session exposures lasting more than an hour due to time constraints. Fortunately, for many individuals anxiety decreases fairly quickly. Furthermore, there is evidence that briefer exposures are still potentially useful, especially if the client returns to the phobic situation later for additional exposure (de Silva & Rachman, 1984; Rachman, Craske, Tallman, & Solyom, 1984).

Graduated versus Rapid Exposures

Evidence regarding the best rate for progressing through the exposure hierarchy items has been mixed, with one direct comparison finding few differences in outcome following gradual versus more rapid exposure or flooding (Everaerd, Rijken, & Emmelkamp, 1973), and another finding that rapid exposure is more effective than a more graduated exposure schedule (Fiegenbaum, 1988). In practice, exposure seems to work regardless of whether steps are taken gradually or more quickly. An advantage of taking smaller steps is that anxiety is not as overwhelming during the practices. However, if steps are too small, gains occur more slowly, which can increase the length and costs of treatment, and be a blow to the client's motivation (often, nothing is more motivating than seeing quick improvements). Generally, we recommend that clients take steps as quickly as they are willing to; if they find a particular practice more difficult than they can handle, they can always try something easier.

Preventing Safety Behaviors and Rituals

People with anxiety problems often engage in a wide range of behaviors designed to protect themselves from threat. These may include subtle avoidance behaviors (e.g., distraction, wearing extra makeup to hide blushing, or wearing gloves to avoid contact with a potential source of contamination), carrying safety objects (e.g., carrying medication in case of a panic attack), overusing alcohol or drugs (e.g., having a few glasses of wine to manage anxiety at a party), or engaging in compulsive rituals (e.g., checking, cleaning, or counting in obsessive–compulsive disorder). Generally, these behaviors can undermine the effects of exposure, and eliminating them often leads to improved outcomes (Morgan & Raffle, 1999; Craske, Street, & Barlow, 1989; Wells et al., 1995). In fact, in the case of obsessive–compulsive disorder, ritual prevention is generally viewed as an essential component of treatment (see Chapter 8, this volume).

Intensity of Exposure

Typically, we recommend that the intensity of fear experienced during exposure start in the moderate to high range (e.g., a rating between 70 and 100), though a practice need not be a horrific experience to be of benefit (Foa, Blau, Prout, & Latimer, 1977). In fact, if fear levels are too high (to the point of being overwhelming), the individual will be less likely to stay in the situation and may start to engage in a variety of subtle avoidance behaviors. Of course, if fear levels are two low, exposures will not be all that useful either.

Importance of Varying Context and Exposure Stimuli

People with anxiety disorders often fear the environments in which they encounter their feared objects and situations, in addition to fearing the objects themselves. Gunther, Denniston, and Miller (1998) found that conducting exposure practices in a variety of contexts protected clients from experiencing a return of fear after treatment had ended, relative to exposure in only one environment. Therefore, it is recommended that clients practice exposure in a variety of places, such as at home, at work, or in other environments where they tend to encounter the situations they fear. In addition, varying exposure stimuli (e.g., practicing driving on a number of different bridges rather than just one bridge; practicing exposure to several different spiders instead of just one) has been found to be associated with better long-term outcomes (Rowe & Craske, 1998).

Modeling Nonfearful Behavior

Just as fear can be learned through observational learning or modeling (Mineka, Davidson, Cook, & Keir, 1984), clients often find exposures easier when a therapist or other trusted individual shares in the exposure experience or demonstrates the exposure task first. For example, a client with obsessive–compulsive disorder might find it easier to touch a contaminated object after seeing his or her therapist touch it initially. Though some studies have confirmed better long-term outcomes for exposure treatments that include a modeling component (e.g., Menzies & Clarke, 1993), others have failed to find any benefit of adding modeling to exposure (e.g., Bourque & Ladouceur, 1980). Though findings have been inconsistent, in our experience, modeling is often a useful component of exposure-based treatments, and we recommend including it when possible.

Minimizing Danger

Though it is important to conduct exposure practices that are likely to trigger an anxiety reaction, it is at least as important to ensure that the actual risks during exposures are in fact minimal. Clients may not always be the best judges of whether a particular practice is in fact safe. Before planning an exposure, it may be helpful for clients to ask themselves whether the average person without an anxiety problem would consider the practice to be dangerous. If the answer is "yes," then it is probably a good idea to try a different practice.

Assigning and Reviewing Exposure Homework in Groups

Each group session typically begins with a review of homework. Each client takes a turn at describing his or her experience with the homework from the previous week. When a particular client is speaking, the other group members should be encouraged to participate in the process by asking questions and making suggestions. Homework is assigned at the end of each session in much the same way. Each client describes his or her homework plan for the following week. The therapists and other group members provide feedback on the plan, which may lead to some changes in the homework that is finally assigned. Therapists should record each client's homework assignment, so it can be checked on at the next session. In addition, clients should be encouraged to record their homework assignments on paper, so that they are sure to remember what they agreed to do.

BEHAVIORAL SELF-MONITORING

A hallmark of behavioral treatment is careful monitoring of symptoms in behavioral diaries. Self-monitoring helps clients to become more aware of the their behaviors, as well as the triggers for, and consequences of, their behaviors and emotional responses. In addition, completing diaries encourages clients to stay engaged in treatment throughout the week rather than just during their therapy sessions. Finally, diaries can be used to document progress during treatment.

Typically, diaries allow clients to record their symptoms, either in particular situations (e.g., during an exposure practice) or throughout the week. For example, individuals with bulimia are often asked to monitor their food intake during the week, as well as any purging episodes that occur. Similarly, people with panic disorder are typically required to monitor their panic attacks, recording the intensity of each attack, the circumstances under which it occurred, and the symptoms that were experienced. A Panic Attack Record (Barlow & Craske, 2000) is a simple form that can be completed immediately after each panic attack for this purpose (see Figure 4.1).

When using monitoring forms in groups, it is important to spend an adequate amount of time teaching group members how to complete the forms. We recommend that clients turn in their monitoring records at the start of each session (particularly during the first few treatment sessions), so therapists can provide corrective feedback on how the forms were completed. Once cli-

---

Date _____ Time began _____

Triggers _____

Expected _____ Unexpected _____

Maximum fear   0   1   2   3   4   5   6   7   8

               None   Mild   Moderate   Strong   Extreme

Check all symptoms present to at least a mild degree:

Difficulty breathing	_____	Chest pain/	Fear of dying _____
Racing/pounding heart	_____	discomfort _____	Fear of losing
Choking symptoms	_____	Hot/cold flashes _____	control/going
Numbness/tingling	_____	Sweating _____	crazy _____
Trembling/shaking	_____	Feelings of	
Nausea/abdominal		unreality _____	
distress	_____	Unsteadiness/	
		dizziness/faintness_____	

FIGURE 4.1. Panic Attack Record. From Barlow and Craske (2000). Copyright 2000 by Graywind Publications. Adapted and reproduced by permission of the Publisher, Oxford University Press. All rights reserved.

ents have a good understanding of how to complete their diaries appropriately, handing in the diaries is less important. Instead, clients can hold on to their diaries, using them to prompt their memories as they describe their experiences with the previous week's homework.

SOCIAL SKILLS TRAINING

Social skills training (SST; e.g., communication training, assertiveness training) is often included as a component of behavioral treatment for a number of different problems, including social anxiety disorder, depression, schizophrenia, and couple distress. Essentially, the process involves teaching clients to identify particular social skills deficits or communication-related behaviors that they would like to change, then targeting those social skills directly in treatment. The goal of SST is to improve the client's functioning in social and performance situations in order to increase the likelihood of a positive response from others, which in turn may lead to other positive consequences (successfully interviewing for a job, getting along better with others, becoming an effective presenter, etc.). Table 4.1 includes a list of behaviors that may be

TABLE 4.1. Behaviors Targeted in Social Skills Training

General category	Examples
Nonverbal communication	• Eye contact • Body language (e.g., personal space, posture) • Facial expressions
Conversation skills	• Tone and volume of speech • Strategies for starting and ending conversations • Asking open-ended rather than closed-ended questions
Presentation skills	• Refraining from reading a presentation to an audience • Developing effective slides and audiovisual aids • Using humor in the presentation • Strategies for answering audience questions without seeming defensive
Dating skills	• Asking another individual out for lunch or dinner • Strategies for following up after a date
Assertiveness skills	• Asking for something in a direct manner, without coming across as overly passive or aggressive • Asking another individual to change his or her behavior • Refusing an unreasonable request
Conflict skills	• Learning how to defuse an argument • Learning how to deal with situations that may lead another individual to become angry
Listening skills	• Listening to other people instead of planning what one is going to say next in a conversation • Asking for clarification when a statement is unclear

worked on in SST. Detailed strategies for improving social and communication skills are available elsewhere (e.g., McKay, Davis, & Fanning, 1995).

In some ways, presenting the rationale for SST is more straightforward in a group setting than in individual therapy. In individual therapy, a client may respond negatively to the suggestion that he or she needs to work on his or her social skills. However, in a group setting, these strategies can be brought up more generally, so that no particular client is likely to take the suggestion personally. In addition, it is helpful to begin by having clients identify social behaviors that they would like to work on, rather than having the therapist point out social skills deficits of which the client may not even be aware. As treatment progresses, it is often useful for the therapist to suggest additional behaviors that the client may wish to target.

SST is often accomplished in the context of exposure practices or behavioral role plays. After identifying particular behaviors to change, clients are encouraged to practice replacing problem behaviors with more adaptive behaviors, perhaps after modeling by the therapist or other group members. For example, clients may be taught to make appropriate eye contact or to give a presentation without having their voice drop off. It is often helpful to videotape the role-play practices, and to play the tapes back, so the client can evaluate his or her performance and group members can provide objective feedback.

PROBLEM-SOLVING TRAINING

Impaired problem-solving skills are a feature of depression (Davila, Hammen, Burge, Paley, & Daley, 1995). In addition, although problem-solving impairment may not be a significant feature in generalized anxiety disorder (GAD; Ladouceur, Blais, Freeston, & Dugas, 1998), frequent worry is associated with impaired confidence in one's problem-solving abilities (Belzer, D'Zurilla, & Maydeu-Olivares, 2002). Because of the possible relationship between impaired problem-solving skills and problems with depression and anxiety (as well as other conditions), treatments for these disorders sometimes include problem-solving training as a component (e.g., Brown, O'Leary, & Barlow, 2001; Bieling & Antony, 2003). Problem-solving training targets two types of problem-solving deficits (Meichenbaum & Jaremko, 1983): (1) a tendency to view problems in vague, general, and catastrophic ways, and (2) a failure to recognize and implement possible solutions. In addition, treatment may target related issues, such as time management skills and general organizational skills.

Problem-solving training involves teaching clients to use a structured, step-by-step approach to solving problems that involves five steps:

1. *Defining the problem.* The first step involves identifying the specific problem to be solved. Clients are encouraged to replace problems that they describe in vague or general terms (e.g., "I hate my job") with a list of more specifically defined problems (e.g., "I would like to find a job that will allow me to use my background in design"). If the client identifies multiple problems, he or she is encouraged to prioritize the list and to use the problem-solving strategies to work through each problem, one at a time, starting with the most important problem.

2. *Brainstorming possible solutions.* This stage involves having the client list as many solutions to the problem as possible, without filtering, censoring, or judging solutions that come to mind. All possible solutions (good and bad) should be recorded at this stage. When teaching problem solving in groups, all clients in the group should be encouraged to generate possible solutions to problems raised.

3. *Evaluating possible solutions.* At this stage, clients are taught to evaluate the advantages and disadvantages of each solution generated in step 2. Through this process, clients work at reducing the length of their lists by eliminating solutions that are impossible or impractical to implement, that are unlikely to work, or that can only be implemented at great cost. The remaining list should include only those solutions that are reasonable options.

4. *Choosing the best solution.* Next, clients should select the best solution (or solutions) from their list, based on the evaluation completed in step 3.

5. *Implementing the solution.* The final step involves implementing the selected solution. Upon implementing the solution, the client may encounter various obstacles. If this occurs, he or she should use the same problem-solving approach to get around any problems that arise along the way.

In group treatments, problem-solving skills are usually introduced didactically. The entire group may then participate in working through one or two sample problems presented by the therapists, followed by some actual problems that group members may be experiencing in their lives. Clients should then be encouraged to practice their problem-solving skills throughout the week, as problems arise in their day-to-day lives.

CONCLUSIONS

This chapter has provided an overview of how to administer behavioral strategies in a group format. We began with a discussion of some of the advantages and obstacles to administering behavioral treatments in groups. Much of the chapter has focused on exposure-based treatments. In addition, suggestions for implementing other strategies (e.g., behavioral self-monitoring, social skills training, problem solving) were provided.

CHAPTER 5

Basic Structure and Implementation of CBT Groups

The delivery of group CBT involves many details related to patient selection, therapist stance and style, as well as within-session and between-session structure; considerable energy must go into planning and organization of CBT to achieve maximum efficiency and clinical effectiveness. Therapists who move from working with individuals to a group format are often surprised to discover the number of factors that are introduced when therapy relies on the presence of more than two individuals for a therapy hour. The need to gather a group of people in one time and place for regularly scheduled meetings for the length of a treatment protocol may seem like an easily achievable task, but it actually requires that many specific elements work in concert. This chapter aims to cover this territory and provide information about some of the basic underpinnings of any CBT group. Time spent in thinking through these issues carefully before conducting any group pays dividends; when structural issues are not planned or anticipated well, these components can be distracting, even undermining, to the delivery of the treatment.

We describe four factors that are critical to the organization and structure of CBT groups: patient selection, therapist factors, between-session structure, and within-session structure. These do not represent all of the relevant domains that actually need to be considered to conduct a group. Several very concrete considerations are also important. These include physical space, scheduling of groups, clinical documentation, outcome measurement, and approaches to treatment noncompliance or dropouts, and are not considered here. These issues vary widely from one clinical setting and problem focus to another, but they are still important details to be considered. A room that is too small (or too large) for the number of occupants, lack of patient handouts when needed, follow-up with patients who do not attend sessions, and patient scheduling problems (e.g., a patient needs to leave a group because child care arrangements fall through) can all impact significantly on the group experience for therapists and patients.

PATIENT SELECTION

As in any psychotherapy pursuit, accurate and complete diagnosis using DSM-IV criteria is likely to be both useful and necessary prior to any CBT group. This is a given when a specific disorder protocol is to be implemented, but it is also helpful in more heterogeneous group settings. Axis I diagnoses can help therapists anticipate the most pressing symptoms and problem areas that group members will need to address and allow for appropriate treatment planning. Axis II diagnoses, in addition to anticipating focal areas, can also help therapists to prepare for distinct interpersonal styles and contemplate how a personality disorder diagnosis may impact on group processes. More explicit consideration of comorbidity issues is provided in Chapter 16.

In addition to basic Axis I and II diagnostic screens, a group suitability interview can be an important tool to ascertain fit with a group CBT approach. Suitability interviewing provides an assessment that can not only be useful in making treatment decisions but may also have the added benefit of enhancing a client's readiness for a brief, focused treatment such as CBT. Such an interview can also offer numerous opportunities to socialize the patient to the group experience, describing the process and helping to set realistic expectations. In the process of completing a suitability assessment for CBT, patients may make significant progress in understanding their difficulties from a biopsychosocial perspective, simply by answering questions about their compatibility with the cognitive model. At the same time, if the patient has a different view of his or her disorder, for example, a biological perspective, this interview can suggest an alternative approach.

Although originally developed as a screening tool for individual CBT in depression, the CBT suitability interview described by Safran and Segal (1990) can readily be adapted for a group setting. Ten dimensions are assessed, including (1) the client's ability to notice automatic thoughts, (2) the client's awareness of emotions and ability to discriminate between various emotional states, (3) the degree to which a client accepts responsibility for change, (4) the compatibility between a client's understanding of his or her problem and the CBT model, (5) the length of difficulties with depression, (6) the ability of the client to maintain focus on a particular problem, (7) the client's optimism that change is possible, (8) the ability of client and therapist to form an initial therapeutic alliance, (9) the ability of the client to have trusting relationships in his or her life, and (10) the degree to which various interpersonal, disruptive processes may interfere with therapy. The scores on this instrument have shown moderate correlations with both client and therapist ratings of success in treatment of depression (Safran & Segal, 1990). These various domains likely tap at least four distinct factors that are likely to predict treatment outcome: a capacity to reflect on one's own mental experiences and the ability to engage in "metacognitive" processing in a therapy setting, compatibility with the rationale of CBT, clinical variables such as chronicity and levels of hopelessness, and interpersonal process factors. The two sets of factors most relevant to all CBT group approaches are interpersonal style and the patient's "fit" with a CBT model.

Formal assessment of interpersonal style, and explicit criteria for inclusion and exclusion in a CBT group are theoretically possible to develop. However, in practice, real-world suitability assessments are likely to take place without the benefit of time and resources to gain a complete understanding of all possible interpersonal factors that might influence group processes. Instead, therapists selecting patients for groups could use the alliance and relational style that has been demonstrated in the interview process as a proxy for the kinds of relationships the patient might form with group leaders and other patients. This may involve observation of a greater than desirable frequency of potentially disruptive behaviors (e.g., tangentiality, overt expressions of suicidality, extreme neediness or need for reassurance, expressed hostility or mistrust) or a less than desirable frequency of positive behaviors (e.g., inability to engage in self-disclosure, lack of appropriate affect or humor, lack of fluctuation in affect). The strength of friendships and family relationships can be an important indicator of a person's ability to maintain and benefit from interpersonal interactions. Similarly, patients with an absence of any significant positive relationships, or a long history of destructive relationships in which the patient played a key role, are unlikely to benefit the group or group process.

Useful questions for therapists to ask themselves about potential group members include the following:

1. What kind of relationships will this person wish to form with other group members?
2. What kinds of interpersonal behaviors of this person will support group cohesion and process?
3. What kinds of interpersonal behaviors have the potential to undermine group cohesion and process?

It may also be useful to contemplate commonly used techniques, such as thought record work or behavioral activation, and consider how the individual might interact with other group members working collaboratively on his or her own examples and examples offered by other participants.

In terms of "fit" with the CBT model, ideally the model of intervention resonates with the patient. For example, patients who are ready and willing to make changes in their "normal" means of coping or dealing with their difficulties are more likely to respond to suggestions made in group. Patients with an exclusively biological view of their difficulties, or those who believe it is imperative to focus on insights about their early life, will not be well served in a CBT group. Similarly, patients who take little responsibility for helping themselves with their problems may not be successful in a CBT group. On the other hand, suitable patients tend more readily to understand the CBT model and have less difficulty seeing how the model fits them. Such patients may, with little or no prompting, fit their particular difficulties with the generic model described in the interview.

Therapists can discover patients' level of compatibility with the CBT approach in suitability interviewing by discussing sample techniques such as thought records or behavioral exposures. Although it cannot be assumed that patients will completely understand these procedures, their desire to learn more, or their level of acceptance of these interventions, can be important indicators. At a more practical level, patients need to be informed about the expectations for the group, including duration, length of sessions, nature of the group process itself, and the need for homework. Patients who know what the group involves, and who state a commitment to those expectations, will be less likely to drop out of treatment later.

PATIENT DEMOGRAPHIC FACTORS

In addition to diagnostic and suitability variables, the group modality also requires that consideration be given to other patient factors, including age, culture, language, and gender. There are no universal rules for dealing with these issues; some types of problems and settings might lend themselves to more or less heterogeneity. For example, a CBT group for performance anxiety in a college counseling center will draw from a more homogeneous group than an inpatient CBT program for depression. This leads to a natural question: Is it preferable for group members to share features such as age and gender? In general, we advocate for not only allowing but indeed selecting for some amount of heterogeneity in group members, although with some limits. At the outset of a group, heterogeneity can sometimes be seen as an impediment. Certainly, individuals who, superficially, have a great deal in common are more likely to get along spontaneously and identify with a similar "looking" group. However, in a more heterogeneous group, other beneficial factors are also operative; for example, patients learn that their problem is shared by people from apparently different walks of life. This facilitates group processes such as universality. Moreover, because each member of the group brings his or her own experiences to bear when asking questions, giving feedback, or volunteering examples, each group member will receive multiple points of view, and the wisdom of different cultures and age groups. This would not be equally true in a group of same-gender, same-culture, similar-age individuals. On the other hand, very large differences in age can result in a gap that is difficult to overcome. Indeed, older and younger adults require different kinds of intervention strategies and use of language in a group (Thompson et al., 2000). Also, if cultural factors and differences make it difficult for group members to relate in even the most basic ways, such as differences in fundamental values, it may be preferable to aim for somewhat more homogeneity. Also, language can be problematic if a group member has trouble speaking or understanding the chosen language of the group. In individual therapy, language issues are more readily overcome, because the therapist can take this into account and take the necessary time to explain concepts. This is unlikely to be possible in group treatment.

THERAPISTS

Therapist Preparation

Because of the challenges and complexity that the group format adds to CBT, therapists who take primary responsibility for conducting a group should first have adequate training in individual CBT and previous exposure to group CBT as well. Because of the success of CBT in randomized, controlled trials and various systems pressures to implement evidence-based treatments, many new practitioners from various mental health professions continue to be trained in this approach. Often this occurs in relatively short workshops or through self-directed learning. Indeed, given the specificity of most group protocols and the prevailing notion that CBT is a straightforward approach that is readily learned, it is possible to foster the illusion that group CBT is simple to learn and do, and requires minimal training. We advocate that group therapists have a combination of previous experiences in CBT before leading a group. Ideally this would consist of the following elements:

1. Didactic training/coursework in CBT models and techniques.
2. Direct (ideally hour for hour) supervision on multiple individual cases of CBT.
3. Observational participation in a CBT group led by another therapist.
4. Taking on the role of a coleader.

Each of these elements adds a distinct type of knowledge, first establishing a basis for a CBT orientation to treatment and then experiencing, observing, and finally working with group process issues as well. Also noteworthy is that preparation for CBT in treating one kind of disorder does not necessarily prepare a group therapist to treat another kind of disorder. For example, the relative weighting of different strategies in anxiety and mood disorders requires different skills sets and experience, and may not be sufficient for another area without more specialized training.

Therapist Stance in Treatment

Relatively little has been written about the interpersonal style or leadership qualities required for CBT group therapists. White (2000) has made several very useful suggestions about the leader of a group:

1. Models active participation.
2. Models tolerance and openness to individual differences.
3. Uses collaboration and Socratic dialogue.
4. Communicates the universality of experiences using "we" language.

In addition to these important issues, which are illustrated in sample dialogues in this volume, other important structure and process factors have important implications for group therapists. Clearly, CBT requires a combination of both didactic and process work, and each requires a distinctive style. The didactic portion (e.g., presenting the concept of an automatic thought or the nature of an exposure hierarchy) draws heavily on public speaking/presentation skills of therapists. Communication must be simple, clear, and direct, and it is imperative that therapists stay "on message" to complete these tasks, so that the agenda is fulfilled in a timely fashion. Once the more process-oriented portion of a session begins (e.g., helping patients to articulate their automatic thoughts or to develop their own hierarchies), the therapist can take a much more traditional, less directive CBT therapeutic stance, using questions and feedback to deepen understanding and disclosure in patients. This also translates into nonverbal behavior; most therapists stand when presenting didactically and are more likely to sit when an example is being discussed and group process is coming to the fore.

In this sense, the therapist acts much like a coach or guide teaching a new skill. Using the analogy of teaching golf, at first the therapist presents information and frequent "hands-on" feedback about skills, just as a golf coach may help the novice with many minute and directive suggestions around grip, stance, or swing. As time goes by and skills develop, the coach steps back and allows the student to make more independent decisions while playing the course, offering corrective feedback only when the student goes in a non-helpful direction. So a CBT group therapist, over the course of sessions, can step back and allow the group to do more of the therapeutic work. Even at that stage, the therapist's few suggestions are still very important, just as a coach is still important, even to a professional golfer.

Thus, therapists in CBT groups should observe the following general principles, and competence in this area should be defined accordingly:

1. The CBT group therapist embodies the CBT principles of collaborative empiricism, guided discovery, and Socratic learning (described in detail in Chapter 3, this volume).
2. The CBT group therapist is sensitive to process factors (described in detail in Chapter 2, this volume), observing important connections between group members, encouraging openness, and encouraging supportive (and therapeutic) feedback between group members.
3. The primary CBT group therapist is responsible for keeping the group on track through the agenda, redirecting the group as needed to stay on that agenda.
4. The CBT group therapist uses a warm, empathic, directive style that balances group cohesion with group learning.
5. The CBT group therapist observes any obstacles or problems in process and structure, and actively attempts to solve these issues within the group (see Chapter 6).
6. The CBT group therapist is sensitive to the stage of group development, respecting the evolution of group dynamics and allowing the group enough autonomy for members to work with one another.

Number of Therapists

Generally, two therapists are preferred in most applications, and most often the arrangement involves a primary therapist and a cotherapist. The primary therapist takes a greater share of responsibility for leading the group discussion and making the central decisions about following the agenda and process issues. The cotherapist, who has fewer immediate responsibilities, can cover some of the material, and, very importantly, offers a second set of clinical "eyes and ears." While the primary therapist is occupied with presenting material and working examples, the cotherapist is able to note group interactions and process factors about which the primary therapist may need to be informed.

Typically, therapists meet briefly before each session to discuss what material each will be responsible for and to anticipate any potential issues with the material and group members. Equally important, therapists should debrief for a short time after the session. Here the cotherapist and therapist can share any important observations related to use of techniques or process and plan for whatever necessary corrective action that is needed. For example, the cotherapist may be observing a group member who is struggling to keep up with the material, something the group leader may not yet know. It may then be determined that the cotherapist follow up with a phone call to the patient to determine what the difficulties are. This raises a second benefit of having two therapists. The workload of calling patients who miss sessions, assessments, progress notes, and termination reports can also be split. Debriefing can also be useful as a form of peer supervision relative to using techniques, optimizing strategies, or examining whether important opportunities were missed in the session.

The context of CBT groups also has much to offer in terms of training. Advanced trainees can be very effective cotherapists, and acting in such a role is often the final preparation for becoming a primary group therapist. It may also be desirable, especially in teaching settings, to have a third therapist/learner who is a participant/observer in the group. This role will likely be more flexible; some learners may need simply to observe the model in action, whereas others may wish to present some material formally or lead the questioning to gain a working familiarity with the techniques. The learner would participate both in preparation and therapist debriefing, and perhaps would also be involved in an additional period of supervision with the primary therapist to discuss his or her own learning.

A final consideration in examining the number and makeup of therapists is the extent to which this context changes CBT practitioners into a CBT team. It is imperative that the two or more therapists involved in a CBT group see themselves as, and act like, a team; that is, therapists should display a unified front and message to the group at all times. This can be challenged when the two therapists have different ideas about where a group should go; for example, in a Socratic dialogue, the primary and cotherapist may each have a different sense of which questioning strategy is ideal. While it is sometimes possible for each therapist to take a turn in the questioning, therapists need to be very careful about contradicting, or even appearing to contradict, one another. This can send a very confusing message to the group and possibly undermine the group's esteem for one, and often both, therapists. We have noted in our setting situations where two therapists had a very clear difference of opinion on a clinical matter; in essence, both thought they had the "correct" information about a patient question, and neither therapist (both were in training) was willing to cede on the point. The resulting, open disagreement had a far more deleterious impact on the group than if a therapist had said something technically incorrect. Such information can always be corrected in a subsequent group; a clash between therapists cannot be so easily undone. Similarly, therapists can differ about how much time or emphasis to put on any particular topic or example; in the end, this should always be the primary therapist's responsibility during the session itself. The debriefing is the proper forum for therapists to have a full discussion of any differences about the direction of the group or approach to any specific clinical scenario. In many cases, the two therapists might reach a similar conclusion once a full discussion takes place; such discussions obviously cannot happen during the group itself. Resolution of therapist differences can sometimes require taking additional, new information back to the group, especially if it is determined that some countertherapeutic, or at the very least nonoptimal, information or process has taken place. Specific troubleshooting around leadership and cotherapist issues are discussed in greater detail in Chapter 6 of this book.

GROUP STRUCTURE

Structure of Group Sessions

Unlike traditional group approaches, almost all CBT groups are likely to be closed; that is, group members are preselected and are all present for each of the sessions. One potential exception to this general rule might be inpatient treatment programs in which patients may be hospitalized and discharged within a relatively short period of time. In such groups, the principles of CBT are likely to be kept simple and repeated frequently, so that even with a short hospital stay of a few days, patients are exposed to some of the basic ideas.

Group sessions tend to be either 90 minutes or 2 hours in length. The former can be more efficient, whereas the latter allows for more time. A 2-hour group session can allow for a brief break, whereas a 90-minute session typically does not allow for a break. We suggest a 2-hour length for several reasons, first because it allows for needed flexibility in starting the group; it can often take extra time to start the group as members assemble and complete their symptom checklists. Also, a 2-hour length allows for more opportunities to include as many individuals as possible in the discussion and examples; this length may also be necessary for groups doing exposure exercises (see Chapter 4, this volume). Groups that last for more than 2 hours can seem overlong, both from the therapists' and patients' perspectives. More than 2 hours tends to stretch the capacity for patients to attend to material.

Selecting a Protocol

The most common approach to selecting a protocol is to determine the predominant or primary diagnosis of group members. This approach, reflected in Chapters 7 to 15, describes specific approaches to panic disorder, obsessive–compulsive disorder, social phobia, depression, bipolar disorder, eating disorders, substance abuse, personality disorders, and schizophrenia. These protocols have tended to be developed for randomized, controlled trials and thus have considerable specificity for only one disorder. However it is also possible to create more general protocols, for example, in the case of groups that include members with comorbid conditions (described in Chapter 16). In other clinical applications, for example, community mental health settings, group members have a variety of primary disorders that therapists must consider when determining what techniques should be implemented. This may involve selecting specific techniques from single disorder protocols and adapting these to a broader range of difficulties. For example, any anxiety condition will benefit from some type of controlled exposure, elements of which could be taken from social phobia, obsessive–compulsive disorder, or panic treatments.

Before a group begins, a session plan should be laid out to describe the overall plan for what techniques will be taught and to what level of detail and depth. In creating "customized" protocols, special attention needs to be given to the flow of material, so that it is logical and provides a steady progression of learning. One important area to consider is homework, because homework gives patients an opportunity to practice skills learned in one session and at the same time serves as the basis for new learning in the subsequent session. Once this process is completed, it is useful to create a package of materials to be distributed to group members. This can be as formal as constructing a comprehensive manual or as informal as a set of handouts that includes homework sheets. This package should also include any necessary contact information for therapists, dates, and times of sessions.

Group Rules

An important point of departure, usually covered in the first session, is to discuss group rules. These rules cover important areas, including confidentiality, attendance, compliance with homework, and what to do if unable to attend the group. Consideration should also be given to a therapy "contract" that outlines an agreement for group members to attend a minimum number of sessions and a commitment to completing homework. The rules of confidentiality, which may be slightly different in various jurisdictions, should be explicitly discussed in the group, just as they would be in individual therapy. Although these legal and ethical bounds to confidentiality are unlikely to be flexible, group members should discuss the extent to which what they learn in the group could/should be shared with loved ones. In individual therapy, this is rarely a problem, because any experience in that setting is the patient's own and can be readily discussed as the patient deems fit. However, in discussing the group experience with others in their lives, patients may be sharing anecdotes and describing conversations between themselves and other patients. Thus, there is some potential for the listener to receive identifying, personal information about other patients in the group. These issues should be discussed by the group, and some consensus should be reached. Usually this involves a compromise in which patients agree that, when discussing group with others, they allude only vaguely to others' anecdotes or to any of their own discussions with copatients, and most importantly that no identifying information (i.e., copatients' professional status, place of residence, marital status) be discussed outside the group.

Discussion of group rules is also an excellent time to introduce and socialize group members to the model of intervention and expectations about group interaction. Members enter groups with widely varying assumptions and expectations about what the group will be like, ranging from a process-oriented group (e.g., 12-step programs) to something resembling a "course," in which learning is the only goal. The introduction to group rules should thus make plain that a CBT group combines elements of learning, like a course, with elements of experience and group support. The group rules should be explicit about the desire for group members to provide feedback to one another and ask questions of each other. This process will certainly evolve as the group develops, but it is helpful to establish from the outset that group members can and should interact among themselves, not just with and through the leader.

Individual Needs

It is necessary in any group to address the different needs of individuals, but it is also important to emphasize clinical issues in the group whenever possible. Sample scenarios in which individuals need attention include times when patients must miss a group session and would benefit from an update, or when patients have concerns that they prefer to express privately to therapists. When patients do need to miss a session, planned or not, one of the cotherapists should at least make telephone contact with the patient, if possible, providing an update on what occurred in the group and a summary of new material.

More complex decisions need to be made when patients appear to be struggling in a group; we consider this issue specifically in Chapter 6 on troubleshooting. There are certainly times when, for the sake of the individual, as well as other group participants, it may be necessary to provide individual treatment and withdraw someone from the group. It is preferable to do this as openly as possible. Similarly, patients sometimes feel that they cannot or should not bring up certain issues in the context of the group. In such cases, they may ask to speak to therapists privately, which is certainly acceptable, so long as the therapist keeps in mind the priorities of the group. In most cases, it is preferable to bring that issue directly to the group and to help the patient to see the benefits of taking that course of action.

Homework

An absolute priority before beginning a group is to have a structured plan for the assignment and review of homework, as well as preparation of any handouts, worksheets, and exercises that go with the homework. When the homework assignment is left until the last minute or is otherwise cursory or ambiguous, compliance rates fall sharply. We also advocate that at the beginning of each session homework be handed directly to the therapists, who quickly review it. This procedure has several advantages. First, when patients are made aware that homework is to be "handed in," they are more motivated to attempt to complete it. Second, therapists can ascertain directly how well each group member is understanding the material, because they review each individual's work. Third, by surveying the homework, therapists can make a preliminary plan around which examples they will use in the group. Once the homework has been surveyed, and this is often done while participants complete their symptom inventories, it can be returned to each person for use during the session. Also, before openly discussing any homework example in the group, the therapist should ask the permission of the group member to use his or her example.

Choosing Examples

An everyday but important decision that group therapists face is selecting which of many possible examples they might use from the group to illustrate a new technique or to make some other important therapeutic point. For example, if the group as a whole completed 15 thought records, which thought record(s) should be explored in further detail and receive the feedback of the entire group?

Three factors are important to consider. First, group members should be asked whether they have an example that they struggled with or one that they found particularly useful. This reflects a collaborative approach, and allows patients to follow up on examples about which they have important unresolved questions.

A second factor to consider when selecting an example is the intent behind the discussion that the therapist hopes to trigger. In some instances, examples are chosen because they illustrate a point particularly well, or were completed by the patient and had a successful outcome. We term these "positive examples"; they help model how a technique can work well or demonstrate a successful outcome of a problem using a CBT technique. "Positive examples" should be chosen to emphasize the benefits of strategies being taught, because this encourages other group members to use the same strategies in their own situations. However, it should be noted that these examples do not necessarily lead to in-depth discussion, because of the very fact that they do involve an issue that is already fully and positively resolved. A second kind of example that we term "in-progress" involves an item that is as yet unresolved or on which the patient is stuck. These examples can take more time and be more challenging; however, they demonstrate to the group important aspects of working through techniques using Socratic dialogue and other specific CBT techniques, and tend to deepen group process, adding to cohesion and the group's ability to work together. In-progress examples illustrate the therapeutic principles in action and help to move the person toward a successful resolution. A third kind of example, the "transition example," is similar to in-progress examples because it is unresolved; however, transition examples are chosen because they illustrate how the new material for the session can be applied in a specific instance. To return to the thought record homework example, if the goal of the session is to discuss underlying beliefs for the first time, the therapist might select an example in which a belief, more than an automatic thought, seems to be maintaining negative affect or impairment. Good transition examples help group members to understand why a new strategy is being taught and illustrate these new techniques in action in a "real" situation encountered by a group member.

A third factor to consider is "generalizability" of an example. All other things being equal, the examples that generate the most useful discussion are those that are most likely to be shared experiences for many, or most, group members. For example, in depression, examples that involve self-deprecating themes are most likely to resonate with all group members. Such examples are more useful than more idiosyncratic, or complicated, scenarios that lead to difficulties for only one group member.

WITHIN-SESSION STRUCTURE

CBT can be distinguished from many other therapeutic approaches simply by the fact that each session of a course of therapy follows a rational and comprehensive sequence. Even as the content of each group session advances, the basic structure of the sessions is predictable for both therapists and group members. This structure is of central importance for two main reasons. First, the effectiveness of CBT is based primarily on the extent to which the patient learns to use the skills conveyed in therapy. Thus, CBT places a priority on creating an interactive learning forum. Also, an emerging body of research evidence supports the notion that structural elements of CBT, particularly homework, are important as "effective ingredients" in therapy.

If learning is to occur, what is the best means by which to facilitate this process? Two extremes probably define the spectrum of possibilities, and these can also be found in approaches to education in general. At one extreme would be highly structured, rote exercises; education-based examples would be drills to teach spelling or multiplication tables. At the other extreme would be a highly unstructured and undirected, experiential approach, in which principles are said to be discovered rather than learned. Both of these extreme approaches have drawbacks. The former is mechanistic and repetitive—perhaps even boring—and is experienced as a chore rather than learning; a CBT group that is too structured would resemble a course with "lectures." On the other hand, the experiential extreme is inefficient and could result in missing out on important principles; a CBT group based on experiential learning would resemble an encounter group. The approach to group CBT sessions we advocate represents a middle ground between these two extremes. The therapists ensure that during each group session, and over sessions of therapy, the important skills and principles of CBT are covered. At the same time, real problems are discussed and integrated in a way that is not preplanned, and that allows for flexible learning. This approach represents the concept of "guided discovery," a term that describes both the directive and explorative nature of CBT.

The structural elements of CBT sessions described here include seven distinct components that are also present in individual CBT: status check, clarification, the session bridge, the agenda, capsule summaries, session summary, and homework. Each is described in detail below.

Status Check

This usually represents the starting point of the session and has several goals. The first is to understand the patient's clinical status relative to the previous session and to determine whether any improvement has occurred. In many instances, this is most efficiently done using a self-report measure that patients complete while waiting for the group to begin. It is also important to gather some information on the person's functioning, because behavioral change is likely to be part of most therapy goals as well. Second, this is an important opportunity to ask for feedback concerning the homework and the experience of the homework. Third, the status check can reveal whether an important crisis or other event has occurred that needs to be considered during the group.

Typically, this is accomplished via a "go-around," with a member volunteering to go first and then following around with each member. Group therapists often learn a considerable amount from this brief weekly review, including to what extent patients seem to be learning and implementing techniques, their level of compliance, ongoing stressors and impairments, as well as questions group members have about the material. Group therapists may make notes to themselves about issues that they can integrate into that day's session in addition to the material they had planned to review. For example, if one of the planned agenda items is to review avoidance of anxiety-provoking situations and a group member mentions an avoidance decision, the therapist might refer back to that example when presenting the material later in that session. This obviously makes the material more "live" and relevant to the group members.

The status check is also an important time for group members to learn about one another. Review of the week's events often gives group members considerable personal information about one another's lives, and this is important for developing mutual understanding and cohesion. The difficulty with this step tends to be that it can take too much time; thus, it is important to socialize group members to provide their review in a couple of minutes or less.

Clarification

The next area of inquiry relates to the previous session and concerns any clarifications that need to be made. Because much information is provided in each session, group members may well be unclear about a concept or issue from the previous session. Ensuring that such questions are answered is critical for the process of group therapy; patients who do not understand important concepts are likely to be left behind, both by new material and by the group process. To perform the clarification, therapists typically inquire whether group members have questions about material covered in the last session as well as questions that may have arisen around the homework, which often puts skills learned in the last session into practice.

Bridge

The "bridge," the next structural element, is essentially an encapsulation of the last group session, followed by some indication of what is to come in the session. The bridge is important in that it not only introduces the topic for the session but it is also a second opportunity to check learning from the previous session. The bridge is most essential for creating the "story" of therapy. Without it, sessions may seem disconnected, operating in isolation from one another. A bridge is particularly effective when it includes some examples from group members and the homework that was just reviewed. A bridge should be relatively brief, perhaps only a minute or two, and requires careful planning and review of the previous week's notes.

Agenda

The agenda, the next component of the session, involves setting up the "plan" for the session. This is perhaps the most collaborative and formal aspect of beginning the session. It is also here that therapists ask group members directly about their priorities for the session. Much of the information gleaned from the status check, clarification, and bridge can be used to help set the agenda relative to group members' needs. Therapists typically record the agenda on the white board and leave it there, so that group members can follow and anticipate where the session is going. Leaving the agenda on the board can also help therapists explain their need for time management when examples threaten to run over time limits.

The new material for the session is largely determined by the protocol the therapist is following, and this represents the other half of the collaboration. Establishing a balance between patients' wishes and the material that needs to be covered to continue learning is sometimes challenging, but it is more easily accomplished as group leaders gain experience with the process. Compared to individual CBT, an agenda for a group is likely to have fewer items, because each area requires input from multiple individuals. Also, there are circumstances when it is necessary to deviate from the agenda, and this can be guided by both process and technique issues. Sometimes group members may struggle with a certain concept, and this may need to be communicated clearly before it is possible to move on. Other times, the group may need to focus on process issues before moving on. On the other hand, if the group leaders allow too much "drift" from the agenda, they risk falling behind in the protocol. When considering a deviation from the agenda, group leaders should ask themselves, "Will the deviation we are considering be as helpful for this group in the long run as the material we had planned to cover?"

Summaries

A considerable amount of new learning takes place for group members in each session of CBT. To facilitate and check learning, it is necessary occasionally to summarize the points just covered. Summarizing is distinct from Socratic dialogue; it is a more didactic exercise that involves interleaving CBT concepts and elements of group members' disclosures to make the therapy "real." Summaries are best used after a concept has been explained and applied to a problem from a group member's life. The summary is a succinct recapitulation of the concept (e.g., a thought distortion is a biased way of interpreting things) and perhaps one or two examples of this concept in the different group member's lives (e.g., the person was "mind reading" in an interaction, or "catastrophizing" after receiving some form of feedback). The most important summary occurs near the end of the session and involves a recapitulation of the most important points in the session. Many of the skills in summarizing are the same as those required for bridging; that is, the therapist must translate principles into understandable language and include group members' examples to illustrate these principles. Summaries, which test understanding, also may involve questions to and from group members. Summaries also form turning points or transitions in therapy that mark the movement of the discussion from one agenda point to the next.

Homework

The final, critical portion of the session is homework discussion and assignment. Ideally, homework planning is based on both the content of the session and the protocol, and group members' examples whenever possible; that is, good homework assignments blend the concepts learned in therapy with patients' unresolved problems. It is important that sufficient time be left in the session to discuss the homework, rather than having homework be an afterthought. As a rule of thumb, all other session business should be closed, with 10 minutes left free for homework. This leaves time to describe, discuss, and finalize homework plans. Process issues also come into play here. Therapists should encourage group members to provide feedback to one another about the type of homework that would be most helpful for each person.

CONCLUSIONS

Group CBT combines learning and experience in equal measure, with the goal of relieving symptoms and reestablishing the best possible functioning and quality of life. The structure of the experience is critical for optimizing both techniques and process. Before one contemplates a group program, administrative details are important to consider. We have highlighted the issue of patient selection, offering specific suggestions for evaluating the suitability of patients for a group. This can make a critical difference; some groups, from the very first session, feel much more cohesive and positive than others. Most often this reflects a good mix of individuals who "fit" the protocol and also complement one another. Some amount of homogeneity among group members is therefore clearly desirable, but some differences between group members can actually be very positive. We also discussed some issues regarding therapist training and stance, keeping in mind that all CBT is provided through the conduit of the group leaders. The approach they take dictates a great deal about the success of the group. Finally, it is important for therapists to construct protocols and plans for a group carefully, paying special attention to flow of concepts, sessions structure, and creating homework that ties sessions together.

In this chapter, we have also proposed that good group CBT expertly balances the learning objective of a protocol with the experiential needs of group members. Of course, this ideal balance may occasionally be challenged by difficult clinical dilemmas. In some cases, therapists must choose between spending more time to explore and deepen understanding and making sure that they get through the planned didactic material. In day-to-day clinical work, this most often comes to a head when a group member is experiencing strong affect in response to an example, has just made a significant personal disclosure, or has made an important cognitive–affective discovery. When time is short, as it so often is in structured protocols, what a therapist chooses to do represents the influences of many factors simultaneously. But, fundamentally, therapists must analyze the pros and cons, and make a critical decision. Do the advantages of staying with the "experience" or affect outweigh the costs of falling behind in the protocol? What is more important in the short and long term, one group member's current experience and potential for a therapeutic breakthrough or the groups' long-term benefit? What course of action would increase group cohesiveness? What course of action might put cohesiveness at risk? Perhaps most important, can I use what is happening with this client right now to support the point of learning that this group needs? Skilled therapists typically answer "yes" to this final question, and doing so often resolves the apparent tension between dealing with the experiential and the didactic in CBT structure. In well-functioning CBT groups, good techniques and good process are synergistic and always in balance.

CHAPTER 6

Overcoming Obstacles in CBT Groups
CHALLENGES AND PROBLEMS IN GROUP STRUCTURE

Conducting CBT group therapy may appear straightforward in terms of following a preset format and protocol; however, putting protocol into practice, particularly in a group setting, is a dynamic, evolving process that will change with each group as a function of the group members, the clinical picture, and therapist style and skill. Each disorder-specific chapter in this book includes a section to address disorder-specific obstacles and challenges associated with group CBT. However, it is also helpful to consider the obstacles and challenges inherent in CBT groups from a more global perspective. In fact, when we train learners in group therapy, it is from the vantage point of covering the basic principles of group therapy and process, so that they can apply their knowledge and skills to conducting a range of specifically tailored CBT groups. As such, it is important for trainees to have an appreciation of general obstacles associated with group therapy. With any group, problems may arise with respect to three areas: challenging patients, group process, and leadership. This chapter focuses specifically on some of the more common problems and challenges that occur in each of these three areas.

CHALLENGING PATIENTS

In our experience, each group a therapist conducts is likely to have at least one patient that presents a challenge to group process, to other group members, and to group leadership. Consider the following examples of statements made by patients in a group:

PAUL: I don't have anything to share. Nothing happened this week.

WAYNE: (*Interrupting another group member who started to speak*) I know exactly what that is like. For me, I always have to stop whatever I am doing when I get anxious.

TRACI: We are all putting on a persona. Every one of us is fake and we put on an act to others, so that they don't know what we are dealing with inside. We can only do that for so long before something gives.

LESLEY: (*Interrupting group leader in an angry voice*) I have tried this type of treatment before and it hasn't been helpful. It has only been three sessions, but I don't find this group helpful either. I am wondering what other group members feel.

These real examples of group dialogue are likely to trigger some degree of recognition for all CBT group therapists, and are clear indicators of trouble that make therapists have their own "hot thoughts!" But more than being examples of group members' ambivalence or resistance, these examples challenge group leadership and can undermine good group process, and thereby undermine effective treatment. Such challenges are most likely to emerge during the transition phase of the group, when the personalities of individual group members start to emerge and exert influence.

Yalom (1995) has described a number of different "problem patients" that present a challenge to the group, including the monopolist, the silent patient, the boring patient, the help-rejecting complainer, the psychotic patient, the characterologically difficult patient, and the borderline patient. Although these different "problematic presentations" have not been a focus of empirical study, it is our experience that within each CBT group, one or more prototypical problem group members may present a challenge to group functioning. The group leader can use group process and specific interventions to help manage these challenging group members and facilitate group functioning. The common prototypes for challenging group members within a CBT group are presented in Table 6.1, along with strategies for management.

It is important for the group leaders to work through conflicts that may arise from challenging group members and build group cohesiveness. Group leaders need to be sensitive to a number of domains that may signal process difficulties. These areas include being alert to nonverbal behavior and body language (e.g., if one group member is doodling on a paper when another group member is talking, it is a sign that he or she is not engaged in the group), and being sensitive to initial resistance that may occur in a number of subtle ways (e.g., a group member not participating or volunteering information, showing up late, missing sessions, having a difficult time being open to the information presented, such as wanting to hold on to a biological explanation, or having a negative attitude about the value of group or the treatment). It is important to address these types of resistance that may have an impact on other group members' attitudes and commitment to the treatment.

TABLE 6.1. Challenging Group Member Prototypes and Strategies for Management

Prototype	Description	Therapeutic management
Quiet and silent type	• Group participation is minimal. • Prefers to sit in silence.	• Use group to help draw out. • Ask direct questions to help facilitate interaction. • Try to link experiences to other group members' experiences. • When appropriate, process thoughts and feelings about being in the group.
Overbearing type	• Monopolizes group time. • Has no difficulty sharing information.	• Use containment strategies to help balance group time. • May use subtle management strategies (i.e., not reinforcing continued talking with questions or eye contact). • May eventually require more overt management strategies, such as stopping the person midstream (e.g., "I am going to stop you there so we can hear from others").
The helper	• Always giving advice that may or may not be helpful. • May talk in generalities using "we" and not "I." • May focus on others and not on own issues.	• Encourage the person to reflect on personal experience and speak in the first person. • If advice is helpful, then reinforce and direct the person to how he or she can focus on his or her own issues. • If advice is not helpful (e.g., "If you are anxious about going, then don't go"), then process within the group (e.g., "What do group members think about that idea?" or "How does that idea fit with the goals of the group?").
The disbeliever	• A pessimistic person who doesn't really buy into treatment. • May have already tried CBT a number of times. • May challenge the therapist and the therapy.	• "Roll with resistance" (Miller & Rollnick, 2002): Do not engage in argument; agree/validate member's feelings, then shift direction to emphasize personal responsibility and choice. • Use strategies for working with resistance in the group covered in the transition phase from Chapter 2.
The drifter	• Sometimes shows up and sometimes does not. • Does not appear to be committed to the group.	• Address in group. • May need to have an individual meeting.

(continued)

TABLE 6.1. *(continued)*

Prototype	Description	Therapeutic management
The not-appropriate-for-group member	• Somehow this member made it through screening. • Problematic in group because his or her issues may be different from those of the rest of the group. • Often due to problematic personality features (e.g., paranoia) or other conditions that require immediate attention.	• Use management and containment strategies. • Acknowledge that his or her needs may be different from those of the group and shift focus to what the individual may gain from group participation. • May need to discontinue group and find alternative treatment option if the person is too disruptive or treatment needs have shifted.

Group leaders also need to understand that resistance to change may be driven by a number of factors, as described by Leahy (2001), including the need for validation of feelings before moving to an action-based approach, and the inability to manage intense emotions that may be elicited by active therapy. Change required by treatment may be inconsistent with past experience or self-schemas and incompatible with moral beliefs and values. Also, change required by an action-based treatment such as CBT may undermine the benefits of not changing and may be seen as risky in terms of "rocking the boat" or creating instability. Finally, change may lead to a focus on problems that may appear overwhelming and insurmountable.

Incorporating motivational interviewing principles (Miller & Rollnick, 2002) to manage resistance may be helpful in these instances. These strategies include expressing empathy to help normalize ambivalence, developing discrepancies between group members' goals and their present behavior, and "rolling with resistance" by empathizing, validating, and giving the problem back to the group to discuss. Possible microtherapeutic interventions to facilitate these include the following:

• Giving responsibility back to the patient by highlighting the choice of being in the group.
• Normalizing doubts and emphasizing the importance of keeping an open mind and trying the strategies.
• Discussing the importance of homework and the empirical base of the treatment approach.
• Encouraging a wait-and-see attitude (e.g., "What do you have to lose?").

- Containing negativity to prevent contamination of the group.
- Clarifying or providing education by examining your role as group leader and determining what you can do to work through resistance.
- Focusing the group member on his or her own feelings and experience.
- Exploring obstacles that may be in the way of involvement.

What happens when these strategies are put into action? Management of the challenges presented at the beginning of this chapter is illustrated below. Note that these categories are not mutually exclusive. For example, the disbelieving member may be either quiet or overbearing. Although these descriptive categories are based on clinical experience and not on empirical data, they are useful in that they provide the group leader a set of strategies that may help to guide clinical intervention and to manage group function.

The Quiet and Silent Type

The "quiet and silent" prototypical group member is the member is the individual who prefers to sit quietly, providing minimal participation in the group. This individual may be shy and uncomfortable in a group format. Alternatively, and presenting a greater challenge, is the individual who is silent because of a lack of openness to the treatment, as reflected in guarded participation and involvement in the group. It is helpful for the group leader to ascertain the underlying reason for the lack of participation based on observation or through gentle probing in the group. In many cases, as the group sessions progress, the shy group member may become more comfortable and participation may increase. Similarly, the guarded group member may become more open to the therapy and more involved in the group over time.

There are a number of interventions the group leader may use to facilitate the involvement of a quiet and silent type member. The group leader can use the group to help draw the person out. For example, when the individual shares something, the group leader can link that experience to other group members' experiences, with the aim of increasing comfort level in the group. Alternatively, the group leader may use direct questions to help facilitate interaction. Consider the following example:

THERAPIST: Paul, we haven't heard from you yet. How was your week?

PAUL: I don't have anything to share. Nothing happened this week.

THERAPIST: Did you have any anxiety this week?

PAUL: No, not really.

THERAPIST: So that sounds like it was a good week.

PAUL: No, it wasn't. I just didn't go out of the house.

COTHERAPIST: It sounds like it was not a good week. Paul, can you tell us what made it difficult for you to leave the house?

PAUL: I just didn't feel good.

COTHERAPIST: (*taking it to the group*) Have other people had that experience of not feeling good and having trouble going out?

In this case, Paul has sat silently in the group with minimal participation while others reviewed the homework and how their week went. The group leader attempts to draw Paul out with some direct questions. Paul continues with short answers and is not forthcoming with information. The coleader steps in to provide backup and empathizes with Paul ("It sounds like it was not a good week"), then gently draws him out further. Although Paul's reply was short ("I just didn't feel good"), it provided enough for the coleader to take the issue back to the group to see if other group members could relate to Paul's experience. In this way, the coleader is attempting to highlight the similarity between Paul and the other group members, so that Paul feels more comfortable.

Another intervention for facilitating participation by a quiet group member is to process the individual's thoughts and feelings about being in the group. This strategy may raise issues that other group members can relate to, thereby increasing cohesion and comfort in the group.

The Overbearing Type

The "overbearing" group member is the individual who continually tries to monopolize group time with his or her own experience. This type of member shifts the balance of group participation and may also sidetrack the agenda of the group leaders. Strategies for managing this type of group member may involve subtle or overt containment strategies. Subtle strategies may be used at first, such as not reinforcing continued talking by asking questions, nodding, or making eye contact. If these subtle strategies are not enough, then more overt management strategies may be required. More overt strategies require a considered approach that balances the needs of the individual with that of the group. For example, in each of the following cases the group leader jumps in midstream:

> "Jack, I am going to stop you there. You have raised a good point and I want to see how others have managed."
>
> "Susan, I need to jump in here. Those are interesting issues you have raised. We have a few more things to get through and I am just aware of the time, so we need to move on."
>
> "Katie, let me stop you there. Why don't we hear from others on that point?"

Although waiting for the individual to pause is a better place to jump in, sometimes this does not happen, and interrupting the person is necessary.

Letting the person continue on without containment is not good for group process, because other members may disengage or become frustrated with the overbearing, dominant group member. In addition, the group leaders may not be able to cover the items on the agenda for the group if too much time is taken up by one group member. Development of containment strategies is an important skill for the group leader, and one that takes practice and comes with some experience. These are the most challenging of interventions, and trainees often struggle to become comfortable and skilled in their use.

Consider the following example:

WAYNE: (*interrupting Paul, another group member, who started to speak*) I know exactly what that is like. For me, I always have to stop whatever I am doing when I get anxious.

THERAPIST: Paul, can you tell us what you did at that point?

In this example, the therapist uses a subtle containment strategy by not responding to Wayne by reinforcing his point, which might lead Wayne to continue his personal focus. Instead, the therapist redirects the group's attention back to Paul, so that he has time to discuss his experience.

The Helper

The "helper" is the group member who is always giving advice to other group members and in some cases to the group leaders as well (how to run the group better, etc.). Consider the following example:

TRACI: We are all putting on a persona. Everyone of us is fake and we put on an act to others so that they don't know what we are dealing with inside. We can only do that for so long before something gives.

THERAPIST: Is that how it feels for you, Traci?

TRACI: Yes, it feels like I am wearing a persona.

COTHERAPIST: Can you tell us a bit more about what you mean when you say that "something gives"?

TRACI: Well, I feel like I could just freak out from the pressure. I mean, to everyone around me I look normal and confident. They don't know the struggle that is going on inside me every day trying to fight this anxiety.

THERAPIST: I wonder what other group members think about this?

In this example we see that Traci is trying to be helpful by summing things up and making statements that generalize to the whole group. The group leaders could have let this go, without addressing it, but doing so would have passed up the opportunity to encourage Traci to focus on her own thoughts and feelings. Traci often tried to be helpful in the group by providing suggestions and capturing group experience based on her own framework. It is great to have a helpful group member, and often the feedback and advice is very useful to other group members. However, if an individual is helpful to the point that he or she is unable to reflect on his or her own experiences in a specific manner, this behavioral style inhibits the benefit that comes from group treatment. In addition, broad generalizations made by one group member may capture some of the other group members' experiences but likely are not accurate for everyone in the group. Some group members may not feel comfortable speaking up and dissenting. Or in some cases, group members may feel like they do not belong, because their experience is different.

It is important to socialize group members early on to share their experience from their own personal perspective and to avoid speaking in generalities. Highlighting the symbolic importance of the language that group members choose is a key tool for revealing underlying thoughts and feelings, thus increasing awareness and identifying targets for intervention.

Another issue that may arise is not so much that a person takes on the "helper style," but rather that, invariably, in each group, some group members may provide "help" that is not helpful in many cases, and even worse, is detrimental or counter to the therapeutic aims of the group. This problem may arise whenever a group leader or group member takes an issue to the group for suggestions or feedback. For example, in anxiety groups, a common piece of "unhelpful advice" is one group member's suggestion that another group member avoid an anxiety-provoking activity, thus encouraging behavior that reinforces anxiety and is counter to the aims of the group. In such a case, the group leader can take the advice back to the group by asking group members what they think about it, or how the suggestion fits with what they have learned in the group so far. In this way the "unhelpful" or counter-therapeutic suggestion is dealt with in a constructive manner that is processed in the group to enhance or reinforce the underlying principles or objectives of the therapeutic approach. The group leader could also ask the member who volunteered the suggestion what he or she thought the benefits or costs of taking the advice would be (e.g., reducing anxiety in the short term, but reinforcing it in the long term).

In rare cases, a group member may make a comment that is not helpful at all but is hurtful. In one obsessive–compulsive disorder (OCD) group at our center, we had group members do a go-around in which they shared something about their symptoms and what brought them to treatment. After one group member, who had aggressive obsessions, finished her turn, another group member, who had contamination obsessions, stated to the group: "That's crazy." In this case, the group leader had to stop the group member from saying anything more by jumping in and making a general statement about norms for the group: "We need to remember that although individual group members' symptoms may vary, each person here has the same pattern of symptoms in common, and it is important for us to try and understand each other, even when things seem very different from your own experience."

The group leader then took the issue to the group, so that the member who was singled out could have feedback indicating that not everyone thought her symptoms were crazy: "What do other members think?" In this case, two other group members jumped in to say that they had experienced aggressive obsessions before, and that doing so was not crazy, it was just a representation of OCD symptoms.

The Disbeliever

The "disbeliever" is the pessimistic group member who does not really buy into treatment. He or she may have previously tried CBT or many other different approaches. The disbeliever may be a silent member or an overbearing member. In either case, this individual may challenge the therapist and the therapeutic approach, undermine the treatment, and have a negative effect on the group. Consider the following example:

LESLEY: (*In an angry voice.*) I have tried this type of treatment before and it hasn't been helpful. It has only been three sessions, but I don't find this group helpful either. I am wondering what other group members feel.

THERAPIST: (*Jumping in before group members can respond.*) It is too bad that you aren't finding this treatment helpful, Lesley. It sounds like you have tried a number of treatments before and haven't had relief. That must be very frustrating for you. We know that although this treatment is effective for many people, it does not work for everyone. We would completely understand if you decided that you did not want to continue with the group.

GROUP: (*Silence.*)

LESLEY: Well, I didn't mean that this group wasn't helpful. I am actually enjoying the group, and I do want to continue. I just sometimes feel like I will never get better.

THERAPIST: Do other members sometimes feel discouraged about ever feeling better?

WAYNE: Yes, I sometimes feel that way.

THERAPIST: What about for others?

TRACI: No, I am just hoping that this treatment will work.

COTHERAPIST: That is good, Traci. That is what we ask from people—that they keep an open mind and try the strategies. It is normal to feel discouraged or hopeless at times, and it is helpful for us to talk about these feelings in the group. Why don't we find out how everyone did this week with the homework?

In this example, Lesley jumped in at the start of the group to express her anger, frustration, and dissatisfaction. Although it is entirely acceptable for group members to express their feelings in the group, the issues of timing and type of expression were relevant in this case. With regard to the first issue, the leader of the group had just gotten the group started and was about to do a check-in regarding homework. Lesley's demand at the outset of the group overshadowed the group's focus. In addition, this was only the third group meeting. Group norms were being established, and group cohesion was in the early stages of development. Both processes could potentially have been jeopardized or undermined by an aggressive group member. With regard to type of expression, Lesley expressed her anger in a hostile and aggressive manner that was not appropriate for the group.

The leaders had two options in this situation. One option would have been to let the group respond to Lesley directly, without any intervention on the part of either group leader. Although this is what Lesley wanted, the group leaders felt that it would not be helpful for the group for the following reasons: It could serve to contaminate the group with negativity; once started, it could sidetrack the group from focusing on more productive material; and it could send the message that this type of aggressive expression within the group was acceptable. The second option, and the one that the group leader chose, was to utilize specific containment interventions. First, the leader did not allow Lesley to take her issue directly to the group. Second, she rolled with Lesley's resistance by validating her feelings, then giving her the choice to continue with the treatment or not (highlighting her personal responsibility and choice). Then the therapist took Lesley's issue to the group, but on the therapist's terms. As one can see from the interchange, this option effectively defused Lesley's anger and shifted her toward expressing her feelings in a more appropriate manner (i.e., instead of attacking the group, she was able to voice her feelings of hopelessness about recovery). Instead of potentially contaminating the group with negativity, this exchange promoted group interaction on the feelings of frustration associated with recovery. The group leader then normalized these feelings and shifted back to the task of homework review.

The Drifter

The "drifter" is the group member whose attendance at the group is inconsistent. Sometimes the drifter shows up, and sometimes not. The presence of a drifter can interfere with the therapeutic process by affecting group morale and cohesion. The rest of the group demonstrates commitment by making the group a priority and attending each session, save for an emergency. The drifter may miss sessions for a number of reasons, including lack of commitment to the group (e.g., motivation, doubts about treatment, "disbeliever" type personality), symptom severity (e.g., severe agoraphobia, such that the individual relies on another person to accompany him or her to each session), practical issues (e.g., transportation, child care, work schedule), and social anxiety (discomfort in the group).

It is important for the group leader to address the issues of a drifter early on. It is of no benefit to the drifter to let him or her participate in the group in such a manner, missing important material which future sessions are based. The drifter will likely realize little therapeutic benefit upon group completion. More importantly, if a drifter completes treatment in this manner, he or she may do so with the belief that CBT group treatment was received and was a failure, when in fact an adequate trial of therapy was not completed. In addition, other treatment providers will be led to the conclusion that the individual did not respond to CBT, when in fact this determination is not substantiated.

Minimizing the likelihood of a drifter in the group can start right at the pregroup meeting, when the importance of attendance and commitment to the group is emphasized. Each group member should have the opportunity to discuss with the group leader how he or she can make treatment a priority, problem-solving obstacles that may get in the way. In addition, the pregroup meeting is a last chance to screen group members for their appropriateness for the group. If a potential group member is so impaired that questions are raised as to whether he or she will be able to participate fully in the group, it is more helpful to reconsider the suitability of a group intervention. A severely impaired individual may be better served with a course of one-on-one therapy to prepare for group participation. For example, we had a case in which an individual waiting for group OCD treatment was given six sessions of CBT targeting his social anxiety to ready him for participation in the group.

At the start of the group, the issue of attendance and commitment to the group should be emphasized when reviewing group norms. Group members should be encouraged to inform the group in advance if they know that they will have to miss a session. In these cases, it is helpful to have a makeup session in which one of the group leaders meets with the group member to briefly review material that was missed. If a group member misses a session and does not notify the group leaders, it is important for the group leaders to follow up with a phone call to check in. If a missed session is ignored by the group leaders, it undermines the importance of participation in the group. It is helpful to set a rule up front regarding the number of missed sessions allowed before an individual will not be able to continue participation in the group. This should be reviewed in the pregroup meeting, as well as in the first group session, when the group norms are covered. In short-term treatments that consist of 10–15 sessions, a limit of two missed sessions is reasonable.

Once the group is under way, the group leader can manage a drifter by reviewing the issue of attendence with the group as a whole. For example, group leaders can check in with the individual in the go-around regarding difficulties that he or she is having in coming to the group. These difficulties can then be discussed within the group setting. If the problem is practical in nature, a problem-solving approach can be used within the group. Periodically, it is helpful to ask the group as a whole about thoughts and feelings about the group experience (e.g., "How are people feeling about being in the group? What do people think so far?"). In this way, group members can relate to one another, and expectations can be clarified.

If the issue is not resolved within the group, the group leaders may have to meet with the drifter individually to discuss continued participation in the group. This meeting would involve presenting the group leaders' concerns about the inconsistent attendance at group and the effect this has on the individual, the group, and the effectiveness of treatment. Continued participation may be contingent upon no further missed sessions. In some cases, it may be concluded that now is not the right time for the individual to be participating in the treatment, or that this treatment is not suitable. In the latter case, efforts should be made to consider alternative options.

The Not Appropriate for Group Member

The "not appropriate for group" member is an individual who has made it through the screening and into the group, but once the group is under way, it becomes evident that the individual is not appropriate for the group, or that the group is not appropriate for the individual. This occurs primarily due to issues of diagnosis and personality. With the exception of more recent advances in CBT targeting comorbidity (e.g., Barlow, Allen, & Choate, 2004), traditional CBT is based on protocols designed to address single disorders. Thus, it is not surprising that problems may arise when comorbidity is present.

When a coexisting condition becomes a primary concern, the group may no longer be the appropriate treatment intervention. In addition, occasional misdiagnosis may lead to inclusion of a member who is not appropriate for the group. Consider the following example: Ellen presented for treatment at an anxiety clinic, and following the assessment, it was determined that panic disorder and agoraphobia was her primary diagnosis. An additional diagnosis of posttraumatic stress disorder (PTSD) was assigned. Ellen was placed in a group treatment for panic disorder. In the third session, it became quite clear that Ellen's panic attacks really were not out of the blue but were triggered by thoughts that she could be in danger or be assaulted. Her panic attacks were really encompassed by the diagnosis of PTSD, and a diagnosis of panic disorder was not supported. This posed a dilemma for the group leaders. It was clear that Ellen found it difficult to relate to the other group members, because her experience was quite different. In turn, it was also hard for the other group members to relate to Ellen for the same reasons. After the third session, the group leaders met with Ellen to discuss options. They decided that Ellen would benefit more from individual treatment for her PTSD. Ellen agreed that this option made more sense for her and she discontinued her participation in the group. This issue was addressed at the next group session. Ellen came to say good-bye to the group, which allowed her closure. Following her departure, group members were given the opportunity to discuss any thoughts or feelings they had about having a group member leave early.

In addition to issues of Axis I comorbidity, problematic personality traits are another common problem that can lead to a member not being appropriate for group format. Ideally, this would be flagged during the assessment process or the pregroup meeting, but sometimes these traits are missed or are not thought to be of such concern that group format should be excluded as a treatment option. Common personality styles that may pose a problem to the group include paranoid, aggressive and hostile, narcissistic, borderline, and schizotypal. In many cases, individuals with such personality styles can be managed within the group, but their presence is more of a challenge for the group leaders (see Chapter 14, this volume, for a complete discussion of these issues).

To cope with a difficult group member, group leaders can use management and containment strategies. In some cases, this may involve education around appropriate expression of feelings in the group (e.g., for an aggressive and hostile member). Any of the strategies listed at the beginning of this chapter may be useful. If a group member with a co-occurring condition is continuing in the group, it is helpful to acknowledge that his or her needs may differ from group needs, and that he or she may need to focus on what can be gained from group participation rather than what the group does not do. For example, Vincent was in a group for panic disorder, but he also had a diagnosis of irritable bowel syndrome. He found it hard to relate to the idea that nothing bad would happen during a panic attack, because he frequently did experience diarrhea when highly stressed. Vincent's panic symptoms and irritable bowel symptoms were overlapping. He frequently expressed his frustration with the group, his feeling that he was different, and that the strategies did not apply to him. In this case, the group leaders had to address Vincent's concerns by validating his feelings (i.e., he was different), then refocus on what Vincent could gain from the group experience rather than what the group did not give him. Finally, if a group member is too disruptive, the group leaders may need to discontinue the member's participation in the group and find alternative treatment options.

CHALLENGES TO GROUP PROCESS IN CBT

The presence of any of the prototypical problem members discussed earlier may interfere with group process and the smooth facilitation of the group. In this section, we discuss additional factors that may present a challenge to group process.

Didactic Components of CBT

As discussed in Chapter 2, presentation of the educational components of CBT has the potential to challenge group process when material is presented didactically, without the opportunity for group interaction. It is important for group leaders to present educational material in a way that is interactive, and ideally discovered through Socratic questioning of group members and group dialogue. When the group leaders are too didactic, the group takes on the feeling of a classroom rather than a therapy setting that promotes open expression of thoughts and feelings.

Structure of CBT

Having structure and an agenda within the group sessions is an important component of the CBT approach. However, if a session is overly structured to the point that there is little or no opportunity for silence, time for reflection, and spontaneous group interaction, then group process is compromised. Group leaders should budget additional time outside of the structured agenda items to address issues that may arise outside of the anticipated discussion. It is also helpful to plan time at the beginning or end of each session to check on how group members are feeling overall, and any thoughts or feelings they have about the group and how it is progressing. Allowing for unstructured group time promotes feelings of group responsibility and ownership in individual members.

Outside Sessions

In a number of CBT groups, and in anxiety groups in particular, some group sessions may be held outside of the therapeutic setting to provide opportunities for exposure, behavioral experiments, and modeling. For example, a panic disorder group may have a session while riding the bus or going to the mall. An eating disorder group may go to a food court to practice eating risky foods. Sessions held outside the therapeutic setting can be a challenge to group process, because the group may need to split into smaller subgroups to carry out individual exposures (e.g., one subgroup may ride the elevator and another may practice standing in lines). To maintain group cohesion, it is helpful to plan the excursion in advance within the whole group, then to reconvene the whole group at the end of the session, so that each subgroup can report back and progress can be discussed within the group.

Presence of Observers and Trainees

The presence of observers and trainees may also affect group process, because members may feel too inhibited to share when outside individuals are present. It is recommended that group members be informed of observer/trainee participation up front and that the observer/trainee commit to attending each group session in its entirety. In this way, group members become accustomed to the presence of the observer/trainee, and disruption is minimized. It is also a good idea to limit the number of observers/trainees present, so that group members are not outnumbered. For example, in a group of five to eight group members and two group leaders, a maximum of one trainee/observer is recommended.

LEADERSHIP CHALLENGES

Not surprisingly, one of the more common obstacles encountered in CBT groups occurs not because of difficult patient or intervention factors, but because conducting groups involves two or more therapists. Therapists working together may have different approaches to the difficulties they treat, stylistic differences, or different instincts about what is the best intervention for a particular example. We review here some of the common issues encountered and potential solutions.

Ideally, coleaders work together, balancing their interactions, backing each other up, and helping each other out in difficult situations. However, sometimes the styles of coleaders may not be a good fit. For example, you may wonder where your coleader is going with a certain line of questioning or feel like you are doing all of the work and your coleader is along for the ride. In some cases, there may be a coleader conflict due to disagreement on the management of the group. In the worst-case scenario, there may be open disagreement between coleaders in the group. The smooth running of the group requires active participation by both coleaders. It is recommended that part of the time used for planning before and after a group be spent on reviewing coleadership issues and working toward development of a balanced coleadership style. Lines of responsibility should also be clear. When there is a primary therapist, that therapist needs to be empowered to curtail an intervention offered by a cotherapist when the leader is no longer able to recognize the benefit of the intervention or understand where that intervention is going. Cotherapists also need to discuss how to handle a "botched" example. No group we have ever run has gone flawlessly; all therapists can find themselves lost within an example, or have an intervention go awry. It is helpful if cotherapists share a language, code, or nonverbal signal for the other therapist to "rescue" or help redirect the group. It is sometimes necessary for group therapists to acknowledge when they are lost, or when an intervention has not gone in the expected direction. Sometimes it is helpful to take this back to the group, especially in later sessions, to have group members help to troubleshoot an intervention that did not work well initially. Most important, cotherapists should at all costs avoid any overt or covert communication of conflict or dissatisfaction with one another. Finally, in our experience, the more often the same therapists work together, the more smooth and problem free the experience of the group becomes, in part because therapists begin to have a "case formulation" of one another that allows them to better predict their cotherapist's intentions, behaviors, and ways of working with group process.

CONCLUSIONS

In this chapter, we have reviewed some of the common obstacles and challenges to group treatment. Although our list is not exhaustive, we have tried to capture some of the main issues that arise across CBT groups with respect to group membership, group process, and leadership. We have provided specific strategies that may be useful for overcoming these challenges and ensuring that the group is facilitated smoothly.

PART II

Cognitive-Behavioral Therapy Groups for Specific Disorders

CHAPTER 7

Panic Disorder and Agoraphobia

DESCRIPTION OF PANIC DISORDER AND AGORAPHOBIA

Diagnostic Features

A "panic attack" is defined as a discrete episode of intense fear or discomfort that peaks rapidly and involves at least four out of 13 physical (e.g., palpitations, sweating, shaking, nausea) and/or cognitive (e.g., fears of dying, losing control, fainting, going crazy) symptoms (American Psychiatric Association [APA], 2000). *Panic disorder* is an anxiety disorder characterized by the presence of recurrent, unexpected, or "out of the blue" panic attacks and at least 1 month of concern about future panic attacks, worry about the effects of a panic attack itself (e.g., fear of catastrophic outcomes, such as having a heart attack or "going crazy"), and/or alterations in behavior in response to the attacks (e.g., avoidance of situations or physical sensations) (APA, 2000). A diagnosis of panic disorder is not made if the panic attacks are due to the physiological effects of a substance (e.g., caffeine or amphetamine intoxication, alcohol or benzodiazepine withdrawal), a general medical condition (e.g., hyperthyroidism or vestibular condition), or if the attacks are better accounted for by another disorder (APA, 2000). The lifetime prevalence of panic disorder is estimated to be 3.5% based on data from the National Comorbidity Survey (NCS; Eaton, Kessler, Wittchen, & Magee, 1994).

Panic disorder is often accompanied by *agoraphobia*—avoidance or anxiety associated with situations where it may be difficult to escape or get help in the event of panic symptoms or a panic attack (APA, 2000). Common agoraphobic situations include crowds; public transportation; shopping malls or grocery stores; waiting in line; driving in heavy traffic; over bridges, or on highways; airplanes; being home alone; being away from home (e.g., out of town); enclosed places; and confined gatherings where it would be difficult to leave unnoticed (e.g., classroom, movie theater concert, a meeting at work). It is common for individuals with agoraphobia to report a certain distance around their home in which they are comfortable or feel safe. The size of the "safe zone" varies from person to person and may range from just inside the home, to just the driveway, to the block around the house, to the neighborhood in which the person lives. The lifetime prevalence of panic disorder with agoraphobia is estimated to be 1.5% based on data from the NCS (Eaton et al., 1994).

Descriptive Features

The age of onset of panic disorder is bimodally distributed, with development typically in late adolescence (ages 15–19) or early adulthood (ages 25–30) (Ballenger & Fyer, 1996). For descriptive features of a sample of individuals presenting with panic disorder to our center, see Table 7.1. Untreated, panic disorder is often a chronic condition (Keller et al., 1994) accompanied by high social and economic costs (Hofmann & Barlow, 1999). It is not surprising that individuals with panic disorder report a significantly reduced quality of life (Keller et al., 1994) and increased health care utilization (Klerman, Weissman, Ouellette, Johnson, & Greenwald, 1991; Roy-Byrne et al., 1999) compared to those without panic disorder. In comparison to other psychiatric disorders, panic disorder is the leading cause for seeking emergency room consultations (Weissman, 1991) and mental health treatment (Boyd, 1986).

There are gender differences in both the prevalence and phenomenology of panic disorder. Women are more than twice as likely to suffer from panic disorder as males (e.g., Eaton et al., 1994). In addition, women are more likely to experience increased agoraphobic avoidance symptoms (Turgeon, Marchand, & Dupuis, 1998) and respiration-related symptoms (difficulty breathing, feeling faint, and feeling smothered) during panic attacks (Sheikh,

TABLE 7.1. Characteristics of Individuals with Panic Disorder with or without Agoraphobia (N = 231) Presenting for Treatment to a Specialized Anxiety Clinic

	PD (n = 41)	PDA (n = 190)
Percent N	17.7%	82.3%
Age	38.24 (12.50)	36.13 (10.35)
Age of onset*	28.29 (12.85)	25.07 (11.29)
Sex	70.7% female	70.0% female
Number of additional diagnoses	1.51 (1.21)	1.64 (1.32)

Note. PD, panic disorder; PDA, panic disorder with agoraphobia; N, total number of patients presenting for treatment with PD or PDA. Adapted from McCabe, Chudzik, Antony, Summerfeldt, and Swinson (2004). Adapted by permission of the authors.
*p < .05.

Leskin, & Klein, 2002). Finally, compared to men, women tend to have more severe and chronic forms of panic disorder with agoraphobia (Yonkers et al., 1998).

Panic disorder is often comorbid with other anxiety disorders and depression (e.g., Brown, Antony, & Barlow, 1995), hypochondriasis (e.g., Furer, Walker, Chartier, & Stein, 1997), alcohol abuse and dependence (e.g., Leon, Portera, & Weissman, 1995), and personality disorders, most commonly avoidant, dependent, and histrionic (e.g., Diaferia et al., 1993). In addition, individuals with panic disorder report a higher rate of gastrointestinal symptoms, including symptoms of irritable bowel syndrome, compared to individuals without panic disorder (Lydiard et al., 1994).

Cognitive Features

Cognitive-behavioral models of panic disorder place central importance on the role of cognition in the development and maintenance of panic, and in particular, the degree to which an individual is fearful of arousal sensations (anxiety sensitivity). Other cognitive features include attention to physical sensations and threat-related cognitions.

Anxiety Sensitivity

The tendency to make catastrophic interpretations of the physical symptoms of arousal is a stable, individual difference variable called *anxiety sensitivity* (Reiss & McNally, 1985). Individuals with high levels of anxiety sensitivity have a tendency to make catastrophic appraisals of physical sensations (e.g., interpreting a palpitation as a sign of a heart attack), whereas individuals with low levels of anxiety sensitivity do not have a tendency to view uncomfortable physical sensations as dangerous. Although a number of anxiety disorders are associated with heightened levels of anxiety sensitivity (e.g., posttraumatic stress disorder, generalized anxiety disorder) panic disorder, with or without agoraphobia, is associated with the highest levels of anxiety sensitivity (e.g., Reiss, Peterson, Gursky, & McNally, 1986). More compelling is evidence suggesting that anxiety sensitivity predicts vulnerability to the development of panic attacks (e.g., Schmidt, Lerew, & Jackson, 1997; Schmidt, 1999).

Attention to Physical Sensations

Individuals with panic disorder display enhanced attention to physical sensations, particularly bodily sensations associated with arousal. Although evidence is mixed, studies appear to support the finding that panic disorder is associated with a heightened awareness of the bodily sensations of arousal (e.g., Ehlers & Breuer, 1992, 1996), although increased sensitivity does not appear to correspond with increased accuracy of perception (e.g., Antony et al., 1995).

Threat-Related Cognitions

Panic disorder is associated with characteristic threat-related cognitions, including catastrophic thoughts, expectancies of danger, information-processing biases, and underlying beliefs about personal control (for a review, see Khawaja & Oei, 1998). In addition, individuals with panic disorder have a tendency to overpredict their fear level for anticipated exposure situations (van Hout & Emmelkamp, 1994).

Behavioral Features

Key behavioral features that play a role in the development and maintenance of panic disorder include escape, avoidance, and safety behaviors.

Escape

Faced with a panic attack or panic symptoms, individuals with panic disorder often escape from the situation that they are in. Once out of the situation, they typically find that their panic attack has ended, and they are left with an enormous sense of relief. A negative reinforcement contingency is established, such that the urge to escape becomes greater as the frequency of escape increases, and it becomes more difficult for the individual to stay in the situation and tolerate the panic attack. This pattern may lead to complete avoidance of situations associated with panic.

Avoidance Behaviors

In the context of agoraphobia, avoidance behaviors may be overt and involve a range of situations (described earlier) with which an individual has difficulty either when alone or when accompanied. Avoidance behavior may also take more subtle forms as individuals avoid activities (e.g., exercise, sexual intercourse) and substances (e.g., caffeinated beverages, medication) that evoke physical sensations associated with panic.

Safety Behaviors

Individuals with panic disorder, with or without the presence of agoraphobia, often engage in *safety behaviors* designed to help manage or reduce anxiety in an effort to feel more comfortable or to prevent panic symptoms. Safety behaviors play a role in the maintenance of anxiety by preventing individuals from gaining evidence that would disconfirm their fears. Elimination of safety behaviors has been shown to reduce catastrophic beliefs and anxiety (Salkovskis, Clark, Hackmann, Wells, & Geldner, 1999). Common safety behaviors include carrying certain items (e.g., cell phone, water, medication), chewing gum, distraction, traveling accompanied by a familiar person, always offering to drive to maintain control and to avoid being a passenger, and taking a substance to prevent physical symptoms (e.g., antidiarrhea or antinausea medication) or to reduce anxiety (e.g., alcohol or recreational drugs such as cannabis). Individuals may not be aware of their safety behaviors, so these may be difficult to detect upon initial assessment. Careful assessment requires asking specifically about the presence of various safety behaviors, which typically become more evident as treatment progresses and the individual develops an awareness of the function of certain behaviors.

COGNITIVE-BEHAVIORAL APPROACHES TO UNDERSTANDING PANIC DISORDER WITH OR WITHOUT AGORAPHOBIA

A number of cognitive-behavioral approaches to understanding and treating panic disorder have been developed (e.g., Barlow, 1988; Clark, 1986; Margraf & Ehlers, 1988). These models are very similar in their emphasis on the key role played by catastrophic misinterpretation of physical symptoms (e.g., interpreting dizziness as a sign of fainting) and interoceptive anxiety or fear of physical sensations (for review, see Margraf, Barlow, Clark, & Telch, 1993). Many studies provide empirical validation for cognitive-behavioral models of panic disorder with or without agoraphobia (for review, see Taylor, 2000). Two of the most common models are reviewed here.

In 1986, David Clark published "A Cognitive Approach to Panic," an article that put forth one of the first cognitive-behavioral models of panic disorder. According to Clark, panic attacks are caused by catastrophic misinterpretation of the benign physical symptoms of arousal typically involved in the normal anxiety response (dizziness, palpitations, etc.). For example, an individual who misinterprets a random heart palpitation as a sign of a heart attack is likely to become anxious. The experience of anxiety leads to physical sensations of arousal (e.g., dizziness, lightheadedness, sweating) that are then misinterpreted as further evidence of impending catastrophe. Thus, a vicious cycle of anxiety is created, such that catastrophic misinterpretation leads to fear and anxiety, which in turn leads to increased physical symptoms that provide further evidence for the initial misinterpretations. This cycle of anxiety may escalate into a full-blown panic attack.

Similar to Clark's model, David Barlow's integrated model of panic disorder (1988) also highlights the role of psychological responses to physical sensations. However, Barlow's model places greater emphasis on biological and social factors in the development and maintenance of panic disorder. According to Barlow, the initial panic attack is due to a misfiring of the fear system in a psychologically and physically vulnerable individual, usually at a time of stress. Psychological vulnerability is conferred by beliefs that bodily sensations are dangerous (heightened anxiety sensitivity), and that the world in general is dangerous (uncontrollability). Physiological vulnerability is proposed to be due to an overly sensitive autonomic nervous system. The traumatic nature of the initial panic attack leads to interoceptively conditioned fear responses to bodily sensations and the situational context, thus leading to a cycle of panic and anxious apprehension of panic.

TREATMENTS FOR PANIC DISORDER

Evidence-based treatments for panic disorder include pharmacotherapy and CBT. This section reviews both treatments, including evidence for their efficacy alone and in combination, as well as evidence comparing group and individual modalities of CBT.

Pharmacotherapy

A range of medications have been shown to have good treatment efficacy for the management of panic disorder, including selective serotonin reuptake inhibitors (SSRIs), tricyclic antidepressants (TCAs), monoamine oxidase inhibitors (MAOIs), and benzodiazepines (Ballenger, 1993; Toni et al., 2000). A review of meta-analytic studies examining drug treatments suggests that SSRIs are the most effective drugs for treating panic disorder (Taylor, 2000). The SSRIs tend to have fewer side effects and lower rates of attrition than do tricyclic antidepressants such as imipramine (Bakker, van Balkom, & Spinhoven, 2002). Both non-SSRI antidepressants and benzodiazepines are more effective than placebo for treatment of panic disorder (Taylor, 2000). One concern associated with pharmacotherapy treatments is the high relapse rates following medication discontinuation, which may be as high as 50% (Toni et al., 2000) and even higher for benzodiazepines (Noyes, Garve, & Cook, 1991).

Cognitive-Behavioral Therapy

CBT developed by Clark et al. (1994; Clark, Salkovskis, et al., 1999) involves increasing patients' awareness of their appraisal of bodily sensations associated with a panic attack. Treatment then focuses on fostering noncatastrophic interpretations about physical sensations and phobic situations that are tested through dialogue and behavioral experiments. This treatment has been empirically validated in numerous studies (e.g., Clark et al., 1994).

CBT developed by Barlow and colleagues has also been well validated (for review, see Antony & McCabe, 2002). Treatment focuses on targeting the fear of bodily sensations, apprehension of panic, and agoraphobic avoidance through a combination of psychoeducation, cognitive restructuring, breathing retraining (where indicated), exposure to feared bodily sensations, and *in vivo* exposure to the extent that agoraphobia is present (e.g., Barlow & Cerny, 1988; panic control treatment [PCT]; Barlow & Craske, 2000); sensation-focused intensive therapy; Heinrichs, Spiegel, & Hofmann, 2002). However, preliminary evidence suggests that adding *in vivo* exposure to PCT for individuals with panic disorder with agoraphobia does not confer additional benefit over PCT alone (Craske, DeCola, Sachs, & Pontillo, 2003).

A typical course of CBT for panic disorder ranges from 8 to 16 weekly sessions depending on the protocol followed, with the presence of agoraphobia warranting longer treatment time. CBT for panic disorder with agoraphobia is well received by patients who are receptive to developing active strategies to overcome their anxiety. This is evidenced by data showing a high degree of patient satisfaction with CBT for panic disorder with agoraphobia (Cox, Fergus, & Swinson, 1994).

The efficacy of CBT for panic disorder is well established in research settings (e.g., Barlow et al., 2000; Clark et al., 1994), and initial findings in community mental health settings suggest a comparable treatment response (e.g., Wade, Treat, & Stuart, 1998). For a comprehensive review of meta-analytic studies of treatment outcome in panic disorder, see Taylor (2000). Outcome studies demonstrate that CBT leads to a reduction in the main features of panic disorder (e.g., anxiety symptoms, anxious cognitions, agoraphobic avoidance), reduction in general psychological symptoms (e.g., Hahlweg, Fiegenbaum, Frank, Schroeder, & von Witzleben, 2001), and reduction in the severity of comorbid conditions such as depression, generalized anxiety disorder, and specific phobia (Chudzik, McCabe, Antony, & Swinson, 2001; Tsao, Mystkowski, Zucker, & Craske, 2002). In addition, CBT for panic disorder has been shown to lead to improvement in physical health symptom ratings, independent from its impact on anxiety symptoms (Schmidt et al., 2003), as well as improvement in quality of life (Telch, Schmidt, LaNae Jaimez, Jacquin, & Harrington, 1995). The presence of personality psychopathology has been found to affect treatment outcome for panic disorder negatively (see Mennin & Heimberg, 2000, for review).

Individuals with panic disorder and agoraphobia presenting for CBT often have a goal of discontinuing their medication. CBT has been shown to reduce the risk for adverse reactions following withdrawal from benzodiazepines (e.g., Otto et al., 1993; Spiegel, Bruce, Gregg, & Nuzzarello, 1994) and antidepressants (e.g., Schmidt, Woolaway-Bickel, Trakowski, Santiago, & Vasey, 2002; Whittal, Otto, & Hong, 2001).

Group CBT

When given a choice, patients will likely choose individual treatment over group treatment. In one study, 95% of the sample chose individual treatment over group when asked for their preference (Sharp, Power, & Swanson, 2004). However, the higher costs of providing individual treatment, combined with scarce resources, often make group treatment a more cost-effective and practical option. CBT for panic disorder has been extensively evaluated in both individual and group format with similar results, suggesting that group treatment is clinically equivalent to individual treatment (e.g., Cerny, Barlow, Craske, & Himadi, 1987; Craske et al., 1989; Evans, Holt, & Oei, 1991; Lidren et al., 1994; Telch et al., 1993).

Very few studies have been designed to compare directly group and individual formats of CBT for panic disorder. One study comparing group and individual CBT for panic disorder found that although both treatments were comparable for measures of panic and agoraphobia at posttreatment and at 6-month follow-up, the individual treatment resulted in greater alleviation of generalized anxiety and depressive symptoms (Néron, Lacroix, & Chaput, 1995). In another study comparing individual and group format directly in a primary care setting, Sharp and colleagues (2004) found that both group and individual CBT for panic disorder with agoraphobia were superior to a wait-list control group but did not differ significantly from each other. However, individual CBT was associated with greater clinical significance than either group CBT or wait-list control immediately following termination of treatment, as reflected by the larger proportion of patients in the individual treatment group who achieved clinically significant change (i.e., outcome scores at least two standard deviations below the pretreatment mean for the entire sample). However, this advantage for individual treatment was not detectable at 3-month follow-up.

Combining Pharmacotherapy and CBT

Studies examining combined pharmacotherapy and individual CBT do not provide evidence of a synergistic benefit associated with providing both treatment modalities. For example, in a large, multicenter trial comparing CBT, imipramine, and CBT combined with imipramine, Barlow and colleagues (2000) found that the acute response rate for combined treatment had only a limited advantage on some measures compared to CBT alone, but not when compared to CBT plus placebo. At the end of the 6-month maintenance phase, the combination of CBT plus imipramine was associated with a significantly lower panic severity score than CBT alone, CBT plus placebo, and imipramine. However, the combination treatment was associated with the highest relapse rate at 6-month follow-up. The authors concluded that the long-term effects of CBT were reduced by the addition of imipramine.

There is some evidence that adding pharmacotherapy following CBT in a sequential manner may improve efficacy for poor CBT responders. For example, one study found that the addition of an SSRI (paroxetine) following unsuccessful treatment with CBT was associated with further clinical benefit compared to placebo (Kampman, Keijsers, Hoogduin, & Hendriks, 2002). Similarly, adding group CBT following nonresponse to pharmacotherapy has been found to be associated with good treatment response (Otto, Pollack, Penava, & Zucker, 1999; Pollack, Otto, Kaspi, Hammerness, & Rosenbaum, 1994).

Comparing the Effectiveness of Pharmacotherapy and CBT

Numerous comparative treatment trials (e.g., Barlow et al., 2000) and meta-analytic studies (e.g., Gould, Otto, & Pollack, 1995) demonstrate that CBT is as effective as antidepressants or high-potency benzodiazepines in the short term. In a thorough review of the meta-analytic studies of treatments for panic disorder, Taylor (2000) found that CBT and pharmacotherapy (antidepressants, high-potency benzodiazepines) had comparable treatment efficacy, with both treatments significantly more efficacious than placebo control conditions. However, it is worth noting that CBT appears to be associated with less risk of dropout than pharmacotherapy treatment. Another advantage of CBT over pharmacotherapy is the lower risk of relapse and evidence suggesting more enduring effects of treatment following discontinuation. However, there is a lack of studies examining long-term follow-up outcome (Nadiga, Hensley, & Uhlenhuth, 2003), and studies reporting panic-free rates greater than 80% at 1- to 2-year follow-up (e.g., Clark et al., 1994; Craske, Brown, & Barlow, 1991) are limited by cross-sectional assessment that does not accurately reflect the fluctuating nature of residual symptoms (Brown & Barlow, 1995).

An additional advantage of CBT over pharmacotherapy appears to be greater cost-effectiveness. In a study examining the costs and outcomes of CBT and pharmacotherapy, Otto, Pollack, and Maki (2000) found that CBT was a more cost-effective treatment option than pharmacotherapy, with essentially equivalent acute treatment efficacy and greater maintenance of treatment gain, without requiring ongoing treatment. Moreover, group treatment was more cost-effective than individual treatment, with an average total cost over a 1 year period of $523 per person for group treatment compared to $1,357 per person for individual treatment. In contrast, the cost for pharmacotherapy over the same time period was $2,305. Thus, in addition to substantial cost savings relative to pharmacotherapy, group CBT also appears to be particularly cost-effective compared to individual CBT.

ASSESSMENT ISSUES

Comprehensive assessment should be used to establish an accurate diagnosis, to plan treatment, to assess eligibility for group CBT, and to determine treatment outcome. Several factors should be considered when making a differential diagnosis, including medical conditions that may mimic panic symptoms (e.g., hyperthyroidism, hypoglycemia) and use or withdrawal of certain substances that may cause panic symptoms (e.g., caffeine, alcohol, medications, illicit drugs). We recommend that any potential physical causes of panic be ruled out through medical examination before treatment for panic disorder is considered. To rule out other anxiety disorders that present with panic attacks and avoidance, the nature of the panic attacks (i.e., cued vs. uncued), focus of apprehension during a panic attack, and reasons for avoidance should be assessed. For a more detailed discussion of these issues, see McCabe (2001).

Comprehensive clinical interviews such as the Structured Clinical Interview for DSM-IV (SCID-IV; First, Spitzer, Gibbon, & Williams, 1996) and the Anxiety Disorders Interview Schedule (ADIS-IV; Brown, Di Nardo, & Barlow, 1994; Di Nardo, Brown, & Barlow, 1994) are excellent measures for obtaining the information required to make diagnostic decisions, to establish a diagnosis of panic disorder, and to assess comorbidity.

Monitoring Progress and Assessing Treatment Outcome

A comprehensive assessment should also include measures that target the key features of panic disorder: interoceptive anxiety, panic cognitions, and avoidance. Severity of the core features of panic disorder is a strong prognostic indicator of outcome (for a review, see McCabe & Antony, 2005). The widely used Panic Disorder Severity Scale (PDSS; Shear et al., 1997) is a clinician-administered interview that assesses the core features of panic disorder, including panic attack frequency, distress during panic attacks, anticipatory anxiety, agoraphobic fear and avoidance, interoceptive fear and avoidance, and impairment in work and social functioning. A self-report version of the PDSS has been developed that displays good reliability and treatment sensitivity in initial research (Houck, Spiegel, Shear, & Rucci, 2002). The self-report PDSS is advantageous in that it does not require a trained interviewer. In addition to clinician-administered interviews, we recommended including self-report measures that assess the core features of panic disorder. These measures supplement information obtained in the clinical interview and are useful for monitoring treatment progress and outcome. We briefly review some of the common self-report measures here. For a more detailed review of assessment tools for panic disorder the reader is referred to Antony (2001a).

Interoceptive Anxiety

Measures of interoceptive anxiety are useful to identify feared physical symptoms to plan interoceptive exposure, as well as to determine treatment efficacy. Common self-report measures include the Body Sensations Questionnaire (Chambless, Caputo, Bright, & Gallagher, 1984) and the Anxiety Sensitivity Index (ASI; Peterson & Reiss, 1993). Change in anxiety sensitivity (particularly as measured by the Physical Concerns subscale of the ASI) has been shown to be a significant predictor of symptom change following CBT treatment (Schmidt & Bates, 2003).

Panic Cognitions

Common self-report measures of panic cognitions include the Agoraphobic Cognitions Questionnaire (ACQ; Chambless et al., 1984), the Panic Attack

Cognitions Questionnaire (Clum, Broyles, Borden, & Watkins, 1990), and the Catastrophic Cognitions Questionnaire (Khawaja, Oei, & Baglioni, 1994). These measures are useful for identifying targets for cognitive restructuring (e.g., beliefs such as "I will have a heart attack" or "I will be paralyzed by fear") and for determining treatment efficacy. Increased severity of catastrophic agoraphobic cognitions has been shown to be a significant predictor of poor treatment outcome (Keijsers, Hoogduin, & Schnaap, 1994).

Avoidance

The best way to assess avoidance is to develop during a clinical interview a detailed list of situations that the individual fears. A sample is provided in Figure 7.1. Group members can then rate their fear and avoidance levels on their exposure hierarchy at the beginning of each therapy session (see Figure 7.2 for a sample). These ratings provide a useful tool for guiding treatment and for monitoring progress. Exposure hierarchy ratings have been shown to be sensitive to treatment change following CBT for panic disorder and correlate with clinical improvement assessed by standard panic measures (McCabe, Rowa, Antony, Swinson, & Ladak, 2001). Self-report measures such as the Mobility Inventory (MI; Chambless et al., 1985) are also useful for assessing common agoraphobic situations. Increased agoraphobic avoidance has been related to poorer outcome at 6-month follow-up post-CBT (Sharp & Power, 1999).

Name: _____	Session: Preteatment	Date: _____
Item	Fear (0–100)	Avoidance (0–100)
1. Go out without Ativan	100	100
2. Go to movies and sit in the middle of the row	100	100
3. Stay alone at home in the morning	99	100
4. Drive to city alone	95	90
5. Go to the mall when crowded	90	80
6. Go out without cell phone	80	80
7. Drive on the highway alone outside of safe zone	80	60
8. Go to the gym	70	90
9. Drive to city as a passenger	70	40
10. Go to the mall when it is uncrowded	70	0
11. Go to the movies and sit on the aisle	60	100
12. Wait in a line	50	0

FIGURE 7.1. Sample exposure hierarchy with initial ratings.

Name: _____	Session: _____	Date: _____

Item	Fear (0–100)	Avoidance (0–100)
1. Go out without Ativan	_____	_____
2. Go to movies and sit in the middle of the row	_____	_____
3. Stay alone at home in the morning	_____	_____
4. Drive to city alone	_____	_____
5. Go to the mall when crowded	_____	_____
6. Go out without cell phone	_____	_____
7. Drive on the highway alone outside of safe zone	_____	_____
8. Go to the gym	_____	_____
9. Drive to city as a passenger	_____	_____
10. Go to the mall when it is uncrowded	_____	_____
11. Go to the movies and sit on the aisle	_____	_____
12. Wait in a line	_____	_____

FIGURE 7.2. Sample exposure hierarchy rating sheet.

From *Cognitive-Behavioral Therapy in Groups* by Peter J. Bieling, Randi E. McCabe, and Martin M. Antony. Copyright 2006 by The Guilford Press. Permission to photocopy this figure is granted to purchasers of this book for personal use only (see copyright page for details).

Finally, given the impact panic disorder may have on emotional well-being, financial independence, and relationships (Antony, Roth, Swinson, Huta, & Devins, 1998), we recommend including measures of functional impairment and quality of life as part of a comprehensive assessment.

STRUCTURING GROUP TREATMENT

Table 7.2 provides details of group composition and treatment format from a number of studies on group treatment for panic disorder with and without agoraphobia. In this section, we make specific recommendations based on the research literature and our own clinical experience with regard to group format, group composition, group inclusion considerations, and the structure of group sessions.

**TABLE 7.2. Format and Composition for a Sample of Group
Panic Treatments**

Study	No. of sessions	Group composition	Session length	Strategies
Sharp, Power, & Swanson (2004) (primary care setting, groups held in community health centers)	8 sessions over 12 weeks (Sessions 1 to 4 weekly, 5 to 8 biweekly)	6 to 8 members (PD/PDA); 1 therapist (clinical psychologist)	1 hour	Exposure Behavioral and cognitive panic management strategies
Beck, Stanley, Baldwin, Deagle, & Averill (1994)	10 sessions over 10 weeks	4 to 6 members (PD); number of therapists not reported	1.5 hours	Cognitive strategies (formal exposure excluded)
Telch et al. (1993)	12 sessions over 8 weeks (Sessions 1 to 8 twice weekly, 9 to 12 biweekly)	4 to 6 members (PD/PDA); 2 therapists	1.5 hours	Panic inoculation training based on PCT strategies plus self-directed ingestion of caffeine
Lidren et al. (1994)	8 sessions weekly	6 members (PD); 1 therapist	1.5 hours	Cognitive and behavioral strategies

Group Format

We recommend at least 12 sessions, each 2 hours' duration. A longer course of treatment is warranted if individuals in a group have more severe levels of agoraphobia. Additional sessions focus on continued therapist-assisted exposures and modification of agoraphobic cognitions, and may be delivered on an individual basis. We recommend that sessions be held on a weekly basis initially, with spacing out of sessions in the latter stages of treatment. At our center, the first 10 sessions occur on a weekly basis and the last two sessions are spaced out biweekly. The increased time between sessions at the end of treatment allows more time for group members to practice managing issues that arise independently of the group. Spacing out of the final sessions also assists group members in adjusting to the group coming to an end.

To prevent relapse and maintain treatment gains, we recommend that booster sessions be planned. Booster sessions provide a place for group members to check in on issues that may arise subsequently to the end of regular group sessions. These sessions can be held at 3 months, 6 months, and 1 year post-acute treatment. At our center, we hold booster sessions on a monthly basis. Booster sessions can be used to check progress, to set continued goals, to troubleshoot obstacles, and to review treatment strategies.

Group Composition

Clinical outcome studies on group treatment for panic disorder typically use small groups, with four to eight participants. At our center we typically include five to eight patients. As the number of participants increases, treatment outcome may be compromised. We recommend the presence of two therapists, so that there is always backup for dealing with any difficulties or issues that arise. The presence of two therapists also ensures continuity of leadership in the case that one therapist is absent from a session due to illness. Effort is made to balance the contributions of the two therapists, so that group members do not respond more to one therapist than to another. However, because our center is a training facility, it is often the case that one therapist is at a senior level and the second therapist is in training. In this instance, the senior therapist takes the lead for planning and running the group, with increasing responsibility given to the second therapist as appropriate. In some cases, we also have a third trainee in the room, but this person would take an observer role, so that the group is not confused by too many therapists.

To promote group process and cohesiveness, certain factors are important to consider when determining group composition, including demographic characteristics, and symptom profile and fit. Group leaders should aim to balance the group in terms of demographic factors and symptom profile. The more balanced a group is, the greater the group cohesiveness, and the lower the risk of dropout. If possible, group leaders should strive to balance the group on these factors, even if it is the addition of just one other member to match the "lone" member with (examples are provided below). If group leaders are not able to match a "lone" member, it may be a good idea to offer this person individual therapy. If that is not an option and the person is included in the group, the group leaders should make special efforts to link the person's experience with other group members and to foster cohesiveness.

Demographic Factors

Because a higher proportion of females than males present for treatment, group leaders may be faced with an imbalance in gender. For example, a lone male in a group with six females may feel isolated and "different," and may not relate to the female experience. The addition of just one more male to the group would make a substantial difference in this group member's experience (e.g., he would feel like he is not the only man with this problem).

Age should also be considered. For example, including one 18-year-old in a panic group composed of four women ages 32–60 and two men ages 36 and 40 may increase the probability of the 18-year-old dropping out. In this situation, the younger group member may not feel like he or she relates to the rest of the group, especially when group members say things like "When I was your age . . . " and "You're lucky you are dealing with this now." The addition of another member close in age would provide some balance for the "lone" member and foster feelings of inclusiveness. Given that the diagnosis of panic disorder is often delayed over the course of years (Ballenger, 1997), it is more common for individuals to present for treatment at an older age.

Symptom Profile and Fit

The more homogeneous the composition of the group, the greater the likelihood that group members will relate to each other and find the group beneficial for their needs. Increased homogeneity leads to increased group cohesion and reduced risk of dropout. Degree of agoraphobia is a factor that should be considered when balancing group composition. Individuals may be frightened by the presence in the group of other individuals with more severe symptoms. Alternatively, the individual with more severe agoraphobia may be overwhelmed by the rest of the group if he or she is unable to progress at a similar pace. In addition, individuals with no agoraphobia may not relate to some of the treatment components utilized for the rest of the group (i.e., *in vivo* exposure). For example, an individual with panic disorder who is included in a group with seven other members who also have agoraphobia may not relate to the treatment when the group is working on *in vivo* exposures. This individual may be better suited for briefer, individual therapy. Alternatively, the group leaders should let the individual know up front that he or she may not relate to certain aspects of the group, because other group members may have varying levels of avoidance. The group member can be encouraged to take what he or she can from the group, and focus on reducing more subtle avoidance or safety strategies that he or she may be practicing. As group members practice situational exposure, the individual can practice further on interoceptive exposures. Again, if possible, it is recommended that the group be balanced by inclusion of at least two members with panic disorder without agoraphobia, or two members with greater levels of agoraphobic severity. If resources allow, it may be better to run a separate group or provide one-on-one therapy for individuals with more severe agoraphobia, who may have difficulty maintaining pace with the rest of the group.

The presence of panic disorder in the context of a medical condition such as diabetes is another factor that should be balanced, if possible. For example, Jake had diabetes and panic disorder with agoraphobia. He often felt like he was "different" in the group, because he had the added complication that his high and low blood sugars often caused panic-like symptoms. Although the group leaders were unable to include another group member with diabetes in the group, they were able to rely on their previous treatment experience—"the patient in the pocket"—to normalize Jake's experience and to help him feel included in the group. The group leaders were able to let Jake know that they had seen other individuals with the same experience and challenges, and to share strategies these "past patients" had found useful for overcoming their panic (e.g., learning to differentiate symptoms of panic from symptoms of high or low blood sugar).

Assessing Eligibility for Group CBT

A number of factors should be considered when determining an individual's eligibility for group CBT for panic disorder: diagnosis, insight, level of motivation, openness to group treatment, interpersonal skills, and personality characteristics. Group leaders need to balance the needs of the individual with the needs of the group in determining eligibility.

Diagnosis and Clinical Severity

Ideally, all group members should have a diagnosis of panic disorder with or without agoraphobia. In some cases, individuals with other conditions may benefit from this treatment approach (e.g., agoraphobia without a history of panic disorder). Symptom similarity and appropriateness of treatment strategies should be considered. When comorbidity is present, panic disorder with or without agoraphobia should be established as the primary diagnosis. When individuals with a secondary diagnosis of panic disorder are included in a group treatment, their primary condition may interfere with their ability to focus solely on their panic symptoms. They may bring up issues in the group to which other members do not relate; consequently, they may feel that the group is not meeting their needs.

Clinical severity of symptoms is also a consideration. An individual with a very mild degree of severity may not need the full course of group treatment and may be better treated with a brief course of individual treatment. At the other extreme, an individual with severe agoraphobia may be too impaired to attend group regularly. For example, we had one person at our center that could only leave the house accompanied by her husband. She refused to attend group unless her husband could sit in on the group sessions. In this case, individual treatment was deemed more suited to her treatment needs.

Comorbidity

Comorbidity is the norm in individuals presenting for treatment with panic disorder. In patients at our center, the average number of additional diagnoses is greater than 1.5 (see Table 7.1). Therefore, the presence of comorbidity does not rule out group treatment. However, panic disorder should be the primary disorder (i.e., the disorder causing the individual the most distress and/ or impairment). In addition, the presence of additional disorders should not interfere with the individual's ability to participate in the group treatment. For example, an individual with psychotic symptoms may not do well in a group setting where treatment is focused solely on panic disorder and would likely benefit from a more individualized treatment approach. The presence of substance misuse, abuse, or dependence may also interfere with an individual's ability to participate in group treatment. These issues should be considered on a case-by-case basis.

Insight

Individuals who have difficulty accepting their diagnosis of panic disorder and instead continue searching for physical causes may be disruptive and difficult to manage in a group. For example, in one group at our center, such a patient refused to do any interoceptive exposure that would raise his heart rate. Despite our best treatment efforts, he was convinced that his problem was physical in nature. It was difficult for other group members to relate to him and vice versa. Although he did make some small gains in the group (his belief rating that his problem was physical reduced from 99 to 75%), he did present a continual challenge to the group leaders.

Patient Motivation and Preferences

Patient motivation for CBT, as well as personal preferences for the group modality, should be considered when determining inclusion in the group. It should be emphasized that most people are apprehensive about group treatment initially, and the therapist should normalize this. Explaining the benefits of group treatment (e.g., meet others with the same condition) versus individual treatment usually helps to increase the individual's openness to trying group treatment.

Motivation for CBT can be determined by explaining the treatment, as well as what will be required (e.g., weekly homework assignments), and asking about the individual's readiness and openness to trying this treatment approach. The expectations for group treatment (e.g., participation) should also be explained to establish whether the individual is motivated and committed to participate in the process (e.g., consistent attendance).

Individuals with low levels of motivation at the outset of treatment will likely not do as well, and their presence in the group may impact morale through homework incompletion, inconsistent attendance, guarded disclosure, and, in some cases, dropout. If not managed appropriately, the presence of such a member can detract from the therapeutic experience for the rest of the group, leading to contamination of other group members (e.g., fostering an attitude that homework or attendance is not important) or threatening the feelings of safety and trust relative to disclosure in the group.

Interpersonal Skills

An individual's ability to interact in the group should also be considered and balanced with the group's needs. An individual with poor social skills may not do as well in a group format for panic disorder. For example, someone who is extremely shy may have difficulty with self-disclosure and anxiety due to the group setting. In this case, group format may actually interfere with treatment progress. A basic level of appropriate communication skills is essential. For example, an individual with an aggressive communication style may compromise the culture of safety and acceptance in the group, and detract from the therapeutic experience of other group members.

Personality Considerations

The presence of certain personality characteristics may also factor into determining an individual's appropriateness for group treatment. An individual with narcissistic or borderline traits may not be suitable for group treatment, because he or she may present a challenge to group leader in terms of management, containment, and protection of other group members.

Structure of Group Sessions

At our center, group sessions typically last 2 hours. Sessions begin with group members' completion of fear and avoidance ratings on their exposure hierarchies (see Figure 7.2). An agenda that includes the goals for the session is then set. The group is given the opportunity to contribute to the agenda with any questions or issues that members would like addressed. A typical session then begins with a homework review, with an emphasis on integration and review of material from the previous week. Group members are asked to take out their homework and go through it with the group. This is important, because it sets a norm that homework completion is important. This can be reinforced by collecting homework at the end of the session, then redistributing it at the beginning of the next session. Following homework review, the session focuses on presenting new psychoeducational material, clinical strategies, or in-session exposure. The session ends with group members planning new homework and discussing details of how they will achieve their homework goals. The group is utilized for problem-solving obstacles to homework completion.

KEY TREATMENT COMPONENTS

This section provides an overview of the main treatment components of CBT for the treatment of panic disorder with and without agoraphobia. For a more detailed description see Craske and Barlow (2001), Clark et al. (1994), and Antony and Swinson (2000a). For a good discussion of clinical strategies to manage treatment issues arising in CBT for panic disorder, see chapters by Huppert and Baker-Morissette (2003) and McCabe and Antony (2005).

Psychoeducation

Psychoeducation, an essential component of CBT for panic disorder, forms the foundation for the development of CBT skills. For individuals with panic disorder, education about panic attacks and the nature of panic disorder often has a substantial role in reducing anxiety. Ideally, material is presented in an interactive format, with the therapists using guided discovery and Socratic questioning to illustrate key concepts. A whiteboard is useful for presenting information. It is recommended that the therapists utilize the group for generating suggestions and ideas about material that is presented, so that the presentation does not become too didactic. Information can be presented in a variety of ways: through handouts, presentation on the whiteboard, discussion of concepts utilizing examples from the group, and discussion of more general examples. Examples of topics covered in the psychoeducational component of CBT for panic disorder include the nature of anxiety and panic (e.g., the role of the fight–flight system), the role of interoceptive conditioning in the development of panic disorder following the initial panic attack, the CBT model of panic disorder, and the three-component model of anxiety (thoughts, physical sensations, and behavior).

Cognitive Strategies

Cognitive strategies for panic emphasize the importance of misinterpretation of bodily sensations in the development and maintenance of panic disorder. Group members are encouraged to monitor their anxious thoughts. Individuals who have difficulty accessing their thoughts are instructed to ask themselves questions when they notice themselves feeling anxious (e.g., "What was going through my mind just before I got anxious" and "What am I afraid might happen?"). The role of information-processing biases and cognitive distortions is reviewed, with an emphasis on the tendency for individuals with panic disorder to catastrophize the consequences of anxiety and panic (*castastrophization*) and overpredict the likelihood of negative events (*probability overestimation*). Group members practice identifying their tendency to engage in these two common distortions. Different cognitive strategies are then used in the group to challenge anxious thoughts and to encourage more realistic appraisals (e.g., evidence gathering, cost–benefit analysis, behavioral experiments).

Exposure-Based Strategies

Exposure-based strategies involve having group members gradually confront feared situations and physical sensations, until fear reduction is achieved. Exposures may be self-directed (completed individually as part of homework) or therapist/group assisted (completed as part of the group).

In vivo Exposure

In vivo, or "real-life," exposure involves the systematic and repeated confrontation of agoraphobic situations and is guided by an exposure hierarchy that comprises individually tailored items. Safety cues should be incorporated into the hierarchy. A sample exposure hierarchy is provided in Figure 7.1. The exposure hierarchy rating form to be completed at the beginning of each group session is provided in Figure 7.2. The majority of exposures throughout the group sessions are self-directed. Each group member selects the situations that he or she will practice in between the group sessions. Repeated, massed (vs. spaced practice) exposure is encouraged, with an expectation of at least three major practices of a selected item per week. The importance of daily exposure is emphasized. Group members are encouraged to conduct exposure at their own pace. For some people, this pace may be gradual, as they work their way up the exposure hierarchy. Other people choose a more intense approach, selecting items near the top of the hierarchy to confront. If warranted, group members are encouraged to have a helper assist them in more challenging exposures (e.g., family member or friend). At least one to two group sessions are used for therapist-assisted exposure. This often involves the group taking a bus ride to a shopping mall, where subgroups are formed to carry out relevant exposures (e.g., waiting in line at the bank, riding the elevator, sitting in the crowded food area).

Interoceptive Exposure

Interoceptive exposure involves having patients bring on the sensations that they fear in a controlled and repeated manner, so that fear reduction is achieved. After review of the rationale for interoceptive exposure, the therapists lead the group through symptom testing to determine what exercises provoke anxiety-related symptoms specific to each group member. After briefly demonstrating each exercise (e.g., hyperventilating, breathing through a straw, spinning, using a tongue depressor, jogging on the spot), the therapist leads the group through the exercise. Group members are encouraged to continue the exercise until they experience intense physical sensations. After each exercise, group members share their experiences (e.g., symptoms, anxiety, similarity of symptoms to panic). After symptom testing, group members are encouraged to practice the exercises that were most powerful for them in triggering physical sensations similar to panic. As these exercises are repeatedly practiced, habituation of the fear response occurs.

Combined In Vivo and Interoceptive Exposure

Upon completion of the interoceptive exposure component, group members are encouraged to practice combining *in vivo* and interoceptive exposure (e.g., wearing a very heavy sweater to the mall, staring at a light in a store, or hyperventilating in the car before entering the mall). Part of a group session may involve the therapists assisting group members in combined practices (e.g., having a group member sit in the food court at the mall and trigger feelings of unreality by staring at the overhead light, then walk around feeling unreal).

Additional Treatment Strategies as Needed

Sometimes, addition of further treatment strategies is warranted (e.g., breathing retraining, relaxation, education of family members). At our center, we do not routinely incorporate breathing retraining (a standard component of PCT) for a number of reasons. Diaphragmatic breathing retraining is based on the rationale that hyperventilation may lead to panic symptoms. However, it may be used as a safety behavior to get rid of panic symptoms, thus undermining the goal of treatment (direct confrontation of panic symptoms). Furthermore, evidence from a dismantling study shows that the addition of breathing retraining does not provide additional benefit over and above CBT without breathing retaining, and may be associated with less complete recovery (Schmidt et al., 2000).

In some cases, when it is evident that marital distress is a factor contributing to the maintenance of panic disorder with agoraphobia, the addition of sessions geared to the marital relationship may be warranted. However, a review of the research examining the marital relationship and CBT for panic disorder indicates that the empirical data results are mixed on whether panic disorder is associated with greater interpersonal and marital problems, whether marital factors predict outcome in CBT, and whether the addition of an intervention geared to improve marital communication yields greater treatment improvement (Marcaurelle, Bélanger, & Marchand, 2003).

If there are group members present who are overly distressed and have difficulty engaging in treatment, it may be appropriate to include a relaxation component in the group treatment. However, the purpose of teaching this skill should be emphasized (alleviate distress versus anxiety avoidance). In some cases, a group member may reveal a problem with family members (e.g., symptom accommodation or interference in treatment) and inclusion of a session for family education may be warranted. This may be difficult in the group setting, so if it is one group member having difficulty, it may make sense to have an individual meeting with the group member and his or her family, separate from the regular group session. The session would provide an opportunity to provide education on the nature of panic disorder and agoraphobia, the role of the family in symptom accommodation. In addition, the session would focus on preparing family members for increased independence and role changes. There is evidence that including significant others in treatment may improve long term outcome for panic disorder with agoraphobia (Cerny et al., 1987).

SAMPLE CBT GROUP PROTOCOL
FOR PANIC DISORDER WITH AGORAPHOBIA

The following 12-session group treatment protocol is based on standard treatments for panic disorder with and without agoraphobia described by Craske and Barlow (2001) and Antony and Swinson (2001). A brief description of what occurs in each session (elaborating on the summary provided in Table 7.3) follows.

Pretreatment Individual Meetings with Group Members

This session involves a meeting between the individual group member and either one or both of the group therapists. The session provides an introduction to the group, the treatment schedule, an overview of what to expect in sessions, and covers issues of confidentiality, the importance of attendance, and expectations for homework. This session also allows an opportunity for group members to have their questions addressed and for the therapist to normalize anxious apprehension about commencing treatment with a group of strangers. The remainder of the session is spent developing the exposure hierarchy (see Figures 7.1 and 7.2) with the assistance of information gathered in the assessment process. The pregroup meeting also increases the comfort level of prospective group members by allowing them to know at least one person who will be in the room at the first session (the therapist).

Session 1: Presenting the Treatment Rationale

Session 1 is the first opportunity for group members to meet each other and the group leaders. Because the therapists have a lot of ground to cover in this session in terms of presenting information, it is important that they aim for a balance between presenting information and allowing space for group interaction and discussion. Promoting group discussion can take place with the introductions. It is helpful to have a group go-around in which group members introduce themselves and say a little bit about themselves (unrelated to panic) as a way to break the ice (e.g., where they grew up, where they live, favorite hobby or leisure activity).

Following the introductions, the therapists should review the structure of the group, including the group format (12 sessions, 120 minutes per session) and session format (e.g., homework review, presentation of new material, homework planning). Key aspects of the pretreatment meeting, such as confidentiality, should be reviewed, and group norms should be discussed, including expectations for attendance, the importance of punctuality and advance notice for missed sessions, and the integral role of homework in treatment outcome.

Almost all group members will be expecting the group to help them get rid of their anxiety. Thus, it is important to clarify expectations for the treatment process and inform group members that they will likely experience an increase in anxiety before they experience a reduction as they start to focus on dealing with the anxiety directly instead of using avoidance. Because of this, treatment can be stressful, so group members should be encouraged to use self-reward and set time aside in their schedules to focus on treatment. It

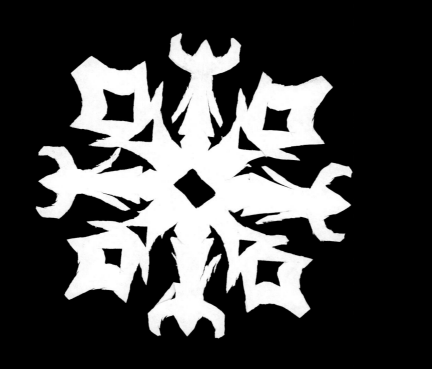

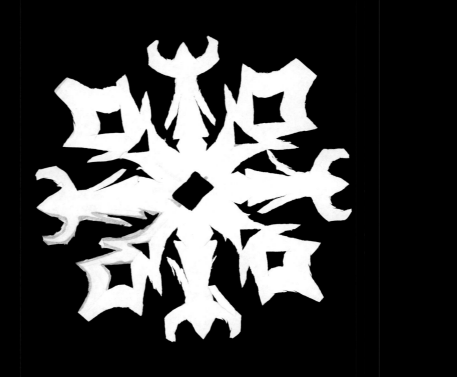

TABLE 7.3. Sample Outline of Treatment Protocol for Group CBT for Panic Disorder

Session	Strategies covered
Pretreatment individual meeting	• Explain how the group will work and what to expect. • Introduce norms and rules for group and provide practical information (e.g., location). • Answer any questions and address concerns. • Develop exposure hierarchy.
Session 1	• Introduction of group members (group members share personal experiences of what brought them to group). • Explain structure and session format of group, and review group norms. • Review what to expect from treatment (clarify expectations). • Review key features of panic disorder. • Present information on the nature of anxiety and panic. • Review three-component model of anxiety. • Present a CBT model of panic disorder. • Homework: Monitor three components of anxiety and fear, read psychoeducational information on the physiological basis of panic.
Session 2	• Homework review. • Psychoeducation: Importance of thoughts and the role they play in emotions. • Review of common anxiety cognitive distortions. • Discussion of group members' examples of their cognitive distortions. • Homework: Monitor three components of anxiety, with a focus on thoughts and identification of cognitive distortions.
Session 3	• Homework review. • Psychoeducation: Strategies for countering anxious thoughts. • Group members practice challenging and countering anxious thoughts, with the goal of realistic thinking. • Introduction to a thought record. • Homework: Monitor anxious thoughts using thought record and practice countering strategies.
Session 4	• Homework review. • Introduce exposure and explain why it works. • Review guidelines for conducting exposures. • Each group member chooses an exposure practice from the exposure hierarchy. • Review exposure monitoring form. • Homework: Conduct exposure practices daily (or confront subtle avoidance or safety behaviors if agoraphobia is not present); continue challenging anxious thoughts.
Session 5	• Homework review. • Group members discuss challenges in conducting exposure practices. • Therapist tracks some examples on whiteboard to illustrate anxiety reduction. • Troubleshooting of obstacles to exposure and review of rationale. • Detailed homework planning. • Homework: Exposure practices, continued challenging of anxious thoughts using thought record.

(continued)

TABLE 7.3. (continued)

Session	Strategies covered
Session 6	• Homework review. • Midpoint of treatment review using exposure hierarchy ratings, highlighting progress made and continued goals. • Rationale for interoceptive exposure presented. • Therapist conducts symptom testing with the group. • Presentation of guidelines for conducting interoceptive exposures. • Homework: Interoceptive exposure practice, situational exposure practice; and continued challenging of anxious thoughts using the thought record.
Session 7	• Homework review. • Group members discuss experiences with interoceptive exposure practices. • Problem solving of obstacles and troubleshooting. • Complete any remaining symptom testing. • Conduct an in-session interoceptive exposure. • Homework: Interoceptive exposure practice, situational exposure practice; continued challenging of anxious thoughts using the thought record.
Session 8–11	• Homework review to facilitate group discussion of concepts, highlight common themes, identify obstacles, and conduct troubleshooting. • The group is used to provide reinforcement and encouragement. • Each group member sets specific homework goals and uses the group to discuss anticipated obstacles. • Combined interoceptive and situational exposure is introduced. • In-session exposure practices are used as needed (e.g., going to shopping mall, riding the bus). • Homework: Interoceptive exposure practice, situational exposure practice, combined interoceptive and situational exposure practice; continue challenging anxious thoughts using the thought record.
Session 12	• Homework review. • Group members review their progress using the hierarchy rating forms, identifying progress as well as continued goals. • Thoughts and feelings regarding termination of the group are processed. • Relapse prevention strategies are reviewed.

should be emphasized that treatment does not eliminate anxiety, but it changes how they react to anxiety and panic, and that the group will give them the skills to manage the panic, so that it does not control their lives. Therapists can build motivation by encouraging group members to use all of the reasons they have for seeking treatment as motivation to challenge their anxiety.

The key features of panic disorder can be reviewed by having group members share their experience with panic, including panic attack frequency, situations avoided because of panic, common anxious thoughts, subtle avoidance, and safety cues. Therapists should make an effort to identify common themes and link group members' experiences to build cohesion.

Therapists should review information on the nature of anxiety and panic, highlighting the fact that anxiety and panic are normal emotions, panic attacks are time-limited, and anxiety and panic are not dangerous. Within this context, a discussion of treatment goals should emphasize that the goal of treatment is to help group members manage their anxiety and panic, not to eliminate fear and anxiety altogether.

The three-component model of anxiety should be presented as a new way for group members to approach their anxiety and panic in terms of its component parts: physical sensations, thoughts, and behaviors (avoidance, escape, subtle avoidance). It is helpful to illustrate this model on a whiteboard and have group members share their symptoms for each component. Therapists can then ask group members for some examples to illustrate how the three components interact with each other to escalate anxiety and panic: For example, a physical symptom is misinterpreted as dangerous and leads to self-monitoring for further sensations (behavior), which then leads to further physical symptoms, increased thoughts of impending catastrophe, and escape and avoidance behaviors.

Therapists present a CBT model for understanding panic disorder, emphasizing the importance of threatening interpretations for physical symptoms and interoceptive conditioning (the pairing of physical sensations with danger). It is helpful to use the example of a conditioned taste aversion to illustrate how the brain can associate danger with a neutral stimulus once the stimulus (e.g., food) is paired with an aversive experience (e.g., nausea), because most group members will be able to relate to this experience.

Homework for this session includes having group members monitor the three components of anxiety and fear whenever they feel anxious or experience a panic attack. Group members are also given readings to review the three components of anxiety and the physiological basis of panic.

Sessions 2 and 3: Cognitive Strategies

Session 2 begins with a check-in to get group members' opinions about the first session. Homework is then reviewed. Group members should be encouraged to pull out their self-monitoring sheets and go through some examples. Therapist should link group members' experiences and identify common themes. It is also useful to use some group members' experiences as examples on the whiteboard to illustrate how the three components interact to escalate the anxiety experience. This model can be used to illustrate the treatment rationale—that although we often do not control physical sensations, we can control how we respond to them (i.e., how we think and behave). Group members should be encouraged to share their thoughts about this model and any questions or concerns that they have about how the model relates to their experience.

The importance of thoughts and the role they play in determining emotion is reviewed, with an emphasis on approaching thoughts as hypotheses and not facts. The two most common types of cognitive distortions associated with anxiety are presented: probability overestimation (i.e., overestimating the likelihood of an event) and catastrophizing (exaggeration of the negative consequences of an event). Group members are encouraged to give examples from their own experience to illustrate these distortions. Homework for Session 2 has group members continuing to monitor the three components of anxiety, while paying close attention to their thoughts and, in particular, to the two types of cognitive distortions.

Session 3 begins with a review of homework. Group members are asked to share examples from their self-monitoring records. Therapists should use the material provided to review the concept of cognitive distortions, and to link group members' experiences and identify common themes. Different strategies for challenging and counteracting anxious thoughts can be presented using the group to generate alternate appraisals and interpretations. The thought record is introduced, and an example is completed on the whiteboard, with the group generating content for each column. Homework in this session includes using the thought record to track anxious thoughts and practicing use of countering strategies. The goal of "realistic" versus positive thinking is highlighted.

It is common for some group members to state that they have done this before, or that they already *know* that their anxious thoughts are not true, but they still *feel* anxious. Therapists should normalize these concerns and feelings, and encourage group members to keep an open mind and practice utilizing the strategies, because countering the anxious thoughts is a skill that takes time to practice. With practice, group members will find that their belief in the alternative appraisal gets stronger.

Sessions 4 and 5: *In Vivo* Exposure

Session 4 begins with homework review. The therapist uses the whiteboard to illustrate some of the group members' more challenging examples, and the group is encouraged to generate questions that counteract the anxious thought. Group members are encouraged to continue practicing their countering strategies for anxious thoughts throughout the rest of treatment. The topic of exposure, with a rationale for how and why it works, is introduced. It is helpful to use an example unrelated to group member anxiety to illustrate the concept of exposure (e.g., asking group members how they would help a child overcome a fear of dogs and what specific steps that they would take), and draw a graph on the whiteboard of what happens to anxiety with repeated exposure practices. The guidelines for conducting exposure, as well as the new exposure monitoring form, are reviewed. Group members choose one exposure practice from their hierarchies as the focus for homework. They are encouraged to practice daily, if possible, but they are asked to engage in a minimum of three exposures over the course of the week. Homework also involves continued challenging of anxious thoughts on a thought record. Individuals in the group who do not have agoraphobia are encouraged to focus on using the exposure principles to confront any subtle avoidance or safety behaviors they might detect.

Session 5 begins with a homework review. Group members are encouraged to share their experiences with practicing exposure. It is helpful for the therapists to track some examples on the whiteboard, using a graph, and to illustrate how anxiety increased then decreased over the course of the exposure. The group provides encouragement, support, and a different perspective (reframing) for individuals who had difficulty with the homework. Group members are encouraged to measure their success by how they coped in a situation (behaviorally) rather than by how they felt (i.e., anxious). This session focuses on problem-solving obstacles to exposure, reviewing the rationale, and setting a detailed homework plan for the week; each group member lets the rest of the group know what he or she will be practicing and how the practices will be conducted. Homework includes exposure and continued challenging of anxious thoughts on the thought record.

Sessions 6 and 7: Symptom Induction Testing and Interoceptive Exposure

Session 6 is the halfway point. After reviewing the homework, the therapists remind group members that they are halfway through and encourage them to use the group time as motivation to really practice their exposures. Group members are given the hierarchies that they have rated at the beginning of each session for the past 6 weeks and asked to reflect on where they were when they started the group, where they are now, and where they have to go. It is important for the therapists to remind the group that each member will be proceeding at his or her own pace.

The rationale for interoceptive exposure is reviewed, with an emphasis on the goal of disconnecting physical sensations from danger through a shift in perspective: viewing physical sensations as an uncomfortable nuisance rather than as a warning sign of impending physical catastrophe. The therapists check to ensure that all of the group members understand the purpose of interoceptive exposure and provide time to discuss any questions or concerns that group members raise. Symptom testing is then conducted, with the therapist first demonstrating each exercise, then leading the group in the exercise. After each exercise, group members are encouraged to share their experience: symptoms, anxiety level, and similarity to their anxiety and panic symptoms. Once symptom testing is completed, group members are asked to share the three exercises that were most effective for them in triggering similar anxiety and panic symptoms. Guidelines for conducting interoceptive exposure are reviewed. Assigned homework includes interoceptive exposure to one of the symptom exercises, continued *in vivo* exposure, and continued challenging of anxious thoughts by using the thought record. Group members are encouraged to let the rest of the group know what they will be practicing over the week for interoceptive and *in vivo* exposure.

Session 7 begins with a homework review. It is helpful to graph out some examples on the whiteboard of how anxiety changes over the course of an interoceptive exposure practice. Any obstacles are discussed and problem solving by the group is encouraged. The rationale for interoceptive exposure is reviewed by group members, with the therapists facilitating the discussion. Part of the session is used to complete any incomplete symptom testing from the previous session and to conduct an in-session interoceptive exposure practice, with group members focusing on the exercise that is relevant to them. The rest of the session is spent carefully planning homework, including interoceptive exposure practices, *in vivo* exposure practices, and continued challenging of anxious thoughts.

Sessions 8–11: Continued Practice of CBT Strategies

Sessions 8 through 11 are used for continued practice of CBT strategies. Homework review is done in a thorough way, and therapists facilitate the group in reviewing concepts, highlighting common themes, providing positive reinforcement and encouragement, and identifying and troubleshooting obstacles. Therapists conduct homework planning in a focused manner by having group members be very specific in setting their homework goals and the steps they will take to meet their goals and overcome anticipated obstacles. The combination of interoceptive and situational exposure is introduced, and relevant practices are developed for homework.

It is also helpful to plan some in-session exposure practice as a group for one or two sessions. At our center, we take one to two sessions to travel by bus to a shopping mall, where we then break up into smaller groups to conduct relevant exposures (standing in line; sitting in the food court area; triggering feelings of depersonalization/derealization by staring at a light, then walking around the mall; walking around without carrying medication; going into a busy coffee shop, etc.). The exposures are planned in the previous session and time is left at the end of the session for group members to debrief and share their experiences. The therapists encourage group members to reflect on and share what they have learned from their exposure practices. Group members also find that this a good opportunity to help each other, and it is generally viewed as a powerful learning experience.

Session 12: Termination and Relapse Prevention

After a homework review, group members are given their hierarchy ratings from pretreatment to the present to examine for patterns and changes. Group members are asked to share the progress they have made by reflecting on where they started and where they are now, as well as their goals for continued recovery. Part of the session allows time for group members to share what they have learned from the group and what important experiences they will take with them, following the worksheet displayed in Figure 7.3. Time is also spent processing group members' thoughts and feelings around termination. Relapse prevention is discussed, and the group generates strategies for managing any flare-up of anxiety or panic in the future. At our center, all group members are offered a monthly booster group that they can attend on a drop-in basis to boost their strategies, review concepts, and share any difficulties. We also give group members the opportunity to decide whether they would like a follow-up group to check on progress and facilitate continued recovery. These sessions are offered at 1 month, 6 months, and 1 year posttreatment if desired by the group.

---

1. Think back to when you first started treatment. What gains or accomplishments have you made over the past 14 weeks? What goals have you achieved? What obstacles have you overcome?

2. What do you need to keep working on after the group ends? What are the situations or experiences that you would like to tackle?

3. What key information or phrases did you learn in the group that you need to take with you to keep you going?

FIGURE 7.3. Posttreatment planning form.

Posttreatment Evaluation

Posttreatment evaluation involves having each group member complete the assessment package he or she completed at pretreatment. It is also recommended that each group member have an individual meeting to update current symptom status (e.g., full or partial remission) and determine any further treatment planning needed for additional difficulties.

PROCESS ISSUES

A number of group processes facilitate treatment for panic disorder with and without agoraphobia. The group provides a sense of collectivity, with members working together on similar challenges. The group proceeds with a sense of momentum, providing a positive and motivating atmosphere to set goals and share experiences. At our center, panic groups tend to be more cohesive than other (e.g., OCD or social phobia) groups, likely due to shared clinical features of the condition (vs. OCD, whose symptoms may be quite diverse) and the openness of group members to share experiences (vs. social phobia, in which group members may have difficulty with disclosure).

The qualities of the group leaders also play a role in group process and there is some evidence that therapist characteristics may be associated with treatment outcome in panic disorder with and without agoraphobia. For example, Williams and Chambless (1990) found that clients who rated their therapist as more self-confident, and more caring and involved, were more likely to show improvement on a behavioral avoidance test. In addition, level of experience in conducting psychotherapy (but not CBT specifically) has been related to treatment outcome (Huppert et al., 2001).

Challenges to Group Process

A number of issues may present a challenge to group process and require management by the group leaders. One such challenge is "thought/emotion contagion," the group reaction to an anxious thought reported by another group member (Huppert & Baker-Morissette, 2003). Although this is an issue for many groups, it is of particular concern for a group with patients with panic disorder, who are quick to learn associations with feared consequences. Group therapists should be vigilant for this effect and manage it by discussing group members' reactions (thoughts and feelings) and encouraging cognitive restructuring.

Heterogeneity in group membership may reduce group cohesiveness and present a challenge to group process. Individuals who do not feel included in the group may be at risk for dropout. Although this issue is best addressed when the group is formed by balancing group membership, sometimes the heterogeneity does not become evident until after the group has begun, or it may not have been possible to provide alternative options for a "lone member" (described earlier). During group, heterogeneity can be minimized by therapists' promotion of links between group members and highlighting similarities.

Group members who have experienced negative events during panic (e.g., fainting, vomiting) also present a challenge to group process, because they may challenge information presented by the therapists and trigger fear in other group members. In these cases, it is important for group members to roll with the resistance and practice the strategies discussed in Chapter 2, this volume. Therapists should accept the fact that negative events may sometimes happen but shift the group focus to realistic probabilities (e.g., "You fainted once in 200 panic attacks. What is the likelihood of you fainting during a panic attack based on your own experience?" [0.5%]) and decatastrophization (e.g., "What was the outcome of the experience? How bad was it? What are the long-term consequences?").

Participants whose anxious thoughts are resistant to change may also pose a challenge to group process when group members who may be ready to move on become frustrated by a "stubborn" group member. In such a case, it is helpful for the group leaders to encourage the individual to keep an open mind and continue practicing the cognitive strategies. The most powerful change agent is behavior, so moving the group along to the behavioral strategies may help the "stuck" group member.

Noncompliance with exposure homework is also an issue for the group. Noncompliance may be due to motivational factors, lack of understanding of the rationale, or symptom severity (e.g., exposure practice is too overwhelming). Group leaders need to ascertain the reasons for noncompliance, and then manage it accordingly by boosting motivation, reviewing treatment rationale, or troubleshooting exposure practices. A helpful strategy for motivating group members to gear up their practices is to remind them what session the group is working on and how many sessions are left, emphasizing the importance of making treatment a priority.

In some cases, a group member may require individualized attention for issues that cannot be managed in the group (severe agoraphobia interfering with group attendance, exacerbation of comorbid disorders, etc.). This may be handled by having an individual session, in addition to the group session, to address the issues and to reassess treatment needs, including the appropriateness of continuing in the group. For individuals with severe agoraphobia, providing additional sessions after group has ended for those who need further exposure assistance may be beneficial.

Other Issues to Consider

Many patients may taper off medication in group. Therapists can discuss this as a group issue, highlighting the benefits of CBT in managing reactions to possible withdrawal effects. In some cases (i.e., as-needed benzodiazepine use), tapering off medication may be necessary to obtain the full therapeutic benefit of CBT, and reduction of use should be encouraged and incorporated in the exposure hierarchy. This should be discussed within the group in terms of the necessity of experiencing anxiety to achieve the goal of overcoming anxiety.

Over the course of the group, individual group members are bound to experience a setback at one time or another. This experience should be reframed as a learning experience and discussed within the group in terms of strategies to manage setbacks. Being able to handle a setback with the support of the group is good preparation for handling setbacks that may occur once the group is over.

CONCLUSIONS

Panic disorder with or without agoraphobia is uniquely characterized by the presence of unexpected panic attacks. Cognitive features include marked anxiety sensitivity, increased attention to bodily sensations, and the presence of threat-related cognitive biases. Behavioral features include escape, avoidance, and subtle safety behaviors. Cognitive-behavioral models of panic disorder place central importance on the role of catastrophic misinterpretation of physical sensations and interoceptive anxiety. Both pharmacotherapy and CBT are empirically supported treatments for panic disorder with or with agoraphobia. Group CBT provides a cost-effective, efficient format for treatment delivery. Consideration should be given to a number of factors when structuring group treatment, including group format and group composition. We reviewed the key CBT components, along with group process issues and obstacles specific to panic disorder. A sample CBT group protocol was also provided.

CHAPTER 8

Obsessive–Compulsive Disorder

DESCRIPTION OF OBSESSIVE–COMPULSIVE DISORDER

Diagnostic Features

The hallmark feature of obsessive–compulsive disorder (OCD) is the presence of obsessions, compulsions, or both. On the surface, deriving a diagnosis of OCD may seem straightforward. However, diagnosing OCD can often be challenging due to the overlap in features with other conditions, including tic disorders, impulse control disorders, obsessive–compulsive personality disorder, somatoform disorders, generalized anxiety disorder, phobias, eating disorders, psychotic disorders, and depression. This section includes a summary of the key diagnostic features of OCD according to the text revision of the fourth edition of the *Diagnostic and Statistical Manual of Mental Disorders* (DSM-IV-TR; American Psychiatric Association [APA], 2000). More detailed discussions concerning diagnosis and classification of OCD may be found elsewhere (Antony, Downie, & Swinson, 1998; Krochmalik & Menzies, 2003; Okasha, 2002).

DSM-IV-TR defines an "obsession" as a recurrent thought, image, or impulse that is experienced as intrusive, inappropriate, or distressing, and that the individual attempts to ignore, suppress, or neutralize with another thought or action (e.g., a compulsion). According to the official diagnostic criteria, obsessions are not simply excessive worries about real-life problems, and the individual must recognize that the thoughts, images, or impulses are the product of his or her own mind.

Typical obsessions include contamination fears (e.g., fear of germs, diseases, detergents, chemicals, toxins, and various other perceived contaminants), doubts about actions (e.g., whether doors are locked, appliances have been left on, there are errors in one's written work, one has hit a pedestrian while driving), religious beliefs (e.g., thoughts of a religious nature that are distressing, such as blasphemous images or thoughts about being possessed by the devil), sexual thoughts and images (e.g., irrational doubts about one's sexual orientation, irrational thoughts about sex with a child or some other inappropriate partner), aggressive thoughts (e.g., intrusive thoughts of hurting a loved one), thoughts of accidentally harming oneself or others, and impulses to have things exact, in a particular order, symmetrical, or just right.

A "compulsion" is defined as a repetitive behavior or mental act that a person performs in response to an obsession or according to specific, rigidly applied rules (APA, 2000). Compulsions are aimed at reducing distress or discomfort, or at preventing some negative outcome from occurring. Typical compulsions include excessive washing, cleaning, checking, reassurance seeking, repeating actions, counting, praying, hoarding, and restating things.

A diagnosis of OCD requires that the individual have insight into the fact that the obsessions and compulsions are excessive or unrealistic, at least some of the time. Individuals who lack insight most of the time (but who do have insight at least some of the time) are said to have OCD with *poor insight* (previously referred to as *overvalued ideation*; APA, 1987). An individual with OCD must also experience clinically significant distress or impairment in day-to-day functioning. For example, cases in which symptoms take up more than 1 hour each day are typically considered to be clinically significant. Finally, as with all of the anxiety disorders, a diagnosis of OCD requires that the symptoms not be better accounted for by another mental disorder, a general medical condition, or the use of (or withdrawal from) a substance (APA, 2000).

Note that OCD is a heterogeneous condition. Although symptom overlap is common, symptoms sometimes shift from one cluster to another over time, and most individuals with OCD do not experience all of the symptoms described in this section. For example, some individuals have symptoms focused exclusively on concerns related to contamination and washing, whereas others may have symptoms that cut across several content areas.

Cognitive Features

Cognitive-behavioral models of OCD emphasize the importance of beliefs, appraisals, and other cognitive features in the cause and maintenance of OCD. The Obsessive Compulsive Cognitions Working Group (1997) identified six belief domains that are relevant to OCD: (1) inflated responsibility, (2) overimportance of thoughts, (3) excessive concern about the importance of controlling one's thoughts, (4) overestimation of threat, (5) intolerance of uncertainty, and (6) perfectionism. In this section, we consider a number of these domains, as well as several related cognitive features (e.g., attention and memory biases, magical thinking, thought–action fusion) that are relevant to the understanding and treatment of OCD. A comprehensive review of the role of cognition in OCD is available elsewhere (e.g., Frost & Steketee, 2002).

Metacognition and OCD

The term "metacognition" refers to a belief that an individual has about his or her beliefs. For example, the belief that one must control or prevent intrusive thoughts is a metacognition, as is the belief that one's thoughts are dangerous or very important in some way. Most cognitive models of OCD emphasize the role of metacognitions, arguing that it is patients' beliefs about their obsessions that maintain the disorder. Researchers have begun to generate data confirming the importance of metacognitive factors for understanding OCD (e.g., Gwilliam, Wells, & Cartwright-Hatton, 2004).

Attention and Vigilance in OCD

Although the literature is somewhat inconsistent, overall there is little evidence that individuals with OCD are biased to attend to *general* threat cues more closely than individuals without OCD (e.g., Moritz et al., 2004). However, there is evidence that individuals with OCD (particularly those with contamination concerns) may be vigilant for information related to their specific obsessions (Summerfeldt & Endler, 1998; Tata, Leibowitz, Prunty, Cameron, & Pickering, 1996).

Memory Biases in OCD

Research results on memory and OCD have also been mixed. Although some studies have failed to find general memory deficits in OCD, a meta-analytic review concluded that OCD checkers are impaired on certain types of memory tasks (Woods, Vevea, Chambless, & Bayen, 2002). There is also evidence that people with contamination obsessions tend to have better memory for contaminated objects than for clean ones (Radomsky & Rachman, 1999), and that individuals with OCD have difficulty forgetting threat-related information when instructed to do so (Wilhem, McNally, Baer, & Florin, 1996) compared to people without OCD. Regardless of whether people with OCD actually have memory deficits, it is fairly clear that patients with OCD with significant checking compulsions have impaired confidence in their memories even in studies showing no actual memory deficits (e.g., MacDonald, Antony, MacLeod, & Richter, 1997). Furthermore, repeated checking seems to reduce confidence in one's memory even further (Radomsky, Gilchrist, & Dussault, 2003).

Magical Thinking

Magical thinking involves assuming that there are associations between events that in reality are not related. Though not everyone with OCD engages in magical thinking, OCD symptoms do tend to be correlated with measures of magical thinking (Einstein & Menzies, 2004). Examples of beliefs that reflect magical thinking include the following:

> "My boyfriend will be in a car accident if I don't finish my term paper by midnight."
>
> "If I do everything seven times, I can prevent bad things from happening."
>
> "If I step on a sidewalk crack, I'll break my mother's back."

Thought–Action Fusion

The term "thought–action fusion" (TAF) refers to the tendency to view thoughts and actions as equivalent. Examples of TAF include the belief that thinking about harming a loved one is the moral equivalent of actually doing it, or the belief that thinking about doing something horrible increases the likelihood of acting on the belief. TAF is a common feature of OCD (Rachman & Shafran, 1999; Shafran, Thordarson, & Rachman, 1996) and, in our clinical experience, is particularly relevant in people with religious, aggressive, and sexual obsessions. Conceptually, TAF may be best thought of as a subtype of magical thinking (Einstein & Menzies, 2004). Recent research suggests that TAF can be corrected through standard CBT techniques, such as psychoeducation (Zucker, Craske, Barrios, & Holguin, 2002).

Perfectionistic Thinking

"Perfectionism" may be defined as a tendency to set standards that are both rigid and unattainably high. It is a feature of depression, eating disorders, several anxiety disorders, as well as certain other psychological problems. Individuals with OCD tend to show higher levels of perfectionism compared to people without anxiety disorders. In particular, they are overly concerned about making mistakes, and they also report excessive doubts about whether they have done things correctly (Antony, Purdon, Huta, & Swinson, 1998). Clinically, some patients also present with excessive attention to detail and a need to have things "just right."

Inflated Responsibility

A growing literature suggests that individuals with OCD often have an inflated sense of responsibility (for a review, see Salkovskis & Forrester, 2002), meaning that they tend to be overly concerned that their actions and thoughts will lead to negative consequences, or that failing to act will lead to negative consequences. The construct of inflated responsibility is closely related to some of the other cognitive features of OCD discussed earlier, including perfectionism, TAF, and magical thinking. Examples of OCD presentations that may reflect a sense of inflated responsibility include the following:

- A person who checks excessively when leaving a room to make sure that nothing has been left behind.
- A person who repeatedly asks for reassurance that others are not offended by something he or she said.
- A lawyer who spends hours reviewing reports and letters to ensure that everything is accurate, so harm will not come to his or her clients.
- A new mother who avoids spending time with her baby for fear of acting on intrusive sexual obsessions.

Overestimation of Threat

As with all anxiety disorders, people with OCD often judge situations to be much more dangerous than they really are. For example, perfectly safe objects may be viewed as contaminated, or the perceived consequences of making mistakes may be exaggerated. The tendency to overestimate threat has been found to be correlated with severity of symptoms such as washing, checking, doubting, obsessing, mental neutralizing, and hoarding (Tolin, Woods, & Abramowitz, 2003). In addition, compared to people without OCD, people with OCD tend to request more information and tend to spend more time deliberating before making decisions about low-risk situations and about situations relevant to their OCD (Foa et al., 2003).

Intolerance of Uncertainty

The inability to tolerate ambiguity and uncertainty has been studied extensively in generalized anxiety disorder, but only recently have investigators begun to study this phenomenon in OCD. Preliminary findings suggest that intolerance of uncertainty is indeed a feature of OCD, particularly among people who check excessively (Tolin, Abramowitz, Brigidi, & Foa, 2003). The heightened desire for certainty is especially problematic given the tendency for OCD patients to be uncertain about things. As reviewed earlier, doubts about actions and a lack of confidence in memories are common features of OCD.

Behavioral Features

The most common behavioral features of OCD may be conceptualized either as avoidance behaviors or as compulsions, both of which are used to prevent harm from occurring or to reduce discomfort. The distinction between avoidance behaviors and compulsions is often blurred. For example, suppression of intrusive thoughts (listed below as an example of an avoidance behavior) can just as easily be conceptualized as a cognitive compulsion.

Avoidance Behaviors

People with OCD often avoid situations that trigger their obsessions and fear. For example, people who fear contamination avoid objects that are perceived as contaminated, and individuals who fear hitting pedestrians while driving may avoid driving, particularly in areas with pedestrian traffic. Avoidance may also be more subtle. For example, people with OCD engage in various forms of cognitive avoidance, including distraction, suppression of intrusive thoughts, and replacing intrusive thoughts with neutral ones (e.g., Freeston & Ladouceur, 1997; Purdon, Rowa, & Antony, in press). Like other forms of avoidance, cognitive avoidance is thought to be counterproductive, serving to maintain anxiety and distress over the long term (Purdon, 1999).

Compulsions and Other Protective Strategies

One of the hallmark symptoms of OCD is compulsive rituals, the most common of which include checking, washing and cleaning, counting, repeating actions, and repeating phrases. Frequent reassurance seeking is another common compulsion used to reduce anxiety triggered by doubts about one's actions, intrusive thoughts, or memories. Reassurance is often sought from family members, therapists, books, and other sources.

People with OCD often engage in other protective behaviors as well. For example, people with contamination fears may wear gloves to prevent contaminants from getting on their skin. People who fear leaving their small appliances on may unplug them and bring them to work each day, just to be sure. Reliance on safety cues (objects or people whose presence engenders a sense of safety) is also common in OCD and other anxiety disorders. Finally, some patients with OCD tend to overrely on substances as a way of managing their discomfort (Denys, Tenney, van Megen, de Geus, & Westenberg, 2004; LaSalle et al., 2004), though alcohol and drug use may be less of a problem in OCD than in certain other anxiety disorders.

COGNITIVE-BEHAVIORAL APPROACHES TO UNDERSTANDING OCD

Early behavioral models of OCD (e.g., Meyer, 1966) were based on traditional learning theories, such as Mowrer's (1960) two-factor model for the development of fear. According to Mowrer, fear is initially triggered through classical conditioning, in which a previously neutral stimulus (e.g., a dog) is associated with some negative event or experience (being bitten), and subsequently becomes an object of fear. Fear is thought to be maintained through operant conditioning processes (specifically, negative reinforcement), in which the avoidance of the feared object or situation maintains the problem over time by reducing the uncomfortable feelings of fear and anxiety, and providing a sense of relief. In the case of OCD, learning models assume that obsessive–compulsive symptoms begin after some sort of classically conditioned negative event. For example, developing food poisoning might lead to a fear of contamination, or losing something important might lead to excessive checking. By engaging in various avoidance behaviors and compulsive rituals, the individual with OCD increases the likelihood that his or her symptoms will continue over time.

Despite their intuitive appeal, learning models of OCD have not been well supported by research. For example, Jones and Menzies (1998) found that less than 13% of OCD washers reported either direct or indirect conditioning events that might account for their symptoms. Therefore, theorists have turned their attention to cognitive and cognitive-behavioral approaches to better understand OCD (e.g., Rachman, 1978, 1997, 1998, 2002; Salkovskis, 1985, 1998). Two core features of current cognitive-behavioral models of OCD are the notions (1) that individuals with OCD have an exaggerated sense of responsibility for causing or preventing harm, and (2) that metacognitions (i.e., beliefs about intrusive thoughts) are key to understanding this condition.

For example, Salkovskis (1998) reviewed research showing that almost 90% of individuals in the general population experience intrusive thoughts that are similar in content to clinical obsessions, and argued that what distinguishes normal intrusive thoughts from clinical obsessions is not the nature of the thoughts, but rather the way in which the individual interprets the thoughts. According to Salkovskis, intrusive thoughts become a problem when they are interpreted as an indication that an individual may be responsible for either causing or preventing harm to oneself or others. For example, if a person believes that the thought "I will stab my child" increases the chances of doing so, he or she might be inclined to make efforts to suppress the thought and to avoid sharp objects such as knives. Behavioral compulsions, attempts to suppress thoughts, and efforts to neutralize obsessions are thought to reinforce the individual's fear of the intrusive thoughts by preventing him or her from learning that the thoughts are not dangerous. The model appears to be best suited to explaining OCD profiles that involve an intense fear of one's intrusive thoughts (e.g., sexual, aggressive, and religious obsessions).

As another example of a cognitive theory, Rachman (2002) published a model of compulsive checking. According to this theory, compulsive checking occurs when people believe that they have a heightened responsibility to prevent harm and are unsure whether the perceived threat has been removed. For example, a pharmacist who has obsessions about giving customers the wrong medications, and who doubts his memory about what medications he has dispensed, may check his work repeatedly. According to Rachman, three factors that contribute to the intensity of checking are (1) the level of perceived responsibility, (2) perceived likelihood of harm, and (3) perceived seriousness of harm.

TREATMENTS FOR OCD

Evidence-based treatments for OCD include primarily pharmacotherapy and psychological treatments such as behavior therapy and CBT. In addition, several long-term follow-up studies suggest that up to half of patients with treatment refractory OCD report significant benefit following psychosurgery (e.g., cingulotomy, anterior capsulotomy), with relatively few side effects (e.g., Dougherty et al., 2002; Jenike, 1998; Kim et al., 2003). However, because of the intrusive nature of psychosurgery and a lack of controlled studies, these procedures are currently used only in the most severe, refractory cases. This section provides a brief review of the current status of pharmacological and psychological approaches to treating OCD. More comprehensive reviews may be found in a number of sources (e.g., Antony & Swinson, 2001; Maj, Sartorius, Okasha, & Zohar, 2002; McDonough, 2003; Menzies & de Silva, 2003).

Pharmacotherapy

Numerous studies have shown that the selective serotonin reuptake inhibitors (SSRIs), as well as the tricyclic antidepressant clomipramine, are effective in reducing OCD symptoms (Antony & Swinson, 2001). For example, in a large study of more than 500 patients, the Clomipramine Collaborative Study Group (1991) found that those taking medication experienced on average a 38% reduction in scores on the Yale–Brown Obsessive Compulsive Scale (Goodman et al., 1989a, 1989b), compared to only 3% of those taking placebo. There have also been numerous controlled studies confirming the efficacy of SSRIs, including sertraline, fluoxetine, fluvoxamine, paroxetine, and most recently, citalopram (Antony & Swinson, 2001). In general, medications other than clomipramine and the SSRIs have not been found to be effective for treating OCD (Antony & Swinson, 2001).

There is no evidence that any single SSRI works better than any other. In addition, although effect sizes have tended to be largest in studies using clomipramine, head-to-head comparisons of SSRIs and clomipramine have found them to be equivalent (see McDonough, 2003, for a review). The decision of which medication to use typically involves considering the evidence regarding efficacy, as well as available information on side effects, interactions with medications that the individual may be taking, possible effects on medical conditions from which the person suffers, previous response to medications taken by the patient, and previous response to medications taken by family members of the patient.

Because SSRIs have a more favorable side effect profile than clomipramine, medication treatment for OCD typically begins with an SSRI. If the chosen medication does not lead to the desired reductions in symptoms after 12 weeks of treatment at an adequate dose, it is reasonable to switch to another SSRI and then to clomipramine. In clinical practice, SSRIs are sometimes combined with other medications, though only limited evidence supports this practice. As reviewed by McDonough (2003), SSRI augmentation has typically been based on case studies and small open trials. Studies have generally found only limited benefits for augmenting SSRIs with drugs such as clonazepam, buspirone, L-tryptophan, lithium, and gabapentin. Evidence supporting the addition of atypical antipsychotics to SSRIs for treatment refractory cases is somewhat better (Bystritsky et al., 2004; McDougle, Epperson, Pelton, Wasylink, & Price, 2000), though findings are mixed (e.g., Shapira et al., 2004).

Psychosocial Treatments

Over the past few decades, exposure and ritual prevention (ERP) has emerged as the psychological treatment of choice for OCD. "Exposure" involves gradually confronting feared situations (e.g., touching contaminated objects; purposely making errors in one's written work; doing things the "wrong" number of times; exposing oneself to anxiety-provoking words, thoughts, or images). "Ritual prevention" refers to the process of eliminating compulsions, rituals, and protective behaviors.

Research supporting the use of ERP for OCD goes back more than 40 years, beginning with the work of Victor Meyer (1966). A large number of controlled outcome studies have demonstrated that ERP is an effective treatment for OCD (for a review, see Franklin & Foa, 2002). Generally, studies support the use of either intensive treatment (consisting of daily sessions for about 3 weeks, administered in either a day treatment or inpatient format) or a less intensive, outpatient-based treatment (often with two or three sessions per week). In one review of 12 ERP studies including about 330 participants, Foa and Kozak (1996) identified 83% of patients with OCD as responders. Furthermore, gains were generally maintained over time, with 76% of patients (from a group of 376 patients in 16 studies) still being considered responders at a mean of 2.4 years following the end of treatment (Foa & Kozak, 1996).

A meta-analysis by Abramowitz (1996) identified several factors that contribute to improved outcomes. Generally, protocols in which strict ritual prevention instructions are given (as opposed to gradual or partial ritual prevention) lead to the best results. Also, protocols that include therapist-assisted exposure appear to be more effective than those that include only self-exposure. Finally, protocols including both imaginal and *in vivo* (i.e., situational) exposure tended to yield better outcomes than those including only *in vivo* exposure. In a subsequent meta-analysis of 16 outcome trials, Abramowitz (1998) found that patients with OCD who had been treated with ERP had scores on standard measures of OCD that were closer to those of individuals in the general population than they were to those of untreated patients with OCD, suggesting that the changes seen over the course of ERP are clinically meaningful. However, after treatment, differences between treated patients with OCD and those in the general population were still significant. In other words, most people continue to struggle with their OCD to some extent, even after successful treatment.

In light of recent cognitive models of OCD, and because ERP only leads to partial improvement in many patients, investigators have begun to examine the benefits of using cognitive strategies. Cognitive therapy involves teaching patients to identify and challenge unrealistic anxious beliefs by examining the evidence regarding the beliefs and conducting behavioral experiments to test out whether negative beliefs are true. To date, studies have mostly focused on comparisons of cognitive therapy to traditional behavioral treatments, and in most cases, cognitive therapy has been found to be an effective alternative to ERP (e.g., Cottraux et al., 2001; McLean et al., 2001; van Oppen et al., 1995; Whittal, Thordarson, & McLean, 2005). Currently, there is a lack of studies investigating the question of whether adding cognitive strategies to ERP leads to improved outcomes compared to ERP alone.

Group Treatments for OCD

Although most studies of psychological treatments for OCD have been based on individual treatment protocols, a number of studies have found that OCD can be treated effectively in a group format (for a review, see Whittal & McLean, 2002). Group treatments that have been described in the literature include cognitive treatments (McLean et al., 2001), behavioral treatments (e.g., ERP; Himle et al., 2001), treatments that combine ERP and cognitive therapy (Cordioli et al., 2003), groups for family members of individuals with OCD (Van Noppen, Steketee, McCorkle, & Pato, 1997), and support groups (e.g., Black & Blum, 1992).

Cordioli et al. (2002) studied a group treatment for OCD that included both cognitive strategies and ERP, provided over 12 sessions, with an average of six patients in each group. In this study, 78.1% of 32 patients showed an improvement of at least 35% in the severity of their OCD, as measured by the Yale–Brown Obsessive Compulsive Scale (Y-BOCS; Goodman et al., 1989a, 1989b). In a subsequent controlled study, the percentage of improved patients was 69.6% for those treated with group CBT and 4.2% in a wait-list control condition, providing further evidence in support of group treatments (Cordioli et al., 2003).

Himle and colleagues (2001) compared a seven-session group ERP treatment to a 12-session group ERP treatment and found both to be equally effective. Both treatments were based on weekly 2-hour sessions. Steketee, Frost, Wincze, Greene, and Douglass (2000) used a combination of group and individual treatment for six individuals with OCD who engaged in excessive hoarding. Treatment included 15 group sessions over 20 weeks plus individual home sessions. Although half of those in the group dropped out early, those who completed treatment experienced a reduction in symptoms.

McLean et al. (2001) compared cognitive and behavioral group treatments for OCD. Both treatment conditions were based on 12 consecutive group sessions lasting 2.5 hours each, with six to eight patients in each group. In this study, the percentage of individuals considered *recovered* at posttreatment was 16% in the cognitive therapy group and 38% in the ERP group, based on a score of less than 12 on the Y-BOCS and a decrease of at least 6 points on the Y-BOCS from pre- to posttreatment. At 3-month follow-up, the percentages were 13% and 45%, respectively, which represented a statistically significant difference. ERP had a slightly higher dropout rate than cognitive therapy, as well as a lower refusal rate.

There have also been preliminary reports on the effectiveness of group interventions for families of patients with OCD. For example, Cooper (1993) reported on a group run with three couples, all of whom had an adult child with OCD. The goals of the group were to provide members with information about OCD and its treatment, to help family members express their feelings about the impact of OCD on their lives, and to enable to them to better manage their affective responses toward the family member with OCD. Members of the group were also taught strategies to deal more effectively with the OCD, including not participating in rituals, managing aggression, and handling resistance. Finally, group members were encouraged to increase the frequency of pleasurable and meaningful activities in their lives. Van Noppen et al. (1997) compared two types of group treatment for OCD—one that included groups of six to eight patients on their own, and another that included groups of six to eight patients along with at least one family member each (usually a spouse or parent). Treatment consisted of 10–12 two-hour sessions. Both group formats led to comparable gains (with 70 to 80% of patients improving by at least 20% on the Y-BOCS). Gains were at least as strong as those in previous studies based on individual therapy. Group therapy was associated with a low dropout rate and with relatively large treatment effects compared to those reported in previous individual treatment studies.

To date, only two studies have compared individual and group treatment for OCD. Fals-Stewart, Marks, and Schafer (1993) treated 93 patients in one of three conditions: (1) 24 sessions of behavioral group treatment over 12 weeks, (2) 24 sessions of behavioral individual treatment over 12 weeks, or (3) 24 sessions of individual progressive muscle relaxation over 12 weeks (control condition). Both behavioral treatments were equally effective overall, and were more effective than relaxation training, which did not lead to significant improvements. Individual treatment worked more quickly than group treatment, though by 6 weeks (Session 12) there were no longer significant differences between group and individual treatment. This study is unusual in that treatment was conducted over 24 sessions.

O'Connor et al. (2005) compared group and individual treatments for patients with OCD who had primarily obsessions without compulsions. The group treatment condition included four individual sessions, followed by 12 group sessions lasting 2 hours each. The individual treatment condition included 16 sessions (14 lasting 1 hour, and 2 lasting 90 minutes). Treatment in both conditions included psychoeducation, cognitive strategies, and ERP. Overall, both treatments were effective, though individual treatment produced the greatest changes in OCD symptoms, as well as anxiety and depression. The large size of the groups (26 individuals were treated in two groups) may have accounted for the weaker effects of group treatment in this study. Follow-up findings were not presented.

A recent meta-analysis found that individual therapy leads to larger changes than group treatment for OCD. Eddy, Dutra, Bradley, and Westen (2004) found that among those who completed treatment, a mean of 44% of patients (averaging across studies) who received individual therapy were considered recovered, compared to an average of 28% for those who received group treatment. These percentages as computed for all patients (based on "intent to treat" analyses that also included patients who did not complete treatment) were 37 and 22%, respectively. However, until a number of methodologically sound studies provide head-to-head comparisons of individual and group treatment, it will be difficult to know which approach is most effective.

Combining Pharmacological and Psychosocial Treatments

Studies comparing ERP to pharmacotherapy have generally found both approaches to be about equally effective (Abramowitz, 1997; van Balkom, van Oppen, Vermeulen, & van Dyck, 1994). In addition, studies examining the combination of pharmacotherapy and psychological treatment (mostly ERP) have generally failed to find any advantage of combining treatments (for a review, see van Balkom & van Dyck, 1998). However, some studies have identified particular conditions under which combined treatments may be warranted. Hohagen et al. (1998) found that the combination of ERP and an SSRI was more effective than ERP alone for reducing obsessions (but not compulsions), and for patients who had depression along with their OCD. O'Connor, Todorov, Robillard, Borgeat, and Brault (1999) found that the combination of CBT and medication was more effective than either alone, particularly when the CBT was added after a period of medication use (rather than introducing both simultaneously). Finally, Kampman, Keijsers, Hoogduin, and Verbraak (2002) found that adding CBT can be useful for patients who do not respond to an SSRI alone.

ASSESSMENT ISSUES

A thorough discussion of issues related to the assessment of OCD is beyond the scope of this chapter. For a detailed review, the reader is referred to chapters by Summerfeldt (2001) and by Taylor, Thordarson, and Söchting (2002). Numerous scales have been developed for measuring various aspects of OCD. Antony (2001b) reviewed the details on more than 20 different instruments (clinician-administered and self-report) currently used for measuring different aspects of OCD symptomatology. These include general scales for measuring OCD severity, as well as scales for measuring particular features of OCD, such as responsibility beliefs, degree of insight, indecisiveness, and beliefs concerning TAF.

In the context of group treatment for OCD, assessment has two main functions. First, a detailed assessment should be completed to indicate the degree to which the individual is suitable for group treatment. Second, appropriate measures should be used to assess treatment outcome. The issue of suitability for group treatment is discussed in various sections throughout the remainder of this chapter, including a review of recommended inclusion criteria for group treatment. Therefore, this section focuses more on measuring symptom severity before and after treatment.

Summerfeldt (2001) reviewed several obstacles in the assessment of OCD. These include comorbidity and symptom overlap (e.g., distinguishing between OCD and obsessive–compulsive personality disorder), heterogeneity of symptom content, upsetting or embarrassing symptom content (e.g., patients may be reluctant to admit to having sexual obsessions), symptom shifting over time, clinical features that affect response style (e.g., avoidance, need for exactness, doubt, obsessional slowness), and lack of insight. Because of these obstacles, it is important that the assessment take a multimodal format, including information from standard self-report and clinician-administered scales (Antony, 2001b), behavioral assessments (e.g., Chorpita & Taylor, 2001), and detailed interviews with patients and perhaps their family members.

With respect to standard scales, we recommend including the Y-BOCS as part of the assessment battery. Ideally, the standard clinician-administered version should be used, though the self-report version (Baer, 2000) may be considered if therapist time constraints are a problem. The Y-BOCS provides not only detailed information regarding the breadth of symptom content but also information about other aspects of severity, including the time taken up by symptoms, distress, and functional impairment. In addition, one or two brief symptom measures may be useful for measuring initial severity and treatment outcome. In our center, we use the Obsessive Compulsive Inventory (Foa, Kozak, Salkovskis, Coles, & Amir, 1998), and a number of other fine options are available (for a review, see Antony, 2001b), including the recently developed Clark–Beck Obsessive–Compulsive Inventory (Clark & Beck, 2002; Clark, Antony, Beck, Swinson, & Steer, 2005).

STRUCTURING GROUP TREATMENT

Group Composition and Format

Table 8.1 provides details from several studies on group treatment for OCD that relate specifically to group composition and treatment format. In this section we make specific recommendations based on existing research, as well as our own clinical experience.

TABLE 8.1. Format and Composition for Group OCD Treatments

Study	No. of sessions	Group composition	Length of sessions	Strategies
Cordioli et al. (2002, 2003)	12 weekly sessions	8 patients 2 therapists	2 hours	Education, ERP, cognitive therapy, group techniques
Fals-Stewart et al. (1993)	24 sessions over 12 weeks	10 patients	2 hours	ERP, imaginal exposure (when appropriate)
Himle et al. (2001)	7 or 12 weekly sessions	Not reported	2 hours	Education, behavior therapy
McLean et al. (2001)	12 weekly sessions	6–8 patients 2 therapists	2.5 hours	ERP, cognitive therapy, behavioral experiments
O'Connor et al. (2005)	16 sessions over 20 weeks	Mean of 13 patients (26 patients in two groups)	2 hours	ERP, cognitive therapy, relapse prevention

Note. Neither Fals-Stewart et al. (1993) nor O'Connor et al. (2005) reported the number of therapists in each group. Himle et al. (2001) did not report the number of patients and the number of therapists in each group.

Number and Frequency of Sessions

The length of group treatments for OCD across research studies ranges from 7 to 25 sessions, with an average of about 13 sessions (Whittal & McLean, 2002). The protocol described in this chapter is based on the treatment used at our center, which lasts 14 sessions (weekly at first, with the last two sessions occurring biweekly). We recommend that treatment typically last between 10 and 15 sessions. Most group treatment studies are based on weekly sessions (the study by Fals-Stewart et al., 1993, was an exception, with two sessions per week). Though it is often most practical to schedule weekly sessions when working with groups, scheduling more frequent sessions may be useful, particularly early in treatment. Studies based on individual treatment protocols are often based on a more intensive schedule (e.g., several sessions per week), and some patients seem to do better when sessions are scheduled closer together.

Composition of Groups

OCD group treatment studies typically include 6 to 10 patients and two therapists. At our center, we try to include four to seven patients in each group. In our experience, the larger the group, the more likely participants are to feel inhibited socially, and early dropouts may be more likely to occur. Smaller groups also allow for more individual attention to participants' needs. An advantage of larger groups is that patients are more likely to have others in the group with similar symptom profiles. As we discuss later, symptom heterogeneity is a problem in group treatments for OCD, and anything that can be done to help patients not to feel alone in the group is helpful.

Group treatment usually involves two therapists. At our center, we typically include two therapists, and sometimes a third therapist, depending on the availability of our staff and students. One therapist takes a primary role in delivering the treatment, and the extent of the second therapist's involvement depends on his or her level of experience (because we are a training clinic, the second therapist is often a student). Including a third therapist can sometimes be useful for larger groups, especially when conducting in-session exposures. At our center, the third therapist is typically a more junior student whose main role is that of observer. Later in the treatment, when the group splits up for in-session exposures, the third therapist may play a more active role in coaching patients through their practices.

Inclusion Guidelines

Diagnosis and Clinical Severity

Ideally, groups should include only individuals with a diagnosis of OCD. There are no studies examining the effectiveness of mixed groups for individuals with a range of anxiety disorders, and in our experience, treatment works best when the focus is on a particular disorder. In our center, we also require that OCD be the principal diagnosis of each participant. In other words, if multiple problems are present, we select for groups only participants for whom OCD is the most distressing or impairing problem. Finally, most research studies require that participants have clinically significant symptoms, based on a Y-BOCS score of at least 16. However, individuals with less severe symptoms may still benefit from group treatment.

Symptom Profile and Fit

Generally, the more homogeneous groups are with respect to symptom profile (e.g., sexual obsessions, contamination obsessions, etc.), the better. If group members have very different symptom profiles, they are less likely to see the similarities between their symptoms and those of others. In practice, it is often very difficult to assemble homogeneous groups. Still, treating some patients individually may be worth considering if their symptoms are very different from those of other group members.

Comorbidity

Comorbidity is the norm in OCD, and most participants in group treatment have difficulties other than just OCD. Depression and anxiety disorders are particularly common comorbid conditions. Generally, comorbidity should not be a rule out for group treatment. However, if a comorbid condition is likely to interfere significantly with a patient's response to treatment, or with the response of other group members, the therapist should consider treating the patient individually. For example, a patient who has very severe depression, severe borderline personality disorder, or significant problems with substance dependence may be better treated individually than in a group format.

Insight

Although no data address the issue of whether individuals with poor insight should be treated individually or in groups, there are reasons to believe that both approaches may have benefits. Some patients with poor insight may respond best to individual treatment, because it provides a better opportunity for more intensive therapy and to tailor the intervention to the individual's needs (individuals with poor insight often respond less well to treatment). Other individuals may benefit more from group treatment. Meeting others who have similar symptoms (except with more insight) may help the individual to recognize that his or her symptoms are excessive. The decision of whether to include a patient with poor insight in a group treatment should be made on a case-by-case basis, taking these and other factors into account.

Patient Motivation and Preferences

Patients with very low levels of motivation may not do as well in group treatments. In such cases, individual treatment may provide more opportunities for the therapist to target issues surrounding motivation more directly. The patient's preference for group versus individual treatment should also be considered when deciding whether a particular individual is included in a group, though the therapist should recognize that individuals who are initially apprehensive about group treatment often still respond well in the end.

Interpersonal Skills

Individual treatment should be considered for patients who seem unlikely to be able to function effectively in a group (e.g., those who tend to be very hostile toward others). Patients who do not function well with other people may benefit less from group therapy and may also have a negative impact on the response of other group members to treatment.

Structure of Group Sessions

Group sessions typically last between 2 and 2½ hours. Sessions should begin with setting an agenda. The therapists should provide a brief overview of what is to be covered in the meeting, and participants should be given an opportunity to contribute to the agenda if there are specific issues they want to discuss. Next, homework is typically reviewed. Each participant is asked to take 5 or 10 minutes to discuss progress with homework and any issues that arose during the week. Therapists should decide whether to have patients hold on to their monitoring diaries during this part of the session (so patients can be prompted with respect to what happened during the week) or to have the therapist collect participants' diaries and monitoring forms (so that corrective feedback can be provided).

Part of the session may also be spent providing psychoeducation to group members. For example, in the early sessions, participants are provided with a rationale for the treatment and are taught various strategies for dealing with their OCD symptoms. In addition, once ERP has been introduced, part of each session is spent practicing exposure.

Finally, most sessions end with assignment of new homework, which typically involves assignments to practice ERP. In addition, participants are reminded to complete their monitoring diaries, as well as any recommended readings.

KEY TREATMENT COMPONENTS

This section provides an overview of the main components of CBT for the treatment of OCD, including psychoeducation, ERP, and cognitive therapy.

For readers seeking a more detailed description of cognitive strategies, we recommend David A. Clark's (2004) book, *Cognitive-Behavioral Therapy for OCD*. A number of excellent resources also exist for information on delivering ERP-based treatments, including Gail Steketee's (1993) manual, *Treatment of Obsessive Compulsive Disorder*, and a chapter by Foa and Franklin (2001). Table 8.2 provides a summary of what might be included in each session, based on standard CBT approaches to OCD treatment.

TABLE 8.2. Sample Outline of Treatment Protocol for Group CBT of OCD

Session	Strategies covered
Pretreatment individual meeting	• Explain how the group will work and what to expect. • Introduce norms and rules for the group and provide practical information (e.g., location and times for group). • Develop an exposure hierarchy. • Answer any questions and address concerns.
Session 1	• Introduction to group members (group members share experiences about what brought them to the group, and describe OCD triggers and key symptoms). • Explain what to expect from treatment. • Review rules for the group (e.g., confidentiality). • Psychoeducation: Model of OCD, define key terms, overview of treatment strategies, recommend self-help readings. • Homework: Complete monitoring forms, read introductory chapters from self-help readings. • Discuss potential obstacles.
Session 2	• Homework review. • Psychoeducation: Review cognitive model, introduce cognitive distortions. • Homework: Monitor cognitive distortions.
Session 3	• Homework review. • Psychoeducation: Review strategies for challenging cognitive distortions. • Homework: Practice challenging cognitive distortions on thought records.
Session 4	• Homework review. • Psychoeducation: Introduction to exposure and ritual prevention. • In-session exposures and ritual prevention. • Homework: Cognitive restructuring, completion of thought records, exposure practices, and prevention of rituals.
Sessions 5–13	• Homework review. • In-session exposures and ritual prevention. • Homework: Cognitive restructuring, completion of thought records, exposure practices and prevention of rituals.
Session 14	• Homework review. • Psychoeducation: Discuss triggers for relapse and recurrence, review strategies for preventing relapse and recurrence. • Homework: Practice relapse prevention strategies.

Psychoeducation

CBT is very much a skills-based approach to treatment, and psychoeducation is almost always included as a component of CBT. In the context of group treatment for OCD, education may occur in the form of didactic presentations, facilitated discussion among group members, demonstrations, assigned readings, or video presentations. Examples of education topics that are often included are as follows:

- Information about the nature and treatment of OCD
- Guidelines for conducting ERP
- Theories regarding the causes of OCD
- CBT models of OCD
- Information regarding the impact of OCD on the family
- Family factors that can influence treatment
- Making lifestyle changes (e.g., diet, exercise, sleep habits)
- Strategies for improving quality of life (e.g., employment, relationships)

Some of these topics (e.g., CBT models of OCD, causes of OCD) are routinely covered at the beginning of treatment. Others (e.g., lifestyle issues) may be covered later.

Exposure

Exposure to feared situations is believed by many experts to be an important, if not essential, component of treatment for phobic and obsessive–compulsive disorders. Hundreds of studies have demonstrated that exposure consistently leads to a reduction in fear, and much is known about the variables that influence the outcome of exposure-based treatments. In the case of OCD, prevention of the compulsive rituals (discussed after this section on exposure) is an important component of any exposure-based treatment.

Because of the wide range of fear triggers that occur in patients with OCD, it is often impossible to generate exposure ideas that are relevant to all group members. Therefore, during in-session exposures, groups are typically divided up, and members practice exposure either in smaller groups or individually. For example, two members may practice touching contaminated objects (e.g., elevator buttons, money, doorknobs), while another practices writing a letter that contains spelling errors.

Exposure practices may occur in the same room as the group sessions, or group members may leave the room to practice elsewhere, depending on the situations that tend to trigger their obsessions and fear. Therapists typically move around the room to check on patients' progress. In some cases, one therapist may accompany one or more patients on an exposure excursion (e.g., going for a drive with an individual who is fearful of hitting pedestrians while driving), while the other therapist(s) stay behind to work with the remaining patients.

Before exposure begins, it is important to present the rationale for the procedures in a coherent and convincing way. Patients are asked to make a commitment to conduct exposure practices despite feeling uncomfortable and frightened. A model is presented to explain how exposure works, and patients are taught about the best ways to implement exposure practices. Chapter 4 reviewed the most important guidelines for maximizing the benefits of exposure. As a reminder, exposure practices should be predictable, controllable, prolonged, and frequent. Patients should not distract themselves during exposures, and the use of safety behaviors should be minimized. The context of the exposure, as well as the types of stimuli used, should be varied. For example, a person who is fearful of becoming contaminated by certain foods should practice eating a wide range of feared foods, in a wide variety of contexts (e.g., at home, in restaurants, at friends' homes). Finally, patients should be encouraged to take steps as quickly as they are willing to progress. The sooner they move on to more difficult practices, the more quickly they see a reduction in the impact of their OCD.

In vivo (i.e., situational) exposure is most appropriate for individuals who are fearful of particular situations, places, objects, or activities. Examples include obsessions about contamination, losing things, and making minor mistakes. Exposure in imagination is most appropriate for patients who are frightened of experiencing particular images or thoughts (e.g., religious, sexual, and aggressive obsessions). Often, a combination of imaginal and *in vivo* exposure can be useful. Table 8.3 provides examples of exposure practices for a wide range of OCD presentations.

Developing an Exposure Hierarchy

In Chapter 4 we reviewed the process of developing an exposure hierarchy. In OCD, it is not unusual for individuals to have a wide range of situations that trigger anxiety or lead to avoidance. In such cases, it can be helpful to generate more than one hierarchy. For example, a patient with obsessions concerning contamination, as well as aggressive impulses, could have a separate hierarchy for each of these two domains. For another patient (e.g., one who experiences different symptoms at home and at work), it may make sense to have one hierarchy for work-related symptoms and another for home-related symptoms. Hierarchies can be generated collaboratively between the patient and therapist in an individual meeting that occurs before the group begins. However, it is also fine to spend time in the group teaching participants to develop their hierarchies, having them generate hierarchy items as a homework assignment, then providing feedback on hierarchies at the next session.

Figure 8.1 provides an example of an exposure hierarchy for an individual who is fearful of encountering objects, situations, or words having to do with the occult, the devil, or other related constructs. As reviewed in Chapter

TABLE 8.3. Sample Exposure Practices for Particular OCD Presentations

OCD presentation	Examples of exposure and ritual prevention practices
Contamination obsessions and excessive washing	• Touch contaminated objects for an extended period (e.g., rub the object over one's hands and face). • Touch food (e.g., a candy) to a contaminated object and eat it. • Set a timer in the bathroom to ensure that showers last no more than 5 minutes. • Turn off the main water source in the basement, so water is not available for washing. • Contaminate everything in the home.
Fear of particular words or images (e.g., religious symbols, colors, numbers, names)	• Stare at the feared word or image. • Repeat feared words or phrases out loud. • Bring a feared image to mind and keep it there for an extended period. • Write out feared words and phrases. • Describe a feared image in detail, either out loud or in writing.
Fear of running over pedestrians	• Drive on bumpy roads. • Describe an image out loud, or in writing, of having hit a pedestrian while driving. • Do not check for bodies after hitting a bump or experiencing a thought of having hit someone. • Avoid watching the news or listening to accident reports (if one's natural inclination is to engage in these activities excessively). • Purposely watch the news or listen to accident reports (if one's natural inclination is to avoid these activities).
Aggressive or sexual obsessions	• For fear of stabbing a loved one, practice handling knives and other sharp objects with loved ones in the room; describe out loud, or in writing, images of stabbing a loved one. • Consider imaginal exposure to images of hurting a loved one. • Be around children (e.g., change one's baby) despite irrational intrusive thoughts of harming children sexually. • For intrusive thoughts involving doubt about one's sexual orientation, practice looking at photos of same-sex individuals, change in a public change room, and so forth.
Need to repeat actions	• Prevent oneself from repeating actions (e.g., leave the situation before having the opportunity to repeat). • If activities have to be repeated a certain number of times or in a specific way, try repeating them in the wrong way in the wrong number of times.
Need to check one's work (e.g., writing)	• Prevent oneself from checking work. • Purposely make mistakes in one's work (but not mistakes that will lead to serious consequences).
Compulsive reassurance seeking	• Instruct family members and other sources of reassurance not to provide reassurance anymore (they can reassure the patient that the anxiety will decrease over time, but they should not reassure the patient about the content of the obsessions). • Tolerate discomfort without asking for reassurance. • Practice imaginal exposure to feared images that trigger the desire to obtain reassurance.
Perfectionism	• Purposely make minor mistakes that trigger anxiety (e.g., pronounce words incorrectly, fold the towels incorrectly, make spelling errors). • Encourage others to make minor mistakes that trigger one's anxiety.

Item	Description	Fear (0–100)
1.	Repeatedly write or say "I am Satan."	100
2.	Repeatedly write or say "I love Satan."	100
3.	Repeatedly read the word "Satan" silently.	95
4.	Repeatedly tell my therapist to "Go to hell."	90
5.	Watch the film *The Exorcist*	90
6.	Look at realistic pictures of the devil on the Internet.	85
7.	Stare at drawings of the devil on various music CDs.	80
8.	Say the word "devil" repeatedly.	70
9.	Say the word "hell" repeatedly.	60
10.	Stare at a "cute" cartoon picture of the devil	50
11.	Say the word "evil" repeatedly	40
12.	Look at the word "hell"	40

FIGURE 8.1. Sample exposure hierarchy for OCD. For each item, ratings assume that the item will be completed without doing any rituals or compulsions (praying, touching a cross, replacing bad thoughts with safe thoughts, etc.).

4, an exposure hierarchy should contain 10 to 15 items. Items should be as detailed as possible, specifying variables that influence the person's fear. In the case of OCD, hierarchy items and their ratings should include (either explicitly or implicitly) an assumption that the exposure to the item will not be followed by a compulsion.

Ritual Prevention

Complete versus Partial Ritual Prevention

As reviewed earlier, ERP appears to work best when strict ritual prevention instructions are given. In other words, it is best to prevent all rituals rather than to implement ritual prevention in a gradual or partial way. For example, in some intensive treatment programs (e.g., inpatient treatment, day treatment), patients are asked to stop all washing except for a brief shower once per week. In outpatient programs, including most group treatment programs, such restrictions may be impractical, but it is still preferable to eliminate all rituals where possible, and to reduce the frequency of normal behaviors that are similar to the compulsion. For example, for someone who washes excessively, a 5-minute shower every day or every other day may be permitted, but all other washing should still be discouraged. If eliminating all compulsion-like behaviors is dangerous, then the goal should be to decrease the frequency of the behaviors as much as possible. For example, a pharmacist who is afraid of giving customers the wrong medications should be encouraged to check once, if that is the standard of practice, but should be discouraged from checking repeatedly.

Presenting the Rationale for Ritual Prevention

Patients should understand that using compulsions to decrease their fear undermines the effects of exposure. The purpose of exposure is to teach the individual that feared objects, situations, thoughts, and images are in fact safe. When patients use compulsions, they are likely to attribute any positive outcomes to the fact that they engaged in a ritual, rather than to the idea that there was no risk in the first place. There are a number of analogies that therapists sometimes use to make this point.

First, OCD can be compared to a car, and rituals, to gasoline. When an individual does a ritual, it is comparable to putting gas into a car. Compulsions keep the OCD alive. It is not until we allow the car to run out of gas that it finally stops running. The same is true of OCD. It is not until rituals are completely prevented that the OCD symptoms die. Even occasional rituals may be enough to keep the OCD alive.

Another analogy involves comparing OCD to a spoiled child, and comparing compulsions to the act of giving in to the child (e.g., giving the child candy when he or she requests it). Consider the following dialogue:

THERAPIST: In some ways, OCD is like a child who is used to getting his own way. What happens when a parent stops giving into a child's requests? What happens when a parent decides not to give the child the toy or candy he asks for?

PATIENT: The child gets upset. He may have a temper tantrum.

THERAPIST: In the same way, your anxiety will probably flare up when you stop doing your rituals.

PATIENT: That's what I am afraid of.

THERAPIST: What happens when parents give in to the temper tantrums of their spoiled child?

PATIENT: The child learns that screaming is the way to get what he wants. It's better not to give in. Eventually, the child will learn to stop using temper tantrums to get his own way.

THERAPIST: The same is true of OCD. When you stop the rituals, your anxiety may hit the roof. However, if you stick with the plan and prevent yourself from doing the rituals, the anxiety will eventually burn itself out. The urge to do the ritual will die down as well. It may take an hour or two, or it may take all night for the fear to come down. Overcoming your OCD will require a decision to tolerate the discomfort, no matter how intense it gets.

Dealing with Resistance

It is not unusual for patients to express apprehension about stopping all rituals. If this occurs, the therapist should try to alleviate the concerns by helping the individual to look at the situation in as balanced and realistic a way possible (e.g., using cognitive strategies). In addition, the patient should be reassured that the therapist will be there for support. In addition to the weekly group meetings, some patients may need extra support by phone or through additional, individual sessions. Group members may also be able to support one another between sessions (e.g., it is not unusual for group members to exchange phone numbers). Patients should also be encouraged to rely on family members for support. At moments when the urge to do the ritual is overwhelming, patients should be encouraged to do whatever they can to prevent the ritual (go for a walk, get away from the situation, talk to a close friend, etc.). Although distraction is generally discouraged during exposure practices, it is preferable to distract oneself than to do the ritual.

If patients cannot commit to preventing their rituals, there are a few options to consider. One option is to have patients agree to delay their rituals. A patient who can delay a ritual for 15 minutes and then reevaluate the situation may find that he or she can then delay the ritual for another 15 minutes, and so on. Sometimes, agreeing to delay the ritual for 15 minutes at a time, until the urge finally subsides, is more tolerable than the thought of promising not to do the ritual at all. Patients may also be willing to eliminate only some rituals (e.g., washing but not checking; home rituals but not work rituals; evening rituals but not daytime rituals), at least to start. If the most a patient will agree to do is eliminate rituals partially, it is better to tie the decision of which rituals to eliminate to factors such as the type of ritual, the location, or the time, rather than tying the decision to the severity of the person's anxiety or urge to do the compulsion.

Eliminating Cognitive Rituals

In addition to eliminating overt rituals, cognitive rituals should be circumvented. For example, if a patient tends to count in 3's, he or she should be encouraged to stop counting. If necessary, the patient can be encouraged to perform a behavior that competes with the cognitive ritual (e.g., counting in 2's) temporarily, but the therapist should be vigilant for the possibility that the competing behavior can itself become a ritual.

Undoing the Effects of Rituals

If the patient cannot resist the urge to do the compulsion, he or she should be encouraged to undo the effects of the compulsion by engaging in additional exposure. For example, after a shower, patients should make an effort to come into contact with contaminated objects. In addition, a number of strategies can be used to circumvent the urge to do the compulsion. For example, eating a candy that has come into contact with contamination may help to prevent the urge to wash (there is no point in washing, if the contamination has already been taken into the body). Similarly, purposely making mistakes in a letter, then mailing it may circumvent urges to check the letter for mistakes.

Cognitive Strategies

There is some controversy in the literature regarding whether it is appropriate to use cognitive strategies when treating OCD. For example, Stanley and Averill (1998) argue that (1) ERP alone is an established way of changing beliefs in OCD; (2) there is significant overlap between the behavioral experiments used in cognitive therapy and the exposure component of ERP, calling into question the unique contribution of cognitive therapy; and (3) the evidence regarding cognitive restructuring in the treatment of OCD is still fairly limited compared to the amount of support for ERP.

There are other, more clinically based reasons to use caution when trying cognitive strategies. First, cognitive restructuring may be viewed by the patient as a form of reassurance. If the patient's compulsions include reassurance seeking, some forms of cognitive restructuring may serve to maintain the need for reassurance. Second, some patients tend to think in a very detailed, compulsive way, and they sometimes get lost in their thoughts (ruminating about a wide range of thoughts that enter their heads). For these patients, cognitive restructuring may simply be impossible, and the most effective way to change their beliefs may be through less cognitive means, such as ERP alone.

Despite these issues, evidence has emerged in recent years that cognitive treatment can be useful for the treatment of OCD. Cognitive therapy emphasizes strategies such as normalizing intrusive thoughts, correcting faulty appraisals, generating alternative beliefs, examining the evidence for particular beliefs (e.g., beliefs concerning responsibility), preventing efforts to neutralize intrusive thoughts, and testing beliefs through behavioral experiments. In addition, cognitive therapy for OCD often emphasizes changing metacognitive beliefs (i.e., beliefs about beliefs), such as the belief that one's intrusive thoughts are dangerous and should be controlled, as well as beliefs about the overimportance of one's thoughts.

When using cognitive strategies in groups, it is useful to have members of the group help one another with the process of cognitive restructuring. For example, all members of the group can be invited to generate alternative beliefs to challenge a particular group member's intrusive thought. Group members can also be encouraged to role-play how a therapist might respond to a particular concern raised by a patient in the group. By helping patients to develop their skills at challenging one another's intrusive thoughts, they may become better able to apply the skills to their own obsessions.

SAMPLE CBT GROUP PROTOCOL FOR OCD

This 14-session group treatment protocol is based on standard treatments for OCD described by Steketee (1993), Foa and Franklin (2001), Clark (2004), and other sources. The first 12 sessions occur weekly, and the last two sessions, biweekly. After a thorough assessment, and before the treatment begins, each patient meets individually with one of the group therapists to provide an opportunity for the patient to meet one of the therapists, to have any concerns or questions addressed, and to develop an exposure hierarchy. Therapy begins with presenting the rationale for treatment, which is mostly based on an ERP model. In addition, some sessions emphasize cognitive strategies. All sessions last 2 hours. The content of each session is summarized in Table 8.2.

Pretreatment Individual Meetings with Group Members

This session involves an individual meeting between one patient and one or more of the group therapists. At this session, a basic introduction to the group is presented, including the group schedule (location, times, and dates), a brief overview of what will occur during group sessions, the importance of maintaining confidentiality, the importance of regular attendance, and expectations regarding homework. Patients are given an opportunity to ask questions and to have their concerns addressed. Next, an exposure hierarchy is generated using items previously endorsed on the Y-BOCS, as well as any feared objects or situations mentioned by the patient during the appointment.

Session 1: Presenting the Treatment Rationale

This session has several purposes. First, it is an opportunity to introduce group members and therapists to one another. In addition, ground rules for the group are reviewed to remind participants of some of the issues raised during the pretreatment meeting. Patients are provided with a model of OCD and an overview of the treatment strategies. Possible obstacles to improvement, and ways of overcoming these obstacles, are discussed. Homework for the first session typically involves reading introductory chapters from an ERP-based self-help book (e.g., Foa & Wilson, 2001; Hyman & Pedrick, 1999). Components of the first session are as follows:

1. Introduction of group members and therapists.
2. Group rules and overview: confidentiality, group structure, importance of regular attendance, expectations regarding homework (60–90 minutes per day), importance of being honest about symptoms and completed homework, reminder to have realistic expectations, reminder to expect treatment initially to cause increased discomfort.
3. Definitions of key terms: "obsessions," "compulsions," "OCD,"

"cognitive rituals," "cues," "triggers," "avoidance," and "neutralization."

4. Presentation of the cognitive-behavioral model of OCD, including the effects of compulsions and neutralizing on maintaining obsessions over time.
5. Having each patient review his or her key obsessions and compulsions, followed by discussion to ensure that all group members understand how their symptoms fit into an OCD profile, which of their symptoms are obsessions, and which are compulsions (including mental rituals).
6. Discussion of treatment procedures, including cognitive strategies, exposure, and ritual prevention.
7. Discussion about the role of the family, including ways in which family members may be able to help (stopping accommodation, being supportive, being present during homework practices, etc.).
8. Discussion about the costs and benefits of overcoming the problem, as well as obstacles that patients expect to encounter over the course of treatment.
9. Homework: Introductory readings on the CBT model and on an overview of treatment strategies.

Sessions 2 and 3: Cognitive Strategies

Session 2 begins with a discussion of the readings from the previous week. Next, the cognitive model for OCD is reviewed. During sessions 2 and 3, participants are taught to identify examples of anxious thinking (e.g., TAF), and strategies for combating cognitive distortions are presented. Patients are instructed in how to complete cognitive monitoring forms. Homework includes challenging intrusive thoughts (e.g., examining the evidence, conducting behavioral experiments) over the next week rather than neutralizing or suppressing unwanted thoughts. In addition, participants are encouraged to complete self-help readings related to the cognitive strategies.

Session 4: Introducing Exposure and Ritual Prevention

The first 45 minutes of this session are spent reviewing cognitive monitoring forms from the previous week. The rationale for ERP is then presented. Guidelines for exposure are reviewed (e.g., the need for exposure practices to be predictable, prolonged, and frequent). Patients are instructed in how to use exposure monitoring forms. They are also encouraged to stop their rituals immediately. Strategies for dealing with intense urges to engage in compulsions are discussed. In addition to continuing to complete cognitive monitoring records, patients are encouraged to engage in at least 1 hour of exposure per day over the coming week, starting with an item from the bottom half of their hierarchy. They are also encouraged to complete self-help readings on ERP.

Sessions 5–13: In-Session Exposures

Each session begins with a review of homework, lasting about 45 minutes. During the homework review, the therapists take advantage of any opportunities to challenge anxious appraisals that arise. The next hour is spent on in-session exposures, individually tailored to the patients in the group. The final 15 minutes are spent assigning homework for the next week, including exposure to feared situations, objects, and images; prevention of rituals; and cognitive restructuring. Throughout treatment, patients should be vigilant for any new rituals that emerge, as well as any new avoidance behaviors.

Session 14: Termination and Relapse Prevention

After a review of the homework, issues related to relapse and recurrence are discussed. Participants are reminded that the severity of OCD normally fluctuates over time. They are encouraged to tolerate periods of increased severity, without falling back into old habits of avoidance and rituals. Instead, they should engage in occasional exposures to help maintain their gains. Being vigilant for possible triggers of recurrence, including increased life stress, helps to alert patients to the possibility of symptoms worsening, so they can be better prepared.

Posttreatment Evaluation

Patients are invited to complete a posttreatment evaluation. At this stage, the main outcome measures are repeated. Patients who require additional treatment may be offered a series of individual sessions, pharmacotherapy, family sessions, self-help interventions, support groups, or other interventions, depending on their needs and preferences. In addition, we offer all patients the opportunity to participate in a monthly booster group designed to help previously treated patients at our center maintain their improvements.

Variations on the Protocol

There are a number of ways in which this protocol can be modified. First, there are data supporting group treatments of longer (e.g., 25 sessions) and shorter (e.g., 7 sessions) durations. The length of each session can also be extended (e.g., some centers have group sessions lasting 2½ hours). Session frequency can be altered as well. Although we recommend against meeting less often than once per week, there may be benefits of increasing the frequency of meetings to more than once per week. If possible, including family members (e.g., a spouse or parent) in one or more sessions may be useful, particularly for patients who report that their family members "don't understand," or in cases where family members engage in counterproductive behaviors, such as accommodation. Finally, if practical, there may be cases in which group and individual treatments can be combined. For example, it is possible to deliver the early sessions (e.g., psychoeducation, cognitive therapy) in a group format, and the later sessions (e.g., exposure) in an individual format.

ADVANTAGES OF TREATING OCD IN GROUPS

Group treatments are often more cost-effective than individual treatments. They take up less therapist time (on a per patient basis), and the reduced cost per session is often passed on to the patient. Group treatment is particularly useful in settings where the number of patient referrals is simply too large to manage on an individual basis. However, the benefits of group treatment are not simply financial. There are many other benefits to patients, some of which are difficult to measure objectively.

Patients often describe a sense of relief when they discover that they are not alone. They often say that it is very comforting to meet others with OCD and to discover that they seem so "normal." This helps patients realize that to the average person, an individual with OCD would probably not stand out as being unusual in any way. It also helps them to be less embarrassed and secretive with respect to their own symptoms.

In most cases, patients tend to be very supportive of one another during the course of group treatment. For example, they are empathic when a patient is discussing painful symptoms, and they may express worry about a patient who does not show up for a given treatment session. When group cohesion is strong, patients may exchange phone numbers and develop lasting friendships with other group members. It is not unusual for some patients to get together between treatment sessions and to do their homework together. Group members often value suggestions and feedback received from other group members, whose personal experience with OCD gives them a special ability to empathize with patients' symptoms.

In their study of group treatment for compulsive hoarding, Steketee et al. (2000) described a number of advantages of treating this population in groups. During exposures involving sorting and discarding objects, the presence of other group members appeared to provide social pressure on the individual, which increased compliance with the exercises. Also, because many clients felt isolated in their hoarding difficulties, they appreciated the support they received from other group members. Although hearing other patients' beliefs about saving and hoarding was useful in some cases, it reinforced other individuals' own beliefs about saving. We return to this issue and other possible negative effects of group treatment in the next section.

Overall, group members should be encouraged to participate in group discussions and to share their experiences. In addition, it is often useful for participants to take a more active role in one another's treatment, as they become more familiar with the strategies. For example, group members can help with the process of cognitive restructuring and may suggest to one another exposure practices that might be completed for homework.

OBSTACLES TO TREATING OCD IN GROUPS

Heterogeneity in Group Membership

Perhaps the biggest challenge in treating OCD in a group format is the fact that OCD is a heterogeneous condition, and patients often present with very different symptom profiles. For example, an individual who is fearful of contamination may seem to have little in common with an individual who is constantly thinking about stabbing members of his or her family.

Heterogeneity among group members can lead to a number of different problems. First, patients who feel different than other group members or whose symptoms are more "socially unacceptable" may be reluctant to discuss their symptoms in front of the group. In fact, they may refuse group treatment completely. This is particularly a problem for individuals who have aggressive, religious, or sexual obsessions. Therefore, it is useful to have more than one person in each group with these kinds of thoughts. Second, patients sometimes trivialize the concerns of others. For example, a patient might say, "I wish my fear was just of making mistakes at work. I could live with that! My fear of killing my children is much more of a problem." Finally, some patients may not be understanding or supportive toward the other group members. They may give others strange looks or make insensitive comments.

To deal with these issues, it is important early in treatment to educate the group about the various ways in which OCD symptoms are expressed. Right from the start, therapists should emphasize the commonalities across OCD presentations, particularly with respect to the cognitive and behavioral influences. Patients should also be reminded that the distress and impairment associated with OCD can be severe, regardless of the specific symptom profile, and that it is important for group members to be supportive.

A final issue to keep in mind is that because patients tend to have different symptom profiles, parts of the group necessarily have an individualized focus. For example, during exposure practices, patients may end up working on their own.

Symptom "Contagion" among Group Members

Patients who receive group treatment for OCD are often concerned about "catching" OCD symptoms from other group members. In reality, this is something that we have never actually seen occur. What may happen, however, is a tendency for some patients to reinforce avoidance behaviors in others. For example, some patients may suggest ways in which others can neutralize their obsessions (e.g., suggesting a new cleaning product to an individual with contamination concerns). People may also share information that strengthens one another's beliefs about the feared situations (e.g., sharing a story about a friend of a cousin who became ill by forgetting to wash her hands after handling raw chicken) However, after participants have become more familiar with the treatment rationale, they learn to stop encouraging one another's avoidance. With corrective feedback, this issue can usually be dealt with early in treatment.

Other Disadvantages of Group Treatment

A number of other problems may arise during the course of group treatment. First, patients who are progressing more slowly than others may become discouraged and drop out of treatment prematurely. Also, a group format minimizes the amount of individualized attention that each patients receives. As a result, some participants end up having to listen to discussions that are not relevant to their own situations. Others may not receive as much individual attention as they need. In these cases, having the patient attend a few individual sessions, in addition to the group, may be useful, if it is practical and the individual can afford it.

GENERAL OBSTACLES TO TREATING OCD

Although the focus of this chapter is on group treatment, there are a number of obstacles that often arise while treating OCD either in groups or individually. Although these obstacles are not unique to group treatment, they often arise when providing treatment in groups, so they are discussed briefly in this section.

Breadth of Symptoms

Data from our center (Antony, Downie, et al., 1998) suggest that most people with OCD experience obsessions and compulsions of more than one type (washing, checking, repeating, etc.). A challenge that often confronts therapists is how to decide which symptoms to focus on first. Generally, this decision should be made after considering which symptoms cause the most distress and impairment, and which symptoms the patient is interested in working on first. It is often not practical to have the patient work on all symptoms at the same time. Rather, selecting those problems that are most important to overcome first may be a more useful approach.

Symptom Shift

In addition to having a wide range of symptom types at any given time, some patients with OCD report having symptoms that shift from one type to another over time. In some cases, symptoms may change over the course of months or years. However, in other cases, shifts may occur on a daily or weekly basis. For example, an individual may report being concerned about contamination one week, and then return the next week and explain that the exposure homework assigned was not relevant, because contamination concerns were no longer an issue. Instead, during the previous week, the obsessions might have shifted to a focus on appliances being left on, for example. In such cases, the symptoms may seem like a moving target, and it may be difficult to find appropriate strategies to deal with them. For patients whose symptoms shift over time, it is especially important for them to understand the general principles of treatment and how they apply to a wide range of symptoms. In addition, patients may have to adapt planned homework practices to deal with new symptoms as they emerge.

Noncompliance with Exposure Homework

Antony and Swinson (2000a) reviewed the following possible reasons why patients may not complete their exposure homework assignments: (1) not understanding the assignment, (2) not understanding the relevance of the assignment to their goals, (3) homework assignments that are too difficult, (4) other demands on patients' time (e.g., young children to take care of, busy work schedule), and (5) the therapist not checking on homework at the start of each session. To improve compliance, it is important to identify the factors that interfere with completion of homework for each patient in the group for whom noncompliance is an issue.

Depending on the reason for noncompliance, some strategies for improving compliance include (1) making sure that the homework is explained in detail and that the instructions are written down by the patient; (2) ensuring that homework practices are relevant to the individual's goals; (3) simplifying the homework task; (4) encouraging the patient to try something easier, if a particular task is too frightening; (5) arranging for telephone contact or additional individual sessions between group meetings; (6) identifying family factors that may be contributing to noncompliance, or factors that may improve compliance (e.g., including family members in the practice); (7) trying the homework practice in the session before assigning it for homework; (8) encouraging the patient to schedule the practice in a date book or diary, so it is not forgotten; and (9) suggesting that the patient find ways to manage other demands, in order to make time for the homework (e.g., taking a day off work to engage in a prolonged exposure practice, or hiring a babysitter, so the children do not disrupt the homework session).

Transfer of Responsibility

Occasionally, patients will transfer responsibility to the therapist, which can undermine the effects of exposure. In these cases, it is important to transfer responsibility back to the patient. Consider the following dialogue as an example of how this can be accomplished:

PATIENT: The thought of making mistakes at work over the coming week doesn't bother me. Because you asked me to do it for homework, you will be responsible if anything happens.

THERAPIST: Because it is so frightening for you to feel responsible for the possibility of doing harm to someone else, it is important that you take responsibility for what happens during your exposure practices. Although I was the one to recommend this practice, ultimately you need to take responsibility for deciding whether to follow my recommendation.

PATIENT: Even so, I don't feel responsible, because you made the suggestion. Because we spoke about doing this, I feel like you will be responsible if something happens, so it doesn't really scare me.

THERAPIST: In that case, perhaps we should try things differently this week. I would like you to come up with your own homework practice, but not tell me what it is until next week, after you have done it.

PATIENT: Now, that's something that I'm pretty sure will make me anxious. I don't want to do it, but it sounds like it may be helpful.

Issues Surrounding Religion

People who have religious obsessions are on average more religious than individuals who do not have religious obsessions (Steketee, Quay, & White, 1991). One issue that sometimes arises when treating patients with OCD whose obsessions are primarily of a religious nature is trying to distinguish between religious beliefs that are simply part of the person's religion and those that are best conceptualized as part of the OCD. For example, patients with religious obsessions are usually uncomfortable with the suggestion that they expose themselves to frightening thoughts of a religious nature (e.g., "I am Satan"), but it may be difficult for them to know whether it is their OCD that makes them uncomfortable or their religious convictions. In such cases, it may be useful for patients to consult with family members or their religious leader to see which of their intrusive thoughts and compulsive behaviors are excessive in the context of their religion. Getting "permission" to participate in the treatment assignments can also be helpful in some cases. For example, obtaining reassurance from a minister, priest, rabbi, or other leader that it is okay to complete exposure practices can help a patient to move forward with the treatment.

Effects of Functional Impairment

OCD is associated with impairment in a wide range of functional domains, including relationships, work, and quality of life (see Antony, Downie, et al.,

1998). For most patients, overcoming OCD leads to improvement in functioning across the board. However, for others, functional impairment may need to be targeted as a separate issue. For example, a patient who has had OCD for many years, and who has therefore never worked or been in a long-term relationship, may feel overwhelmed as his or her OCD improves and these other issues move to the forefront. In these cases, it is important to work with the patient on overcoming some of the obstacles to improving his or her quality of life (e.g., obtaining relevant job skills, expanding social networks). Group therapy for OCD may not be the best place to deal with these issues, if they are only relevant to one or two patients in the group. If that is the case, it may be more appropriate to provide some individual sessions to address these broader concerns.

Family Issues

Often family members do things that make it easier for the patient to engage in rituals or to avoid feared situations. Such behaviors are often referred to as "accommodation," and they may help to maintain an individual's OCD symptoms over the long term. In a study by Calvocoressi and colleagues (1995), family members of individuals with OCD reported a wide range of accommodation behaviors, including participating in rituals, providing items for rituals, helping the patient to avoid feared situations, and modifying the family routine. In this study, only 11.8% of family members assessed reported no accommodation. About half reported mild levels of accommodation, and the remaining participants report moderate or severe levels of accommodation.

It is often useful to include family members of patients with OCD in the treatment. This can be accomplished in a number of ways. For example, family members of patients can be invited to attend one or more sessions (either with the entire group, or for individual meetings including just the therapist, the patient, and one or more family members). Alternatively, if family sessions are not feasible, patients should be encouraged to share treatment guidelines with their families and to have their families complete relevant self-help readings on OCD. Patients will likely do better in treatment if their family members have a good understanding of the nature and treatment of OCD, are provided with instructions not to reinforce OCD behaviors, and are given skills for interacting with the patient around issues concerning the OCD (for a review of family issues in the treatment of OCD, see Steketee & Pruyn, 1998).

CONCLUSIONS

OCD is a heterogeneous condition associated with a wide range of cognitive and behavioral features. Extensive research supports pharmacological interventions, as well as CBT-based treatments. From a psychological perspective,

OCD is believed to stem from a tendency to misinterpret situations, objects, and one's intrusive thoughts as dangerous. CBT aims to shift anxious thinking through a number of behavioral and cognitive means. Although OCD is usually treated individually, several studies have shown that group treatment can be effective for this problem. Treating OCD in groups is associated with unique challenges, but it also has a number of advantages over individual treatment. This chapter has provided an overview of strategies for treating OCD in a group format.

CHAPTER 9

Social Anxiety Disorder

DESCRIPTION OF SOCIAL ANXIETY DISORDER

Diagnostic Features

Social anxiety disorder (SAD; also known as social phobia) is characterized by an extreme fear of social and performance situations in which a person may be scrutinized or judged by others, embarrassed, or humiliated. Examples of situations that are feared by people with SAD include those involving interpersonal interaction, such as dating, meetings, parties, and conversations, as well as performance situations, such as being the center of attention, public speaking, and eating, drinking, or writing in front of others. According to the text revision of the fourth edition of the *Diagnostic and Statistical Manual of Mental Disorders* (DSM-IV-TR; American Psychiatric Association, 2000), a diagnosis of SAD requires that the phobic situations almost always trigger an anxiety response (e.g., a panic attack). The individual must also recognize that his or her fear is excessive or unrealistic, must avoid the situation or endure it with extreme discomfort, and must experience clinically significant interference or distress as a result of the disorder. Finally, the symptoms cannot be better accounted for by another psychological disorder (e.g., social anxiety due to a fear of having others notice the symptoms of depression or panic disorder), may not be due to a fear of having others notice symptoms of a medical condition (e.g., Parkinson's disease, stuttering), and may not be caused by organic factors (e.g., substance use or a general medical condition). When the individual's fear occurs in most social situations, the SAD is referred to as "generalized."

Cognitive Features

Cognitive-behavioral treatments for SAD assume that anxiety and fear are related to the presence of anxiety-provoking thoughts. In this section, we provide a summary of findings related to cognition in SAD that are particularly relevant to cognitive-behavioral models and treatments for this condition. A full review of the cognitive features of SAD is beyond the scope of this chapter, though recent, comprehensive discussions on this topic are available elsewhere (e.g., Bögels & Mansell, 2004; Hirsch & Clark, 2004; Stravynski, Bond, & Amado, 2004).

People with high levels of social anxiety tend to devote more attention to threat-related social information (e.g., words related to social threat, photos of angry faces) than do nonphobic individuals, though an attentional bias toward social threat has also been shown in other anxiety disorders, such as panic disorder, suggesting that it is not unique to SAD (e.g., Maidenberg, Chen, Craske, Bohn, & Bystritsky, 1996). Studies on memory in SAD have yielded inconsistent results, with some studies finding enhanced memory for socially threatening information in people with SAD (Foa, Gilboa-Schechtman, Amir, & Freshman, 2000; Lundh & Öst, 1996), and others showing either reduced memory for such information (Wenzel & Holt, 2002) or no differences between people with SAD and nonanxious controls (e.g., Cloitre, Cancienne, Heimberg, Holt, & Liebowitz, 1995; Pérez-López & Woody, 2001).

High social anxiety is also associated with a tendency to view one's own social performance negatively, even after controlling for observable indicators of performance quality as rated by independent judges (Ashbaugh, Antony, McCabe, Schmidt, & Swinson, 2005; Rapee & Lim, 1992). In addition, SAD is associated with a tendency to report a higher than normal number of negative thoughts about oneself and about social situations (Stopa & Clark, 1993, 2000), to view negative social events as likely to occur (Uren, Szabó, & Lovibond, 2004), to make unflattering social comparisons of oneself to others (Antony, Rowa, Liss, Swallow, & Swinson, 2005), and to view oneself from an external observer's point of view when exposed to social situations (Hackmann, Surawy, & Clark, 1998; Wells & Papageorgiou, 1999). Finally, people with SAD also score high on measures of perfectionism. For example, they tend to be overly concerned about making mistakes, and they express greater doubt about their actions compared to people without anxiety disorders and to people with certain other anxiety disorders (Antony, Purdon, et al., 1998).

Behavioral Features

By definition, SAD is associated with a tendency to avoid a wide range of social situations. Individuals with SAD may avoid these situations completely, may escape from these situations shortly after entering them, or may engage in a number of safety behaviors to cope with anxiety in social situations. Examples of safety behaviors often observed in people with SAD include the following:

- Wearing extra makeup or a turtleneck sweater to hide blushing.
- Avoiding eye contact in social situations.
- Having several alcoholic drinks before going to a party.
- Eating only in dimly lit restaurants to prevent others from noticing one's symptoms of anxiety.
- Asking another person questions to avoid talking about oneself.

COGNITIVE-BEHAVIORAL APPROACHES TO UNDERSTANDING SOCIAL ANXIETY DISORDER

Though any comprehensive model regarding the *initial etiology* of SAD (e.g., Rapee & Spence, 2004) must take into account a wide range of variables, such as genetic factors, parental and peer influences, negative life events (particularly in the context of social situations), social skills, and cultural influences, models describing the cognitive and behavioral *processes* underlying social anxiety are much more relevant for understanding how the disorder is maintained over time, particularly from a cognitive-behavioral perspective. A number of cognitive-behavioral models for SAD exist, and all share the assumption that social anxiety is maintained by an individual's beliefs, assumptions, and predictions, as well as the individual's tendency to avoid social situations and to engage in various safety behaviors to cope with anxiety.

Among the most frequently cited psychological models of SAD is that proposed by David M. Clark and Adrian Wells (1995). According to this model, SAD is characterized by a number of specific assumptions and beliefs. First, people with SAD are assumed to have a stronger than usual motivation to make a positive impression on others. Second, they believe that they are likely to behave in a way that will be perceived as incompetent and inappropriate when encountering social situations. Third, they believe that they will suffer disastrous consequences as a result of their behavior in social situations. Finally, they tend to view themselves from an observer's perspective when confronting social situations. For example, they focus on what others might be seeing in them rather than on other aspects of the interaction (e.g., how the other person is coming across). As reviewed earlier, research on cognitive features of SAD supports the major components of this model.

The Clark and Wells (1995) model discusses three stages of processing in SAD, beginning with the *anticipatory processing stage*. This stage occurs before a person enters the feared situation. It is characterized by a tendency to worry and ruminate about what might happen upon entering the situation. The second stage, the *in-situation processing stage*, occurs when the person is in the social situation. In this stage, the individual's anxious thinking is fully activated, including negative assumptions, perfectionistic thinking, and negative beliefs about the self. According to the model, the person begins to focus less on social cues and more on how he or she is coming across. There is also an increase in safety behaviors designed to protect the individual from threat or to reduce levels of discomfort. The final stage described in the model is the *postmortem stage*, which begins after the person has left the social situation. In this stage, the person dwells on the negative aspects of his or her performance, having likely missed any signs of social approval due to his or her inward focus while in the situation.

Rapee and Heimberg (1997) published a similar model of SAD from a cognitive-behavioral perspective. Their model shares a number of features with the Clark and Wells model, including the assumption that social anxiety is maintained by biases and distortions in the ways that people think about social and evaluative situations. An additional feature of Rapee and Heimberg's model is the emphasis on beliefs that people have regarding the standards that other people hold. The model suggests that people with SAD assume that others have high standards for them and expect them to come across perfectly. This component of the model is supported by research on perfectionism in SAD showing that people with SAD do in fact assume that others have overly high expectations of them (e.g., Antony, Purdon, et al., 1998).

EFFECTIVE TREATMENTS FOR SAD

Recent reviews on the treatment of SAD provide support for pharmacological treatments, psychosocial treatments (specifically, cognitive restructuring, exposure, and to a lesser extent, social skills training and applied relaxation), as well as a combination of pharmacological and psychological treatments (e.g., Federoff & Taylor, 2001). Research concerning each of these approaches is now reviewed.

Pharmacotherapy

A recent review by Davidson (2003) concluded that monoamine oxidase inhibitors (MAOIs), such as phenelzine, and selective serotonin reuptake inhibitors (SSRIs) such as paroxetine, sertraline, and fluvoxamine, are consistently superior to placebo for treating SAD. Recent evidence suggests that escitalopram is also effective for treating SAD (Lader, Stender, Bürger, & Nil, 2004), but findings with fluoxetine for SAD have not been promising (e.g., Kobak, Greist, Jefferson, & Katzelnick, 2002). Although phenelzine is an effective treatment for SAD, it is rarely prescribed in practice due to interactions with other medications, interactions with foods containing tyramine (e.g., certain wines, cheeses, and cured meats), and a relatively high risk of unpleasant side effects. Therefore, SSRIs are much more frequently used for treating this condition.

There is also now evidence from placebo-controlled trials supporting the use of venlafaxine, a serotonin–norepinephrine reuptake inhibitor (Rickels, Mangano, & Khan, 2004), and research suggests that certain benzodiazepines (e.g., clonazepam) and anticonvulsants (e.g., gabapentin) are effective (for a review, see Davidson, 2003). In addition, SAD has also been found to have a moderately high placebo-response rate (Huppert et al., 2004). A placebo-controlled study of the popular herbal product St. John's wort failed to find any significant benefits of this product over placebo (Kobak, Taylor, Warner, & Futterer, 2005).

Psychosocial Treatments

Evidence-based psychosocial treatments for social phobia have primarily come from a cognitive-behavioral perspective and include various combinations of these four main components: (1) exposure-based strategies, (2) cognitive therapy, (3) social skills training, and (4) applied relaxation (for reviews, see Rodebaugh, Holaway, & Heimberg, 2004; Turk, Coles, & Heimberg, 2002).

In the SAD literature, it is common for CBT to be delivered either in an individual or group format. For example, Heimberg et al. (1990) studied a group CBT program for SAD, including exposure to real and simulated social situations and cognitive restructuring. The study compared cognitive-behavioral group treatment (CBGT) to supportive psychotherapy, and found CBGT to be superior, with findings maintained at 5-year follow-up (Heimberg et al., 1993). Similarly, in a study of individual therapy (including education, social skills training, and exposure, but no cognitive restructuring), Turner, Beidel, Cooley, and Woody (1994) found that 84% of patients receiving individual treatment had improvements, meeting criteria for high or moderate end state functioning following treatment. It is well established that both group and individual treatment are effective for treating SAD.

Comparing CBT Components

Numerous studies have examined the relative and combined effects of various CBT components. At least four meta-analytic reviews (using statistical procedures that combine findings across studies) have examined the question of which treatment components are most effective for treating SAD, including exposure alone, cognitive restructuring alone, exposure plus cognitive restructuring, social skills training, and applied relaxation (Federoff & Taylor, 2001; Feske & Chambless, 1995; Gould, Buckminster, Pollack, Otto, & Yap, 1997; Taylor, 1996). Across meta-analyses, all of these strategies show moderate to large effect sizes in comparison to wait-list control conditions (Rodebaugh et al., 2004). However, the findings differ with respect to the question of whether cognitive restructuring plus exposure is more effective than exposure alone. Feske and Chambless (1995) found no differences between exposure alone and exposure combined with cognitive restructuring. Gould et al. (1997) found that exposure had the largest effect sizes of all the strategies (either when administered alone or with cognitive restructuring). Finally, Taylor (1996) found that only treatments combining cognitive restructuring and exposure were more effective than placebo. Effect sizes for cognitive restructuring alone, exposure alone, and social skills training were not significantly larger than those for placebo in the analysis by Taylor.

Group versus Individual Treatment

Three published studies have directly compared individual and group CBT for SAD in adults. In the first of these, Wlazlo, Schroeder-Hartwig, Hand, Kaiser, and Münchau (1990) compared individual *in vivo* exposure (four 3-hour weekly sessions), group *in vivo* exposure (four 8-hour weekly sessions), and group social skills training (25 ninety-minute sessions, twice weekly). All three treatments were equally effective, though there was a tendency toward superior results with group exposure for a subgroup of participants with skills deficits. Of course, the three treatment conditions differed with respect to content, frequency, number of sessions, and duration of sessions, making it impossible to answer the specific question of whether the group or individual format is superior.

Scholing and Emmelkamp (1993) studied the effectiveness of (1) exposure only, (2) cognitive therapy followed by exposure, and (3) cognitive therapy and exposure integrated from the start of treatment. In addition, all three of these treatment combinations were studied separately in both a group and an individual format. Although there were few differences at posttreatment, by follow-up, the cognitive therapy followed by exposure presented in a group format was the most effective treatment. The integrated group treatment was the least effective option. The effects of the other treatments (including exposure-only in a group format, and the three treatment combinations presented in an individual format) were somewhere in between.

The most recent study to compare group and individual treatment is also the easiest to interpret because of its methodological simplicity (relative to the other two studies reviewed). Stangier, Heidenreich, Peitz, Lauterbach, and Clark (2003) conducted a direct comparison of individual and group cognitive therapy over 15 weekly sessions. Treatment was based on a protocol described by Clark and Wells (1995), including training in shifting attentional focus to external cues, stopping safety behaviors, video feedback to correct distorted self-imagery, behavioral experiments, and cognitive restructuring. Though the treatment was originally developed to be administered on an individual basis, it was adapted for the purpose of this study into a group format.

In this study, individual cognitive therapy was superior to group cognitive therapy, with the percentages of patients no longer meeting criteria for SAD after treatment being 50 and 13.6%, respectively.

Based on these three studies, it is difficult to come to any firm conclusions regarding the relative effectiveness of group versus individual treatment. Methodological limitations make the first of these studies difficult to interpret. The complexity of the second study also makes it difficult to come to any conclusions about the relative effectiveness of group and individual treatment. One problem with all three studies is that none included Heimberg's CBGT, which is often considered to be the gold standard among group treatments for SAD. In other words, direct comparisons of Heimberg's CBGT to a comparable individual treatment remain to be published.

However, results from two unpublished studies suggest few differences between CBGT and individual treatment (Lucas & Telch, 1993; Öst, Sedvall, Breitholz, Hellström, & Lindwall, 1995). In addition, a number of meta-analytic studies have examined the relative effectiveness of group and individual treatments for SAD (averaging findings from across dozens of studies). All three meta-analytic studies failed to find significant differences between these treatment formats (Federoff & Taylor, 2001; Gould et al., 1997; Taylor, 1996). Finally, a study by Manassis et al. (2002) found few differences between group and individual treatment for children with SAD, though for more severely impaired children, the benefits of individual treatment were somewhat stronger than those for group treatment.

Combining Pharmacological and Psychosocial Treatments

There are now a number of studies comparing CBT, medication, and their combination, and overall findings are mixed. In a study conducted in a primary care setting, sertraline, exposure, their combination, and placebo were compared (Blomhoff et al., 2001). Only sertraline and the combined treatment were more effective than placebo, with the largest effects found for the combination of sertraline and exposure. However, exposure sessions in this study were only 15–20 minutes long, and the therapists were relatively inexperienced (family doctors trained to provide exposure therapy for SAD over the course of three weekends), limiting the conclusions that can be drawn from these findings. At follow-up, those who received exposure continued to improve, whereas those in the sertraline and combined conditions showed some deterioration (Haug et al., 2003).

The largest study to date on combined CBT and medication compared fluoxetine, individual CBT, placebo, CBT plus fluoxetine, and CBT plus placebo (Davidson et al., 2004). At posttreatment, all four active treatment conditions were more effective than placebo but did not differ from one another. In other words, there was no benefit of combined treatment over either medication or CBT. Furthermore, although treatment was effective, many patients remained symptomatic. Another study, still unpublished, compared phenelzine, CBGT, and their combination (Heimberg, 2003). Though preliminary analyses suggest a modest advantage of combined treatment over either phenelzine or CBGT alone, final results of this study are pending.

ASSESSMENT ISSUES

Assessment is conducted one-on-one (before group treatment begins) and typically begins with a diagnostic interview to confirm that SAD is indeed the main problem, and to identify any comorbid conditions that may be present. A thorough interview should also be used to assess the most important features of the problem (etiology, triggers, severity, physical symptoms, cognitive features, avoidance strategies, safety behaviors, etc.), and to determine eligibility for group treatment. Issues related to suitability for group treatment are discussed in various sections throughout this chapter.

A number of tools are available for assessing treatment outcome, including monitoring diaries (e.g., thought records), behavioral assessments (e.g., measuring the patient's anxiety level and cognitions during a behavioral role play), and various standard questionnaire measures. We recommend using a clinician-administered scale, such as the Brief Social Phobia Scale (BSPS; Davidson et al., 1991) or the Liebowitz Social Anxiety Scale (LSAS; Liebowitz, 1987), as well as one or more self-report scales. Self-report scales may include general severity measures, such as the Social Phobia Inventory (SPIN; Connor et al., 2000), the Social Phobia Scale (SPS; Mattick & Clarke, 1998), and the Social Interaction Anxiety Scale (SIAS; Mattick & Clarke, 1998), as well as scales designed to measure particular aspects of SAD, such as the Social Thoughts and Beliefs Scale (STBS; Turner, Johnson, Beidel, Heiser, & Lydiard, 2003), which measures cognitive features. A review of these and other scales (as well as information on where to obtain them) is available elsewhere (Orsillo, 2001).

Assessment of SAD often presents a few unique challenges. Perhaps more than any other anxiety disorder, people with SAD are fearful of being negatively evaluated by others, including the therapist, other staff in the treatment setting, and even strangers in the waiting room. Therefore, the assessment is itself a phobic stimulus for many individuals who suffer from SAD. Even filling out questionnaires in the presence of other people can be very difficult for many patients. Patients may also be apprehensive about discussing certain topics, and they may hold back information during the assessment. People with SAD often require extra support and reassurance during the assessment period, and it may be useful to adjust some of the assessment procedures if anxiety is likely to affect the process significantly. For a more detailed review of assessment strategies for SAD, see McCabe and Antony (2002).

STRUCTURING GROUP TREATMENT

Table 9.1 provides details regarding group composition and format from several studies on group treatment for SAD. The best established group treatment for SAD is Heimberg's CBGT (Heimberg & Becker, 2002). The suggestions regarding the structuring of group treatment are based on recommendations from Heimberg and his colleagues, as well as from other relevant research and our own experience in treating SAD in groups.

Group Composition and Format

Composition of Groups

Heimberg and Becker (2002) recommend that SAD groups be run by two therapists, ideally one male and one female. The recommendation of having two therapists is consistent with what generally occurs in studies of group CBT (see Table 9.1), and with our own practice, although studies have typically not commented on the sex of the therapists. Occasionally, we include a third, more junior therapist (e.g., a student), though his or her role tends to be limited primarily to observing the group for training purposes and occasionally helping out with exposures or behavioral role plays.

Though studies vary somewhat with respect to the number of patients per group, most studies include between five and seven patients (see Table 9.1), consistent with Heimberg and Becker's (2002) recommendation to include six participants. In our groups, we typically aim to have five to seven patients per group. In our experience, participants in larger groups (e.g., groups with 9 or 10 participants) tend to feel more socially inhibited, have higher rates of dropout early in treatment, and may not get adequate attention during the session.

Ideally, groups should reflect a balanced mix of sexes, feared situations, and degrees of impairment (Heimberg & Becker, 2002). We have occasionally had groups in which one patient is uncomfortable about being different from all other group members in some noticeable way (e.g., a different sex, much older or much younger, or dramatically different with respect to symptom severity). In such cases, it may be helpful to discuss these differences with the patient before the group begins to assess whether this is likely to be an issue for the individual.

Number and Frequency of Sessions

Most studies of group treatment have tended to include 12 weekly sessions, consistent with recommendations by Heimberg and Becker (2002). In fact, research on individual treatment for SAD suggests that increasing the number of sessions does not lead to better outcomes. Herbert, Rheingold, Gaudiano, and Myers (2004) compared 12 sessions versus 18 sessions of individual CBT for SAD and found that although the two treatments were equally effective by

TABLE 9.1. Format and Composition for Group SAD Treatments

Study	No. of sessions	Group composition	Length of sessions	Strategies
Gelernter et al. (1991)	12 weekly sessions	10 patients 2 therapists	2 hours	Cognitive restructuring, exposure
Heimberg et al. (1998)	12 weekly sessions	5–10 patients 2 therapists	2.5 hours	Education, exposure, cognitive restructuring
Hope et al. (1995)	12 weekly sessions	6–7 patients 2 therapists	2–2.5 hours	Education, exposure, cognitive restructuring
Otto et al. (2000)	12 weekly sessions	3–8 patients 2 therapists	2.5 hours	Education, exposure, cognitive restructuring
Scholing & Emmelkamp (1993)	2 individual sessions and 14 group sessions, twice per week	5–7 patients 2 therapists	2.5 hours	Education, exposure, cognitive restructuring
van Dam-Baggen & Kraaimaat (2000)	17 weekly sessions, plus 3 monthly sessions	5–8 patients 2 therapists	1.5 hours	Education, problem solving, goal setting, cognitive restructuring (but no exposure)

posttreatment, the briefer treatment led to gains more quickly and was associated with fewer dropouts. Although this issue has not been studied in group
treatments, our recommendation is to plan for around 12 sessions, based on
the existing literature. On occasion, we add one or two follow-up sessions
(e.g., at 1-month intervals) if group members express an interest in meeting
again after the period of weekly sessions has ended.

Inclusion Guidelines

The suggestions that follow describe the ideal conditions under which SAD is
treated in groups. Of course, in practice, it is often difficult to assemble the
ideal group, particularly in settings where the number of patients seeking
treatment for SAD is limited. Though it is useful to take these guidelines into
account, there is also room for flexibility. However, the fewer of these inclusion guidelines that are met, the more likely a particular candidate may not be
ideal for group treatment of SAD.

Diagnosis and Clinical Severity

Although treatment studies on children often include groups with a mix of different anxiety disorders, studies of group treatment for adults with anxiety disorders are almost always based on homogenous groups of patients, all with the
same principal diagnosis. Ideally, when treating SAD in groups, it is best to
include only individuals with SAD as a principal diagnosis (i.e., the condition
causing the most distress and/or functional impairment). If working in a setting
where one has no choice but to treat heterogeneous groups, then it may be possible to combine individuals with SAD with people who have certain other
anxiety-based problems. For example, panic disorder with agoraphobia shares a
number of features with SAD. People with both problems often avoid phobic situations, are anxious in social situations, are fearful of particular physical sensations (though often for different reasons), and respond to similar treatment
strategies. In contrast, SAD is sufficiently different from obsessive–compulsive
disorder (OCD) that we would discourage clinicians from combining patients
with SAD and OCD together in the same groups, if possible.

   Ideally, it is best either to have a range of clinical severities among group
members or to have members with a similar severity of symptoms. Problems
may arise when a group is fairly homogeneous with respect to severity, with
the exception of one member. If one member has significantly greater symptom severity or is functioning at a significantly higher level than other group
members, he or she may have different needs than the rest of the group or may
view him- or herself as not fitting in.

   Individuals at the most severe end of the spectrum often do less well in
group treatment (or any treatment, for that matter). In our experience, such
patients may be served best by individual treatment, which allows for more
extensive therapist attention for the opportunity to address issues that may

not be addressed during standard CBT (e.g., social skills deficits). On occasion, we have offered concurrent individual and group treatment for patients who need more attention than the group provides, but who still have much to gain from the group experience (learning that they are not alone, exposure opportunities, etc.). We are aware of no studies investigating the benefits of concurrent individual and group treatment.

Comorbidity

Most studies examining the presence of an additional anxiety, mood, or personality disorder have found that the presence of comorbid diagnosis does not affect treatment outcome for the average patient with SAD (Hofmann, Newman, Becker, Taylor, & Roth, 1995; Hope, Herbert, & White, 1995; Turner, Beidel, Wolff, Spaulding, & Jacob, 1996; van Velzen, Emmelkamp, & Scholing, 1997). However, more severe comorbidity (e.g., higher levels of depression, more severe avoidant traits) may impact upon outcome of group CBT for this condition (Chambless, Tran, & Glass, 1997). In addition, most research on the effects of comorbidity on outcome do not include patients with comorbid substance dependence, schizophrenia, bipolar disorder, or other forms of severe psychopathology, so the effects of these conditions on outcome are unknown.

Generally, comorbidity should not disqualify an individual from group treatment. However, there are certain situations in which comorbidity should lead a therapist to consider individual treatment instead of group treatment, particularly in cases where the comorbidity is likely to impact upon the treatment experience for the patient, or for others in the group. For example, if the additional problems are severe enough that they are likely to be a focus of treatment (e.g., if a patient's marital problems require considerable attention at each session), then individual treatment may be more appropriate. Similarly, patients with current manic symptoms, significant suicidal ideation, or a high likelihood of showing up to sessions intoxicated should probably be treated individually, where attention can be paid to these other concerns.

Insight and Suspiciousness

DSM-IV requires that individuals with SAD have insight into the excessiveness of their SAD symptoms. However, some patients have less insight than others. In addition, a minority of patients with SAD tend to be somewhat suspicious of others, often assuming that others have malicious intentions (e.g., that they are talking behind the individual's back, or undermining the person in some way) and cannot be trusted. In our experience, patients with these qualities present unique challenges in treatment. Although they may do well in group treatment, individual therapy should be considered in cases where insight is particularly poor, or where the individual's suspiciousness is likely to affect his or her ability to get along with other group members.

Patient Preferences

Many patients with SAD prefer individual treatment to group treatment, simply because speaking in front of groups is frightening for people with this problem. Usually, with a bit of reassurance (e.g., being reminded that everyone in the group feels the same way and that the discomfort will decrease as the individual becomes more familiar with the group members), patients often come to recognize the benefits of group treatment. However, a patient's expectations and preferences can affect treatment outcome across a wide range of problems, including SAD (Chambless et al., 1997). If a patient reports a particularly strong preference for individual treatment, it is reasonable to honor such a request, if possible.

Motivation and Availability

Individuals with poor motivation are also often not good candidates for group treatment. Often there is little time to deal with motivational issues during the group, and such patients are more likely to miss sessions, to drop out, or to avoid doing homework, all of which can be disruptive for their own treatment, as well as for others in the group. Individual treatment may be more suitable in such cases, especially if it includes strategies for enhancing motivation.

Individuals with limited availability (e.g., shift workers) should not be treated in groups if they are unlikely to be able to attend all (or most) of the group meetings. If a patient's schedule changes from week to week, individual treatment may be more suitable.

Interpersonal Skills

As reviewed by Antony and Swinson (2000a), there is very little research on social skills deficits in the context of SAD. Though a few studies have found greater social skills impairment (e.g., poor eye contact, impaired conversation flow, visible signs of anxiety) in people with SAD than in people without SAD (e.g., Fydrich, Chambless, Perry, Buergener, & Beazley, 1998), many people with SAD have adequate social skills. Furthermore, there is little research on whether social skills impairment is associated with poorer outcome following CBT. However, one study found a tendency (though not statistically significant) for individuals with greater social skills impairment to do better in a group exposure-based treatment than in either individual exposure-based treatment or group social skills training (Wlazlo et al., 1990).

In our experience, mild to moderate social skills impairment should not be an exclusion factor for group treatment. However, people with very severe social skills impairment sometimes do less well in group CBT, particularly if social skills training is not a significant focus of the treatment.

Structure of Group Sessions

Sessions should be scheduled to last 2 to 2½ hours (see Table 9.1). Each meeting should begin with setting an agenda. Therapists should take 5 minutes to provide an overview of the topics to be covered, and patients should be given an opportunity to add items to the agenda. Next, homework from the previous week should be reviewed. When reviewing homework, the therapist should be sure to look at each participant's monitoring forms, so feedback can be provided, and appropriate questions can be asked to follow up on the material from the forms. Each participant should take about 5–10 minutes to provide an update on his or her progress and to review the week's homework.

Following the review of homework, sessions early in the treatment often include some psychoeducation, which may involve teaching participants about the role of cognitions in triggering anxiety, or about how to use particular CBT strategies (e.g., how to complete a thought record). As treatment progresses, more of the session is spent practicing strategies rather than providing psychoeducation. For example, group members spend increasing amounts of time engaging in exposure practices or behavioral role plays during the group session.

Each meeting ends with assigning new homework. Homework should be planned jointly by the therapists and participants. The therapists should note any planned exposure homework practices, so they can be checked on at the start of the next session.

KEY TREATMENT COMPONENTS

This section provides an overview of the main CBT components for treating SAD. For those seeking a more detailed description of the treatment, we recommend Heimberg and Becker's (2002) book, *Cognitive-Behavioral Therapy for Social Phobia: Basic Mechanisms and Clinical Strategies*, as well as a number of other resources (e.g., Antony & Swinson, 2000a). Table 9.2 provides a summary of what is covered at each session. This outline is based on the treatment provided at our center, which borrows heavily from Heimberg and Becker (2002), with some minor modifications (e.g., we include a session of social skills training, whereas Heimberg and Becker do not).

Psychoeducation

Because CBT is a skills-based approach to treatment, psychoeducation is an important component of the treatment. Education may be in the form of readings, demonstrations, didactic presentations, or video presentations. For example, a video by Rapee (1999), called *I Think They Think. . . : Overcoming Social Phobia*, provides an excellent overview of the nature and treat-

TABLE 9.2. Sample Outline of Treatment Protocol for Group CBT of SAD

Session	Strategies covered
Pretreatment individual meeting	• Explain how the group will work and what to expect. • Introduce norms and rules for the group, and provide practical information (e.g., location and times for group). • Develop an exposure hierarchy. • Answer any questions and address concerns.
Session 1	• Introduction to group members (group members share experiences about what brought them to the group). • What to expect from treatment. • Review rules for the group (e.g., confidentiality). • Psychoeducation: Model of SAD, overview of treatment strategies, recommend self-help readings. • Homework: Complete monitoring forms, read introductory chapters from self-help readings.
Session 2	• Homework review. • Psychoeducation: Review cognitive model, introduce cognitive distortions. • Homework: Monitor cognitive distortions, read self-help chapter(s) on cognitive strategies.
Session 3	• Homework review. • Psychoeducation: Review strategies for challenging cognitive distortions. • Homework: Practice challenging cognitive distortions on thought records.
Session 4	• Homework review. • Psychoeducation: Introduction to exposure. • In-session exposures and role plays. • Homework: Cognitive restructuring, completion of thought records, exposure practices, reading self-help chapter(s) on exposure-based strategies.
Sessions 5–9	• Homework review. • In-session exposures and role plays. • Homework: Cognitive restructuring, completion of thought records, exposure practices.
Session 10	• Homework review. • Psychoeducation: Introduction to social skills training. • In-session exposures and role plays, with attention to rehearsing particular social skills. • Homework: Cognitive restructuring, completion of thought records, exposure practices with social skills rehearsal, reading self-help chapter(s) on social skills training.
Session 11	• Homework review. • In-session exposures and role plays, with attention to rehearsing particular social skills. • Homework: Cognitive restructuring, completion of thought records, exposure practices with social skills rehearsal.
Session 12	• Homework review. • Psychoeducation: Discuss triggers for relapse and recurrence, review strategies for preventing relapse and recurrence. • Homework: Practice relapse prevention strategies.

ment of SAD. Psychoeducation tends to comprise a larger portion of the earlier sessions compared to later sessions, which focus more on practicing the new skills that have been learned.

Examples of topics covered during psychoeducation include the following:

- Information about the nature of SAD.
- Overview of how SAD impacts on a person's life.
- Etiology and processes underlying SAD, from a CBT perspective.
- The relationship among thoughts, behaviors, and anxiety.
- Costs and benefits of overcoming the problem.
- A description of treatment procedures.
- How to complete thought records and other monitoring forms.
- Guidelines for conducting exposure practices.

Cognitive Strategies

Chapter 3, this volume, provided a detailed discussion of how to use cognitive strategies in a group setting. In this section, we provide a brief review of how these strategies can be applied in group treatment for SAD in particular. Cognitive strategies are typically introduced in the second and third sessions, and continue to be discussed throughout treatment (particularly during the review of homework).

As discussed in Chapter 3, cognitive techniques may be grouped into four broad categories: (1) exploring the relationship among thoughts, situational triggers, and affect (e.g., anxiety), (2) exploring evidence and challenging thought distortions to facilitate thinking about situations more objectively, (3) behavioral experiments, and (4) exploring underlying beliefs and assumptions. To complement the material in Chapter 3, we present suggestions for applying each of these strategies in group treatment of SAD.

Exploring the Relationship among Thoughts, Situational Triggers, and Affect

During the early treatment sessions, participants should be encouraged to discuss the triggers for their anxiety, including the types of situations they fear (parties, dating, meetings, public speaking, eating in public, etc.), as well as the variables that influence their fear upon entering these situations. In addition, they should be encouraged to become more aware of the thoughts, beliefs, and predictions that occur in anticipation of encountering these situations (as well as during and after such encounters). Through careful monitoring and discussion in the group, participants learn to become more aware of the situations that trigger anxiety, and the thoughts that are believed to mediate the relationship between these situations and the negative emotions associated with SAD. Examples of typical thoughts include the following:

"The only reason I was invited to the party on the weekend is because the host felt sorry for me."

"I would rather keep a shirt that doesn't fit than return it to the store, for fear that the cashier will give me a hard time or that I will come across as anxious."

"My presentation was a disaster. I am sure everyone noticed my sweating. They probably thought I looked disgusting."

"I should cancel my date. If I don't, my hands will shake so much that I won't be able to hold my fork at dinner."

Exploring Evidence and Challenging Cognitive Distortions

In the anxiety disorders literature, it is common to describe two main types of cognitive distortions: probability overestimations and catastrophic thinking. *Probability overestimations* involve overestimating the likelihood of something bad occurring:

"People will think I am stupid."
"Everyone will notice my shaky hands during the presentation."
"Nobody will talk to me at the party."

Probability overestimations can be challenged through examining both the evidence supporting the thought and evidence that disconfirms it, as described in Chapter 3. Consider the following example:

Probability overestimation:	"I will make a fool of myself during the presentation."
Initial anxiety level:	80 out of 100
Supporting evidence:	1. "I often lose my train of thought during presentations."
	2. "Sometimes people tell me I looked anxious following a presentation."
	3. "I feel like a fool when I am anxious in front of others."
Disconfirming evidence:	1. "I keep getting invited to give more presentations, so I must be doing something right."
	2. "When I collect formal evaluations for my presentations, most people in the audience tend to be happy with my performance."
	3. "Presentations are just a small part of my job. As long as I do the rest of my job well, I can afford to have my presentations be less than perfect."

Revised belief: "Although my presentation may not be perfect, I am unlikely to make a fool of myself."

Revised anxiety level: 40 out of 100

Catastrophic thinking involves overestimating how unbearable or unmanageable a particular outcome would be, if it were to occur. Examples of catastrophic thoughts in SAD include the following:

"It would be awful if the cashier thought badly of me."
"It would be terrible if I lost my train of thought during a presentation."
"I don't think I could cope if my hands got shaky during the meeting."

Catastrophic thinking can be challenged by asking questions designed to put things in perspective:

"What if _____ did happen?"
"Would that really be as bad as I expect?"
"Would it matter the next day? . . . the next week? . . . the next month?"

Behavioral Experiments

A powerful strategy for challenging both probability overestimations and catastrophic thinking is the behavioral experiment. Essentially, this strategy involves setting up a mini-experiment to test the validity of a belief in the way that a scientist might test a hypothesis. Examples of behavioral experiments that can be useful for people with SAD include the following:

- Purposely leaving long pauses in a conversation to challenge the belief that one must always keep a conversation moving along.
- Wetting the forehead or underarms with water before going into a meeting to challenge the belief that sweating in public would be unbearable.
- Spilling water on oneself in a public place (e.g., while drinking in a restaurant or cafeteria) to challenge the belief that it would be terrible to look sweaty in front of others.

Exploring Underlying Beliefs and Assumptions

This strategy involves identifying and challenging more deeply held beliefs, including "rules" that individuals hold, as well as "core beliefs" about the self or others. Underlying beliefs and assumptions can be challenged using a variety of strategies, as reviewed in Chapter 3. Examples of such thoughts that are often found in people with SAD include the following:

"If someone ignores what I say, it means that they don't respect me."
"If I engage in a conversation for too long, I am bound to say something stupid."
"It is terrible to look anxious in front of others."
"I am an unlovable person."
"People are generally cruel."

Exposure

In Chapter 4, we provided detailed instructions for conducting exposures. In addition to exposure to feared situations, treatment of SAD often includes simulated exposure role plays. For example, a patient who is fearful of going on job interviews might be encouraged to practice interview role plays with family members, the therapist, or other group members, before practicing exposure to actual job interviews.

When conducting SAD exposures in a group setting, group members can often contribute in one another's exposures. For example, an entire group can play the role of "audience" for an individual who is fearful of public speaking. Similarly, group members can mingle at a simulated party for a patient who is fearful of making small talk. For some exposures (e.g., those involving one-on-one conversations), group members can be split into smaller groups. Or participants can leave the group to conduct exposures on their own (e.g., going to a nearby coffee shop and talking to the cashier) then return to the group to discuss the outcome. Table 9.3 includes examples of exposure practices that are useful when treating SAD.

Developing an Exposure Hierarchy

Typically, we develop a hierarchy collaboratively with the patient during an individual session scheduled about a week before the group begins. Responses on the standard questionnaires reviewed earlier (e.g., BSPS, LSAS, SPIN, SPS, and SIAS) can be used to generate items for the hierarchy, along with any other feared situations that may come to light during the meeting. In addition to using the hierarchy to plan exposure practices, we use it as an outcome measure. Group participants start each session by providing current fear/avoidance ratings for each item on their hierarchy. Figure 9.1 presents an example of an exposure hierarchy in SAD.

Social Skills Training

Evidence-based protocols for treating SAD vary with respect to the amount of social skills training included. Some effective treatments, including Heimberg and Becker's (2002) CBGT, include no formal social skills training at all, whereas some other investigators (e.g., van Dam-Baggen & Kraaimaat, 2000) suggest that social skills training may be the best way to treat SAD. In our cen-

TABLE 9.3. Examples of Exposure Practices for SAD

Feared situation	Examples of practices
Casual conversation and small talk	• Say hello or ask directions from a stranger (e.g., in line, on an elevator, on the sidewalk). • Attend an art gallery opening. • Attend a party. • Join an ongoing conversation at work.
Meeting new people	• Join a club. • Take a course. • Answer a personal ad. • Attend a party.
Job interviews	• Apply for jobs (even jobs that are not very interesting). • Role-play interviews with friends and family.
Public speaking	• Join Toastmasters (www.toastmasters.org). • Take a public speaking course. • Take a course that involves presentations. • Speak in meetings.
Eating or drinking in front of others	• Have lunch with coworkers. • Eat in a food court at the mall. • Eat a snack while walking around the office.
Writing in front of others	• Complete a contest ballot at a store. • Complete a credit card application in a store. • Write a letter, while sitting in a coffee shop. • Pay for an item by check.
Being the center of attention	• Drop keys in a public place. • Shout out name of coworker or friend from across the room. • Spill water in a restaurant or cafeteria. • Wear an article of clothing inside-out.
Conflict or assertiveness situations	• Return food in a restaurant. • Say "no" in response to an unreasonable request. • Ask someone to change his or her behavior.

ter, we typically include one or two sessions of social skills training, depending on the specific needs of the group members. If social skills deficits appear to be an issue for several group members, then some time is typically devoted to this topic.

Social skills training typically begins with a discussion about how particular types of social behaviors (e.g., poor eye contact, coming across as angry or aloof) can sometimes lead to the negative reactions from others that patients often fear. Patients are encouraged to identify the types of social skills that they might want to work on, sometimes with gentle suggestions from the therapists or other group members. Role-play exercises (often conducted during the course of exposure practices) provide an opportunity both to obtain feedback on social behaviors and to practice new skills. Social skills practices may be videotaped to provide an opportunity for the patient to see how he or

Item	Fear/avoidance (0–100)
1. Have a party and invite everyone from work.	100
2. Give a 15-minute presentation to my department at work.	100
3. Ask someone from my art course to have dinner after class.	90
4. Attend a party being thrown by a coworker.	90
5. Eat dinner in a nice restaurant with a group of six or more coworkers.	80
6. Eat dinner in a nice restaurant with one or two coworkers.	70
7. Ask a question in a meeting at work.	65
8. Tell my boss about my weekend on Monday morning.	50
9. Have lunch in a casual restaurant with one or two coworkers.	50
10. Tell Rick (a coworker) about my weekend on Monday morning.	40
11. Arrive late for an art class.	35
12. Make small talk while standing in line at the supermarket.	30

FIGURE 9.1. Example of an exposure hierarchy for SAD.

she is actually coming across and to give group members an opportunity to provide feedback. Patients should be reassured that it is not essential for them to come across perfectly during the practices.

The following examples of social skills can be targeted during the group:

- Nonverbal communication (e.g., eye contact, body language, personal space, facial expressions, volume and tone of voice)
- Assertiveness training
- Dealing with conflict
- Presentation skills
- Dating skills
- Interview skills

SAMPLE CBT GROUP PROTOCOL FOR SAD

The treatment described in this section borrows from treatments described by Heimberg and Becker (2002) and Antony and Swinson (2001a). It begins with an individual pretreatment session, followed by 12 group treatment sessions. A brief description of what occurs in each session (elaborating on the summary provided in Table 9.2) follows.

Pretreatment Individual Meetings with Group Members

Before the group begins, we recommend that each participant have an opportunity to meet individually with at least one of the therapists. This ensures that
each participant knows at least one person when he or she arrives at the
group. During the individual session, the group is described, and any concerns
or questions are addressed. Information about the location, times, and structure of the group is provided. In addition, an exposure hierarchy is generated.

Session 1: Presenting the Treatment Rationale

The main purpose of the first session is to orient participants to the group, to
provide them with an understanding of their problem, and to introduce them
to the treatment procedures. Some of the topics and issues covered in the first
session include the following:

1. Introductions to participants and therapists.
2. A description of each participant's problem: feared situations and triggers, physical symptoms, thoughts, avoidance behaviors, and safety
   behaviors.
3. Guidelines and overview of the group: confidentiality, importance of
   regular attendance, expectations regarding homework (60–90 minutes
   per day), need to stay focused on SAD and related issues during group
   discussions, and reassurance that coming to the group meetings will
   become easier over time.
4. Description of the nature of anxiety: Participants are taught that anxiety is a normal and healthy response to threat, and that it is designed
   to facilitate survival. Having no anxiety in social situations can be a
   detriment.
5. The three components of anxiety and fear: physical component, cognitive component, behavioral component, and interactions among these
   three components.
6. Discussion of the CBT model of social anxiety (e.g., Clark & Wells,
   1995), with an emphasis on how the model helps to explain the symptom profiles of particular group members.
7. Overview of the treatment procedures and how they relate to the three
   components of anxiety and fear.
8. Discussion of the costs and benefits of overcoming SAD, and strategies for dealing with obstacles that may arise during the course of
   treatment.
9. Homework: recommended self-help readings on the nature of SAD
   (e.g., Antony, 2004; Antony & Swinson, 2000b; Hope, Heimberg,
   Juster, & Turk, 2000), completing monitoring forms that facilitate
   thinking about anxiety in terms of the three components (e.g., for

each episode of anxiety or fear, recording any physical sensations, cognitions, and behavioral responses that occur).

Sessions 2 and 3: Cognitive Strategies

Session 2 begins with setting an agenda, addressing any questions from the previous week's readings, and reviewing the completed monitoring forms. Next, the cognitive-behavioral model of SAD is reviewed briefly, followed by a more thorough discussion of the role of cognitions in maintaining social anxiety. Participants describe how their own beliefs influence their anxiety. Examples of cognitive distortions (e.g., probability overestimations) are reviewed, and participants are encouraged to monitor their own anxious thoughts over the next week (using the first few columns of a thought record). In addition, self-help readings on cognitive strategies for SAD are assigned.

Session 3 begins with setting an agenda, followed by a review of the homework from the previous week. The emphasis of this session is on teaching strategies for challenging anxious thoughts about social situations. Participants are taught to complete a thought record. Strategies for examining the evidence and challenging catastrophic thinking are reviewed. Participants are also encouraged to conduct behavioral experiments to test out the validity of their anxious beliefs and predictions. Homework includes completion of thought records and instructions to complete at least two behavioral experiments over the coming week.

Sessions 4–9: *In Vivo* Exposure and Role Plays

For Sessions 4 through 9, an agenda is first generated, followed by up to one-half hour spent reviewing homework, providing corrective feedback, and helping participants to challenge anxious thinking. Participants are also encouraged to help one another to examine evidence for anxious thoughts that arise during the course of the group.

At Session 4, following the review of homework, the rationale for exposure is presented, including the need for exposure practices to be predicable, frequent, and prolonged (see Chapter 4 for a full description of exposure-based strategies). In the remaining time, participants are provided with an opportunity to try an exposure practice from near the bottom of their hierarchies. Homework includes instructions to practice exposure four to six times over the coming week (in one or more situations), while continuing to use the cognitive strategies learned previously. Self-help readings on exposure-based strategies are assigned.

In Sessions 5 through 9, the review of homework is followed by in-session exposures and role plays. Each session ends with an assignment of homework for the following week (i.e., continuing to practice the cognitive strategies and exposure).

Sessions 10 and 11: Social Skills Training

Sessions 10 and 11 begin with setting an agenda, followed by a detailed review of homework and corrective feedback on the use of cognitive strategies and exposure. In Session 10, participants are provided with an overview of the rationale for social skills training. Over the course of these two sessions, participants identify specific skills that they would like to work on, and they are encouraged to combine the use of social skills rehearsal with their exposure practices. Homework includes continuing to complete thought records and practice exposure, with an emphasis on trying to shift particular social behaviors during the exposure practices.

Session 12: Termination and Relapse Prevention

Homework from the previous session is reviewed. The focus of the remainder of this meeting is on reviewing the progress made by each participant, identifying possible triggers for relapse and recurrence (life stress, a negative experience in a social situation, falling back into old avoidance habits, etc.). Patients are encouraged to be vigilant for these triggers and to notice any changes in their anxiety, before it becomes overwhelming. They are also encouraged to continue occasional exposure practices and to challenge their anxious thoughts on a regular basis.

Posttreatment Evaluation and Planning

At the end of the treatment, group members complete a posttreatment evaluation, including all of the measures that were completed at the start of treatment. For those who are continuing to experience significant social anxiety, we recommend a number of options. At our center, we offer a monthly booster group for patients who have been through one of our treatments and want a forum in which to discuss issues that arise as they continue to work on their anxiety. If the person's anxiety continues to be a significant problem, we sometimes offer individual CBT following the group, or a medication consultation.

ADVANTAGES AND OBSTACLES IN GROUP TREATMENT FOR SAD

Advantages of Group Treatment

Increased Exposure Opportunities

Overcoming SAD usually requires exposure to other people. Group therapy is particularly suitable for treating SAD, because it provides a ready-made context for creating relevant exposures. As reviewed earlier, group members can participate in one another's exposures and role-play practices. In fact, just sitting in the room and talking to other participants can lead to changes in social anxiety, regardless of what is actually talked about in the course of therapy. In contrast, during individual treatment, it is often a challenge to come up with helpful exposure practices that can be practiced during treatment sessions, particularly for situations involving public speaking.

Cost-Effectiveness

Group treatments are less expensive than individual treatments. They take up less therapist time, and can therefore be provided at a lower cost to patients. For clinical settings with long wait lists, group therapy is also a cost-effective way of providing treatment to a larger number of individuals in a shorter amount of time.

Opportunities to Meet Others with the Same Problem

Although patients are often frightened of group treatment (particularly during the first few sessions), by the end of treatment, they are often grateful for having had the opportunity to meet others who have the same problem. For many individuals, the group may seem like one of the first opportunities they have had to speak freely about their anxiety in front of others, without a significant risk of being ridiculed, judged, or misunderstood. In addition, support or advice from another participant in the group (e.g., reassurance that anxiety decreases over the course of exposure) may be perceived by some patients as more credible than the same advice coming from a therapist who has never suffered from SAD.

Obstacles to Treating SAD in Groups
Fear of the Group Setting

For most patients, participating in group treatment requires exposure to a situation (speaking in front of groups) that they almost always avoid because of their anxiety. A significant number of patients refuse group treatment for SAD or drop out shortly after treatment begins, because their fear is overwhelming. In such cases, individual treatment may be most practical, if only to get the individual to a point where group treatment is a possibility. However, note that most patients are initially apprehensive about group treatment, and encouraging them to give it a try usually pays off.

Practical Issues

Group treatment requires that therapists have a large enough referral base to assemble a group of patients with SAD. In addition, scheduling can sometimes be more challenging than is the case for individual therapy, because some participants may not be available at the same time each week. Finally, missed sessions are often difficult to make up. If a patient has to be away during a particular week, we recommend having the person come early to the next group session to meet individually with the therapist for 15–30 minutes to get caught up on any missed material. This is particularly important early in treatment.

CONCLUSIONS

SAD is among the most prevalent of anxiety disorders, and it affects most areas of functioning, including work, relationships, and leisure. From a cognitive-behavioral perspective, SAD is believed to stem from beliefs that it is important to always make a good impression on others, that making a good impression on others is unlikely to occur, and that disastrous consequences will ensue. SAD responds well to CBT, pharmacotherapy, and combinations of these approaches. One of the best studied approaches for treating SAD is group treatment. This chapter has provided an overview of group treatment for SAD from a cognitive-behavioral perspective.

CHAPTER 10

Depression

DESCRIPTION OF UNIPOLAR DEPRESSION

Depression, the most frequently occurring and debilitating psychiatric disorder, causes more disability than any other mental illness. When compared to all medical and mental disease on a common metric, disability-adjusted life years (DALYs), major depression was the fourth leading cause of global DALYs, and by 2020, major depressive disorder is predicted to be the second leading cause of DALYs (Murray & Lopez, 1997a, 1997b). Patients with depression experience more disability than those with hypertension, diabetes mellitus, and chronic pain (Davidson & Meltzer-Brody, 1999), and individuals with depression have more sick days than other patients with physical illness (Kessler et al., 1999; Parikh, Wasylenki, Goering, & Wong, 1996). Because of its prevalence, aspects of depression treatment are relevant to nearly all psychiatric patients seen across different kinds of clinical settings. This chapter first introduces some of the clinical and diagnostic aspects of major depression, followed by a description of a group CBT approach to depression and discussion of relevant group process factors.

Diagnostic Features

A major depressive episode involves at least 2 weeks of depressed mood or loss of interest, accompanied by four or more other symptoms (American Psychiatric Association [APA], 2000), which include changes in weight or appetite, dysregulated sleep, physical agitation or retardation, loss of energy, feelings of worthlessness or excessive guilt, difficulty concentrating or making decisions, and suicidal ideations, plans, or an attempt. Depressive episodes can be categorized by severity as mild, moderate, severe, or severe with psychotic features (i.e., the presence of delusions or hallucinations during the depressive episode). The major depressive episode forms a core component of a number of mood disorder diagnoses. Where such an episode is found to exist in its most simple form, that is, in the absence of other kinds of mood symptoms, the diagnosis of major depressive disorder is the most appropriate. However, a major depressive episode can also be a feature of other mood disorders, including bipolar spectrum disorders and so-called "double depression," described below.

Symptoms of depression may also manifest themselves in a less severe but more long-standing form that falls short of meeting criteria for a full major depressive episode. This diagnosis, dysthymia, is characterized by at least 2 years of chronically depressed mood, accompanied by a minimum two other symptoms of depression, including poor appetite or overeating, sleep disturbance, low energy, low self-esteem, poor concentration or difficulty making decisions, and feelings of hopelessness (APA, 2000). To meet criteria for dysthymia, the person cannot have experienced symptom-free periods of more than 2 months at a time.

Although major depressive disorder and dysthymia are separate diagnoses, they can co-occur within an individual. This phenomenon, typically called "double depression," involves one or more major depressive episodes superimposed on top of preexisting dysthymia. Double depression is distinct from chronic major depression, in which an individual experiences the symptoms of a major depressive episode continuously for at least 2 years. The distinction between these two phenomena is mainly one of *severity* (i.e., periods of dysthymia in double depression are not as severe as chronic major depression), as well as symptom *content* (i.e., the symptoms of dysthymia are similar but not synonomous with those of a major depressive episode; e.g., Keller et al., 1995). For our purposes in this chapter, we focus on depression defined relatively broadly to include major depressive disorder, dysthymia, and double depression, but not bipolar disorder, which is described in Chapter 11.

CBT FOR DEPRESSION

CBT was initially developed for working with depressed patients, and there is a voluminous literature supporting the efficacy of CBT with major depressive disorder and other variants of unipolar depression (DeRubeis & Crits-Christoph, 1998). Some authors have suggested that because CBT teaches the patients a set of skills they can implement after therapy ends, CBT is likely to have a more lasting and potentially prophylactic effect than comparator conditions such as antidepressant medications. More recently, CBT has also been shown to be as efficacious as pharmacotherapy even for severe depression (DeRubeis, Gelfand, Tang, & Simons, 1999).

Evidence for Group CBT in Depression

Depression was the first kind of disorder to which a CBT group format was formally applied and evaluated. These early validation studies conducted by Hollon, Shaw, and colleagues were small but important, in that they compared group CBT not only to medication, but also to individual CBT. Hollon and collaborators found that a CBT group was superior to several other treatments, but seemingly not as effective as individual CBT (Beck et al., 1979).

Subsequently, broader reviews and meta-analyses of psychotherapy for depression have also examined group versus individual treatment, though not always exclusively for a CBT modality. For example, Robinson and colleagues (1990) identified 16 studies using individual treatment and 15 studies using a group approach compared to a wait-list control. Treatment effect sizes, in terms of Cohen's d were nearly identical, 0.83 (SD .77) for individual and 0.84 (SD .60) for group modalities. Although this review focused on short-term treatments beyond CBT only, most of the studies in this analysis were cognitive or behavioral and cognitive. These reviewers also identified five studies that directly compared group and individual treatment. In that smaller set of studies, individual treatment fared better in absolute terms, but the difference in effect size, 0.31, was not found to be significantly different from zero (Robinson et al., 1990). Finally, these reviewers also compared smaller group treatments to larger group treatments, speculating that smaller numbers of individuals in a group might be associated with better outcome. However, they did not identify a significant effect for group size, which ranged from 3 to 12 individuals in the studies they identified.

Specific studies of group CBT have tended to bear out these conclusions regarding individual and group treatments defined more broadly. Individual CBT and group CBT perform at approximately equivalent levels (Burlingame et al., 2004; Morrison, 2001; Scott & Stradling, 1990). Group CBT has also been found to be superior to gestalt group treatment (Beutler et al., 1991; Beutler, Machad, Engle, & Mohr, 1993). On the other hand, much as with individual CBT, evidence that adding group CBT to medication treatment has a more beneficial impact than either treatment alone has been somewhat more elusive (Burlingame et al., 2004). Interestingly, at least four studies utilizing a variety of methodologies have not established that CBT group treatment is more effective than self-help interventions or placebo (Burlingame et al., 2004). One argument that has been advanced to explain mixed findings with CBT groups for depression is that these treatments have not formally taken into account group process factors, and thus do not take advantage of these factors to produce better outcomes (Burlingame et al., 2004).

Taken together, evidence from both meta-analyses and "box-score" reviews points to the overall efficacy of group CBT for depression compared to control and alternative conditions, a conclusion supported by other reviewers of empirically supported treatments (DeRubeis & Crits-Christoph, 1998).

The most pressing question that is not fully answered is whether group and individual CBT can be considered equivalent.

GROUP ASASESSMENT ISSUES

Assessing Eligibility for Group CBT

A thorough description of diagnostic and assessment issues in depression is beyond the scope of this chapter; however, diagnostic screening on both Axis I and II disorders is recommended prior to group CBT. Given the heterogeneity of depression and comorbidity rates, it is important to assess carefully for not only the mood disorder of interest but also other presenting problems. Various clinical settings and clinicians make different decisions about the inclusion of a range of comorbidity; that is, some clinicians elect to treat patients with only major depressive disorder as opposed to patients with dysthymia or major depressive disorder, or a combination of both. The decision on whether to "allow" comorbidity with other common conditions, for example, anxiety disorder(s), is complex, and is considered in greater detail in Chapter 16. In any case, problems are more likely to arise in situations in which diagnostic screening has not been of sufficient depth or breadth, and comorbidity has gone undetected in screening. Once patients are enrolled in a group, the presence of comorbidity often becomes very apparent in both process and application of techniques. Decisions about how to handle this comorbidity are best made before the group starts rather than post hoc. In the instance of previously undetected comorbidity, therapists must all too quickly decide whether and how to alter the group agenda and structure to address this problem. Aside from diagnostic inclusion and exclusion criteria, a group suitability interview process, such as that described in Chapter 5, is an important consideration as well.

Assessing Treatment Outcome

As in individual CBT, the focus of treatment is certainly not only symptoms but also function and reducing vulnerability to future depressive episodes. The assessment of symptoms can be accomplished by a variety of measures, though, for the sake of efficiency, a self-report scale is likely to be preferred. Perhaps the most commonly used scale for the assessment of depression severity is the revised Beck Depression Inventory (BDI). The BDI, described in further detail in Appendix 10.1, is simple to administer and relatively short (21 items taking 5–10 minutes), and at the same time accurately assesses a variety of important domains. Typically, patients are provided with a BDI as they arrive at the group session. The scale can usually be completed while other members arrive, before the start of the group itself. Obviously, a self-report scale that takes a short time has many strengths compared to clinician ratings or assessments that could take up important group time. The BDI also has the advantage of having a specific item concerning suicidality (item 9). Clinicians reviewing the scales (often this would be the cotherapist, while the therapist leads the group), can not only determine overall severity but can also readily recognize any increases in suicidality or hopelessness. Also, the meaning of scores and ranges of scores can be discussed with patients. It is also possible to "plot" scores on a chart, allowing participants to see the pattern of their scores over time. This pattern of scores, and changes in symptoms, likely also form a component of the formal documentation for group members in progress notes or discharge summaries. Finally, the BDI scores can be meaningful for structure and process of the group. Participants whose scores decrease substantially may well be a focus for discussing successful applications of techniques that have been learned. At the same time, participants whose scores have increased can also be a focus in order to better understand why symptoms have increased and what techniques may be useful to control their symptoms more effectively.

Another domain of outcome in treatment includes broader factors, such as functioning and quality of life. Measurement of these domains may not need to occur on a weekly basis, but instead could occur at the beginning and end of treatment. Changes in these domains, in addition to symptoms, can be useful for determining the overall success of the group for the individual; because of the broad nature of these scales, they may also point to areas other than symptoms that need to be addressed. The scales described in Appendix 10.1 focus on different areas of life, in which depression might interfere with normal functioning.

Finally, it may be desirable to measure variables that go beyond observable symptoms and functioning, and assess underlying cognitive vulnerability variables, including dysfunctional attitudes and attributional style. A full discussion of the literature supporting these variables as vulnerability factors is beyond the scope of this chapter; interested readers are referred to comprehensive sources (e.g., Clark, Beck, et al., 1999). A description of the most relevant concepts and measures is provided in Appendix 10.1. Numerous studies have suggested that the types of attributions made for events put an individual at risk for depression. Similarly, presence of activated dysfunctional attitudes has been shown to predict relapse to depression. Thus, the most desirable outcome in the treatment of depression goes beyond symptom reduction and control; it may also be important to assess pre- to posttreatment changes at this level of cognition.

STRUCTURING GROUP TREATMENT

Number of Participants

Importantly, there are few data on optimal group size in CBT for depression. Data that do exist concern groups from a variety of approaches, and these data suggest that group sizes between 3 and 12 participants are equally effective (Robinson et al., 1990). The advantage of a somewhat smaller number, up to perhaps seven participants, is that it is often possible to work on one example with all individuals in each group session. This removes the need to determine, for clinical, technique, and process reasons, which individual's examples, or which individual, should be the focus during session. However, as the number of individuals in a group decreases, efficiency of the group approach also decreases. Thus, more typical sizes for a depression group may well be 10–12 members. When groups exceed 12 members, there is not likely to be sufficient time to work effectively with each person. Moreover, with this many members, participants may have so little time to speak or listen to one another that it is difficult for group cohesion to develop. Group members need to attain a certain level of familiarity with one another's narratives and situations to feel comfortable asking questions or offering important expressions of support. Moreover, it becomes more difficult in a larger group to draw out group members who may be struggling with the techniques, whose depression is more severe, or who have social anxiety about disclosing in the group. In smaller groups, there is more time to draw out group members for the sake of cohesion and to ensure that each individual understands and can implement the techniques that have been taught.

Another important principle is to ensure that group members receive the same amount of attention from therapists. It is not unusual for some group members to volunteer examples consistently or even draw the attention of the group to themselves consistently across sessions. This may be because these individuals are experiencing fewer symptoms and are eager to describe their successes. Focusing on members who are pleased to volunteer their examples can often be the path of least resistance for therapists too, especially if these individuals understand and use the techniques, and other group members seem reticent to put forward their own examples. Although focusing on successfully implemented techniques can be important, it is equally important to ensure that all group participants have the opportunity to have the therapists and the group focus on them. Otherwise, the group risks having some members who understand and use the techniques, and others who may not understand the strategies or feel a sense of belonging to the group. Ensuring equal attention to all members may require being more directive with participants, but it is often the only way to involve group members who are more severely depressed and withdrawn.

Structure of Group Sessions

A closed format for CBT depression groups was first promulgated by Hollon and Shaw in their initial explorations of this approach, and in depression, closed groups have been the norm. The group is typically led by two therapists, either one primary leader and a coleader or two coleaders. The latter approach is suggested only when therapists have previously worked together and have a strong sense of how to divide the material evenly, and whose central message is highly consistent. A primary leader and coleader format is often preferable for clarity, in that one person is primarily responsible for delivery of techniques and leading process, and the other therapist contributes in a planned way. The coleader, having fewer moment-to-moment responsibilities in the group, can also often observe patient and process factors, and point these out to the leader as needed. We suggest a 2-hour session length, because it can often take extra time to start the group, and this length allows more opportunities to include as many individuals as possible in the discussion and examples.

In a number of other ways, aside from length, the overall structure of a group session reflects individual CBT for depression and the generic structure described in Chapter 5. First, the use of a symptom inventory allows for an accurate and efficient assessment of patients' current state. These inventories can be completed in the waiting area or at the beginning of group and be handed to the group therapists. It is also desirable to collect the homework at the beginning of sessions, for reasons described in the group process section of this chapter.

Each group session starts with a review of each person's experiences over the past week. This needs to be done efficiently to keep the session on track. Areas to be covered for each person should include symptom severity, use of techniques (or homework), and any other relevant life events. This is useful both for therapists and for other group members to understand what has occurred in the individual's life in the intervening interval. As in individual sessions, both the content and affect of these summaries are important for determining the nature of the agenda and relevant examples. For example, a number of group members may describe problems doing or understanding the homework. This may be an indication that therapists need to review more and confirm group members' understanding before introducing new material.

The next component of the session involves a description of the previous week's content and how this relates to the planned agenda. It is important to offer opportunities for group members to ask questions at this point, and this bridging between sessions should not be rushed or cursory. Next, the agenda should formally be set; it is preferable to record this on a flipchart or whiteboard for the group to follow visually. This can also be the time to decide which group members' examples, and in what order, should be the focus of the session. Again, there should be explicit time set aside to ask whether group members have items to add to the agenda, and these need to be triaged carefully by the therapists. A large component of the "art" of group leadership is balancing new material to be learned, while also attending to the needs of group members to facilitate cohesion. Too much emphasis on either side of this balance is undesirable; in the former instance, the group may become too much like a "course" or lecture, because members do not feel an affective or interpersonal connection between themselves and the material. In the latter instance, not moving forward with the learning of techniques and skills can result in a group that is stuck on disclosure and affect processing rather than changing problems by applying techniques.

The group next proceeds through the agenda, ideally in the planned order. During this component of the work, therapists need to be acutely aware of their time management. This involves a strong sense of the direction of the group, how much time can be spent on examples, and what is left to cover. As in individual treatment, frequent summaries should be offered by the therapists to consolidate learning. Finally, near the end of the session, therapists must manage one of the most important transitions, setting the stage for homework that is clear, understandable, and related to group members' affective experiences. The single most important factor in accomplishing this is to leave sufficient time for discussion and dissemination of the homework plan. Often, due to time constraints, work on examples can threaten to make homework assignment an afterthought as the group draws to a close. As a result, therapists may not have sufficient time to explain the nature of the homework and its relationship to the session. Similarly, group members may not have time to ask questions about the homework, and any uncertainty very often leads to compliance problems. Ironically, this can lead to a more in-depth discussion of the previous week's homework tasks at the start of the next session—a discussion that should have occurred in the previous session but did not, because time had run out! As a general guide, the last example of the day should be completed with at least 10 minutes of group time left to transition into the homework discussion. This not only allows time for questions and answers but it also emphasizes the central importance of the homework to therapy and group members' progress toward their goals.

OVERVIEW OF CBT STRATEGIES IN DEPRESSION

The 17-session protocol described here (see Table 10.1) was derived from a combination of sources, including Beck and colleagues' (1979) seminal reference and Greenberger and Padesky's (1995) *Mind over Mood*, which is recommended to patients as a companion manual for this group. This protocol consists of 14 weekly sessions based on a linear approach to teaching the various behavioral and cognitive strategies. Sessions 15 and 16 follow, with 2-week intervals between each session. These sessions are also more open-ended in terms of agenda and techniques based on group needs. The final session, a month after sessions 15 and 16, is designed to introduce the concept of relapse and relapse prevention. As an option, booster sessions may continue at bimonthly or monthly intervals, with a focus on retention of gains and relapse prevention.

In this section we review in greater depth some of the unique features of this protocol in the treatment of depression. We focus on not only technique factors in each session but also some of the more common process issues that arise in this protocol for depression.

TABLE 10.1. Sample Outline of Treatment Protocol for Group CBT for Depression

Session	Strategies covered

Session 1	• Introduce therapists and group members.
	• Group "rules."
	  1. Confidentiality.
	  2. Check-in and rating scales.
	  3. Homework.
	  4. Missing appointments.
	• Introduce the CBT approach to depression.
	  1. Behavioral interventions.
	  2. Cognitive Interventions.
	• Describe the biopsychosocial model of depression and introducing the five components.
	  1. Behavior
	  2. Thoughts
	  3. Emotions
	  4. Biology
	  5. Environment
	• Homework: Complete biopsychosocial model and purchase companion manual.

Session 2	• Goal setting.
	  1. Eliciting goals from patients.
	  2. Specifying behavioral changes to meet goals.
	  3. How to track goals and monitor progress.
	• Outline relationship between mood state and behavior.
	• Introduce mood/emotion rating system.
	• Demonstrate relationship between activities and mood (i.e., what activities improve mood, what activities worsen mood).
	• Homework: Complete activity schedule with activities and mood ratings.

Session 3	• Behavioral interventions: Modifying activities to improve mood.
	  1. Introduce the concepts of mastery (sense of accomplishment) and pleasure, using examples from past to illustrate these types of activities.
	  2. Focus on adding mastery and pleasure activities to establish balance of reinforcement.
	• Homework: Complete activity schedule with new activities added in and rate mood.

Session 4	• Examine outcome of behavioral modifications and adjust where needed. • Identify "mood shifts" to target with cognitive interventions. • Label and rate emotion(s) experienced in difficult situations from examples. • Homework: First two columns of dysfunctional thought record (DTR; situation and emotion) to be completed.
Session 5	• Review examples of thought records: Situation description and emotion identification. • Describe interpretation and "self-talk" as the link between situation and emotion, using patients' examples. • Automatic and "hot thoughts": Focusing on the thought most related to the emotion. • Homework: First three columns of the DTR, and identifying hot thoughts.

(continued)

TABLE 10.1. *(continued)*

Session	Strategies covered
Session 6	• Review examples from thought records: situation, mood, and thoughts description. • Identify hot thoughts in the examples. • Introduce the evidence technique, finding evidence "for" the hot thought. • Evaluate evidence that is "for" hot thoughts. • Homework: First four columns of the DTR (adding evidence "for" the hot thought).
Session 7	• Review examples from thought records: situation, mood, thoughts, and evidence "for" the hot thought. • Introduce "evidence against" by asking questions to bring out new facts that do not support the hot thought. • Use patient examples to illustrate questioning to elicit evidence for and against automatic thoughts. • Homework: First five columns of the DTR (adding evidence "against" the hot thought).
Session 8	• Introduce the "thought distortion" list to illustrate that biases in thinking may occur systematically. • Illustrate examples of cognitive errors in examples recorded. • Homework: First five columns of the DTR and identifying the distortion.
Session 9	• Introduce "alternative thoughts," including how to write them. • Troubleshoot alternative thoughts, including ignoring evidence, misspecification of hot thought, activation of core belief. • Homework: Complete DTR (adding alternative thought and mood rerating).
Session 10	• Review thought record examples in which insufficient information exists to draw a conclusion. • Introduce experiments: When there is insufficient evidence to draw a conclusion and more information is needed, devise a way to collect that information. • Create an experiment that is consistent with a patient example. • Homework: Execute the experiment and monitor the outcome.
Session 11	• Review thought records that identify a problem that needs to be solved. • Introduce problem-solving strategies when the evidence suggests a problem that needs to be resolved. • Use a group member's examples to create a problem-solving plan. • Homework: Complete the problem-solving task.
Session 12	• Introduce "deep cognition"; concepts of conditional assumptions and core beliefs. • Illustrate deep cognition using "downward arrow" technique. • Describe downward arrow as used for conditional assumptions about self, others, and the world. • Homework: Complete a downward arrow exercise.
Session 13	• Explain the connection between conditional assumptions and core beliefs. • Illustrate the "continuum" model of core beliefs and emphasize prospective techniques to change core beliefs.

(continued)

TABLE 10.1. (continued)

Session	Strategies covered
Session 13 (cont.)	• Describe evidence gathering, experiments, and problem-solving plans for changing typical patterns of coping and collecting information to support alternative core beliefs. • Homework: Generate a continuum of core beliefs and keep track of evidence concerning alternative core belief.
Session 14	• Introduce coping strategies associated with core beliefs. • Use patients' examples to illustrate the potential self-defeating nature of coping strategies. • Propose alternative coping strategies for patients. • Homework: Implement alternative coping strategies and monitor outcome of the alternatives.
Session 15	• Biweekly booster session to integrate and implement skills learned, as directed by patients.
Session 16	• Biweekly booster session to integrate and implement skills learned, as directed by patients.
Session 17	• Introduce the concepts of lapse and relapse. • Introduce strategies for dealing with lapse and relapse. • Plan patient-specific strategies for coping in relapse. • Wrap-up.

Behavioral Techniques

Perhaps one of the most notable characteristics of the depressed patient is the manner in which his or her life is devoid of gratification and a sense of accomplishment. As a result of loss of reinforcement from usual activities, the depressed person withdraws from many activities. Even those activities that are completed (work or other obligations) are seen to be a chore and not at all enjoyable. In many cases, at the outset of treatment, depressed people may not have enough energy to begin examining their thoughts. They appear sad, and their rate of speech may be slow; impoverished expression of affect is typical. Behavioral activation can increase the depressed person's energy level and set the stage for cognitive strategies.

Because of this "behavioral profile" in depression, CBT usually begins with strategies related to activation. In the protocol, Sessions 2, 3, and a portion of Session 4 address these issues. In Session 2, patients are oriented to the notion of goals, typically translated into behavioral terms, and the steps necessary to reach those goals. This counters hopelessness and helplessness, and specifies reasonable expectations and a way to move in that direction. More formal activation begins by having patients monitor, or record, their daily activities (hour for hour) and rate their mood for each waking hour of the day; this information is processed in Session 3. This is perhaps the most accurate and comprehensive way to understand the patient's level of functioning, and it provides an excellent "snapshot" of the person's life. Also, having patients monitor their usual activities is a quite involving, straightforward assignment that helps to socialize them to the CBT model of homework early in the sessions.

Once the therapists have examined the schedule, they focus on a number of behavioral factors in Session 3. First, how withdrawn is the patient from usual activities of daily living? Are there adequate exposures to potentially reinforcing situations? Perhaps most importantly, is there a balance of pleasurable events and events that lead to a sense of accomplishment (or mastery)? Most often, both a dearth of activity and an imbalance of mastery and pleasurable activities need to be remedied. During this phase of treatment, group members can be encouraged to comment on one another's monitoring homework. This typically represents the first occasion in which group members provide feedback to one another. Importantly, group members usually can readily spot problems with others' activities, seeing stressors, frustrations, and also possibilities for more rewarding activities. It is therefore important for group leaders to point out the ease with which one can fall into routines that involve "blinders" that make it difficult to evaluate behavioral alternatives that might be more rewarding.

The next phase in behavioral activation, again in Session 3, is to explain the notions of mastery and pleasure (or work and play) to the group, and explain that a balance in the perception of these must be in place to achieve satisfaction and happiness. The therapists also explain to the group how the onset of depression can lead to withdrawing from events and activities that actually may improve mood and energy level. The group members are likely to be able to offer many ready examples. Along with this, the group therapists can point to times in the course of the week when a group member was active, and his or her mood was improved. It may be useful to use metaphors, such as the "battery" metaphor, which describes a typical, depressive way of viewing one's energy level. One wakes with a certain level of energy that gets used up by activities and is then depleted. It is always helpful to demonstrate, with group examples, that humans fit much more closely with a "generator" model than a "battery." In other words, engaging in activities draws out more energy that is replenished, for example, by eating and drinking. Only a "generator" metaphor can explain the finding that vigorous exercise results in greater alertness and energy when it is completed.

As a result of this rationale, group members are encouraged to "experiment" with their level of activity, and are asked to introduce new activities in what is termed a graded task assignment. There are a number of ways to identify activities that might be rewarding, and to have group members contribute to one another's list of potential new behaviors to implement. The most commonly used strategies involve asking about past activities, hobbies, and pastimes that were once enjoyable. Group members can learn from this experience not only about the commonalities in pleasurable events but also marked differences in what can be rewarding to one person versus another. This typically reinforces more divergent, creative thinking, allowing all group members to think more broadly and with less self-censoring, pessimism, or criticism of themselves.

Often, even when a group member identifies potentially reinforcing behaviors from the past, it has been a long time since the person engaged in those activities. This is probably a result of the depressed person's pessimism ("This won't make me feel better") and is an excellent opportunity to reinforce the need to always test one's predictions by actually engaging in the behavior. Another strategy is to ask what kinds of things the person has always wanted to try, without ever having had the opportunity to do so. This may also involve brainstorming with other group members to create a set of steps to engage in that activity. Such exchanges need to be encouraged by therapists, and sometimes critical bits of information or questions are all that are needed from therapists to keep a productive dialogue in progress. Indeed, as much as possible, it is desirable to allow group members to work with one another to plan events. This facilitates group cohesion, less self-focus, and efficacy in members who are helping one another. A third alternative for adding behaviors is for the group to examine and discuss the pleasant events list (e.g., MacPhillamy & Lewinsohn, 1982), which contains hundreds of pleasant activities from which to choose. Reviewing this list can also be a component of homework.

Adding such activities has benefits on two fronts. Most concretely, they raise patients' energy level and are likely to lead to better concentration and less fatigue. Second, patients begin to see themselves as more competent and as accomplishing more. Thus, such assignments are likely to produce both functional and cognitive benefits. Group discussion of planned activities, the homework for Session 3, can be very useful for building motivation and a sense of camaraderie in adding to one's behavioral repertoire. Very often, one patient identifying an activity he or she would like to try triggers other members to follow suit. One group member making a behavioral plan can set an important tone for others, and it may be useful to work on as many examples as possible in the time allotted.

Feedback about the outcome of these behaviors is elicited in the first portion of Session 4. Here, too, ample time should be provided for group members to discuss their "findings." Important questions to seed group discussion include "How did things turn out?", "Was the response they got from (themselves, others) what they predicted?", "What lesson do they learn about depression from this exercise?", and "What are the implications of this outcome for the immediate and long-term future?" The goal by the end of the behavioral activation section is for group members to mutually reinforce attempts to change depressive behavioral habits and more actively cope with their illness. As in individual treatment, the increase in group members' physical energy and perceptions of self-efficacy become very useful when the group therapists begin working on the depressive cognitions. This part of treatment also sets the stage for group members to offer each other supportive, encouraging, but also probing feedback. Critically, the behavioral activation aspect of the treatment provides a prototype for positive and collaborative group process prior to working through the more affectively laden, usually very private aspects of the treatment protocol, such as core beliefs.

Cognitive Techniques for Automatic Thoughts

Overview

In depressed patients, thinking reflects the "cognitive triad." Patients have a preponderance of highly salient, negative thoughts and beliefs about themselves, others, and the world (Beck et al., 1979). Since this model of depression was put forward, literally hundreds of carefully controlled studies have been conducted to test its every aspect. Overall, the research evidence points to strong support for these ideas (Clark, Beck, et al., 1999).

Clinically, when depressed patients describe their thoughts, the content of these cognitions is likely to be pervasively pessimistic and negative, especially in response to any problematic or even ambiguous events. The depressed person can be seen as having a set of filters that encodes only "bad news" and pays little heed to the "good news" that occurs. When the depressed person encounters a positive event, he or she is likely to see it as a chance occurrence or a passing event. This cognitive error is usually described clinically as "minimizing" and is also intimately related to the attributional style associated with depression. It is often striking how a depressed person, recounting a seemingly positive event to the group, can turn such a happening (e.g., a compliment, a good work evaluation) into something that is seen as not very important. As a general guide, one theme of cognitive strategies in the protocol is that group leaders, and in time other group members, point out minimizing when it occurs, so that group members pay greater attention to positive events. Another cognitive process that may occur in response to positive events is to deny responsibility for the good outcome. The depressed person is likely to see the positive event as being related to outside factors, such as luck or the result of other people's doing. The aim of the group, then, is to help the patient evaluate more accurately where the responsibility for positive events truly lies.

When encountering negative events (an interpersonal slight, a poor grade, or other difficulties), depressed people have almost the opposite reaction. They see themselves as 100% responsible for the negative outcome. Most of the many specific distortions at work here represent an inability to take into account all of the factors associated with a negative outcome (other than the person's own doing). This represents a second theme in cognitive work on depression in a group. For example, a poor grade may have as much to do with the test as with the test taker, perhaps because the test was written at too difficult a level, or because of other objective factors that account for poor performance. These factors are unlikely to occur to the depressed patient affected by the event; however, with very basic modeling of Socratic dialogue, group members become much more likely to ask one another these critical questions.

Specific Cognitive Strategies

The group protocol described here involves many of the strategies described in Chapter 3 and 4, including the thought record, experiments, problem solving, and the conditional and core beliefs exercise. We focus here on specific applications of these techniques in depression.

An initial point of departure is for patients in the group to begin to monitor their thoughts. The first discussions of "thoughts" occur around specific mood shifts that have been identified by patients following Greenberger and Padesky (1995) in Session 4. By Session 5, group members have completed the first three columns of a seven-column thought record (Greenberger & Padesky, 1995; situation, mood, thought) for discussion. This represents a critical foray by group members into examination of their own and others' thought content. Whereas concepts such as collaborative empiricism and Socratic dialogue have components of the behavioral interventions described previously, these now occur at another level for cognitive strategies. Through specific didactic discussion, but just as importantly, through modeling, group leaders can emphasize the necessary questions that reveal the nature of the thoughts underlying negative emotions.

During initial discussions of thought content, it is important to consider that this is likely the first time that group members have explored the true nature of their negative thoughts. Even more importantly, they are doing so in the context of a group, and are thus disclosing very private, emotionally laden, and possibly frightening material (e.g., suicidal thoughts or ideas). Thus, the protocol allows considerable time, an entire session, for the elicitation of thoughts before moving into disputation and evidence gathering. It is important to emphasize to group members their shared experience of negative thoughts, and the universality of this experience in depression. Another important reason to spend time simply eliciting automatic thoughts is to communicate the need to identify that most salient "hot thought" around which evidence gathering or disputation will occur. It may be useful for therapists to emphasize, as they would in individual therapy, that recording and discussing negative thoughts could well lead to more feelings of depression initially. The need to specify the nature of negative thoughts as the first step to reducing their impact may need to be discussed several times in Sessions 4 and 5.

As discussion of cognitive strategies continues, group interaction becomes steadily more important, especially as therapy progresses toward examining the veracity of thoughts. The protocol focuses on four major themes for exploring the basis of thoughts: evidence gathering (Session 6, 7), labeling of distortions (Session 8), experiments (Session 10), and problem solving, when there is some truth to a negative thought (Session 11). Teaching these techniques should ideally be highly interactive, with group members often questioning one another, pointing out alternative viewpoints to a cognitive distortion or potential ways around a real obstacle in problem solving, or offering feedback that forms the backbone of an experiment. During these sessions, the therapist has four main tasks whose goal is keeping the discussion focused on topic.

First the group leader needs to determine which examples will be chosen for group work. Although each group member should ultimately receive an equal share of focus, particular examples chosen within any one session may depend on several parameters. For example, when using evidence gathering for the very first time, a relatively straightforward example is most useful as a teaching aid. However, if the aim is to illustrate deeper beliefs and their role in negative thoughts, therapists may go out of their way to discuss a complicated thought record that will lead to an examination of these issues. Also, some thought records or experiments are more salient to group members than others because of shared experiences. For example, thought records that involve themes of loss, inadequacy, or unlovability are likely to be relevant to almost all group members. Finally, therapists must determine how well thought records and other tasks are being completed. Participants who are struggling and fall short of completing accurate, meaningful thought records are likely to benefit from having their examples worked on by the group. On the other hand, those examples will take more time to work through and discuss compared to examples that are more complete.

The second task during the sessions on negative thoughts is for group leaders to "seed" questions that stimulate a Socratic dialogue. Once therapists have modeled questions or applied different distortions to several examples, it is preferable to ask group members to begin any example with questions that occur to them. Practically, the therapist might record the example on a whiteboard or flipchart, then ask the group, "What questions do people think we should ask about this thought?" The therapist then simply records the questions and answers. However, it is possible that, on their own, group members may not touch upon areas that the therapist(s) believe are important, or they might have trouble initiating a sequence of questions that productively uncovers evidence. When this occurs, group leaders may need to shape discussions with questions in a way that is both redirective and empathic to the group members. The group dialogue that occurs around thought records is one of the most critical and productive phases of therapy. As group members question one another, they are also learning how to question their own thoughts. Moreover, it is not unusual for group members to ask questions of one another that the therapists might not have thought of; this is the benefit of having many people considering the same problem at once, each with his or her unique perspective.

Similar approaches should be cultivated for experiments and problem solving. It may be most helpful to start with a straightforward example in which the therapist is fairly directive, asking most of the questions and offering input. Subsequent examples shaped by the therapist, for example, may help frame the major question or hypothesis in an experiment that is most relevant to a group member's example. However, the different possible ways of evaluating that hypothesis might be discussed among group members, with only occasional input from the therapist, as needed.

The third task during this part of the protocol is to ensure that the group dialogue stays productive in terms of the techniques being taught. For example, one group member may provide evidence or an observation for another, rather than asking a question. This can be effective in a limited way; that is, the person whose example is being discussed might shift his or her perspective. However, there is an obvious benefit to creating collaborative empiricism among group members as opposed to having group members simply reassure each other. Therapists need to help group members stay focused on the Socratic questioning approach by continuing to emphasize its benefits.

Finally, group leaders need to manage time and the agenda carefully during these sessions. It can be all too easy to spend a great deal of time on one or two examples rather than working through the four or five examples on the agenda. Therapists need to be attuned to making solid progress on examples rather than working them through to completion in every instance. If a member's example requires more work than the group can provide in any single session, then this can form part of the homework for that group member.

Cognitive Techniques for Beliefs in CBT Depression Groups

In depression, the cognitive model suggests that deeply held core beliefs lead to other levels of cognition, including automatic thoughts. Session 12 introduces this concept to the group and marks a return to more didactic work to explain the connection between the readily observable "automatic thought," early life events, and "deep" levels of cognition. The therapist can usually effectively communicate this through an example, possibly focusing on a generic case before moving to group members' examples.

The first of numerous techniques related to deep cognition is the downward arrow. This approach, rather than examining what evidence exists for automatic thoughts, explores the meaning and possible early origins of automatic thoughts (see also Chapter 3). In Session 12, the construct of conditional assumptions, or affectively laden evaluative rules patients have for themselves and others, is also described. Session 13 focuses on core beliefs and early learning, and the therapist works with group members to create a narrative of how they learned their various core beliefs and assumptions. Sessions 13 and 14 also focus on long-term change strategies that can be implemented to help group members move away from rigid, self-defeating rules, and offer an alternative set of rules toward which to work.

Discussion of "deep cognition" can often lead to higher levels of affect than almost any other phase of therapy. However, by this time in the life cycle of the group, cohesion is typically high, and group members are able to provide, and benefit from, mutual support and empathy. In addition, there may be considerable complexity in working with group members to understand how early life events influence their current patterns of automatic thoughts. Therapists can emphasize that changes in these areas may take some time, usually well beyond the time needed to conclude the therapy sessions, and that uncovering these conditional assumptions and core beliefs means that the individual is "on the right track," and that identification of these beliefs is truly the most important step toward moving past them. For example, in Sessions 13 through 16, group members can be asked to rate their degree of belief in both the old belief and the new core beliefs or conditional assumptions. Group members are also encouraged to gather both new and historical information that supports the new, alternative belief.

These deep cognition sessions are in some ways less structured than the earlier sessions. Discussions may involve reflecting on early life events, focusing on the rigidity of certain conditional assumptions, or exploring a core belief, and group discussion can be expected to move between and around these points. At the same time, therapists need to provide opportunities to implement various worksheets and exercises, including the downward arrow, a positive events log, and a core belief worksheet. Sessions 15 and 16 similarly have no specific preplanned agenda. However, a group-driven agenda should be made to review techniques that group members nominate as helpful or for which "refresher" practice may be useful.

The final session is used to discuss relapse and to prepare group members for times when their mood might become worse. It is important to emphasize that some negative affect is a part of living, particularly in response to stressors. Strategies to reduce negative affect that have been learned in the group should be revisited and summarized. At the same time, the notion of relapse needs to be emphasized, so that group members seek proper follow-up should they suffer a relapse. It is therefore important to describe the criteria and signs of a developing clinical depression. It may also be useful to describe possibilities for relapse prevention, such as mindfulness-based cognitive therapy (MBCT; Segal, Williams, & Teasdale, 2002) or self-help relapse approaches (Bieling & Antony, 2003).

GROUP PROCESS FACTORS IN CBT FOR DEPRESSION

Prior to the development of the cognitive model of treatment, conventional clinical wisdom suggested that a group modality was contraindicated in depression (Hollon & Shaw, 1979). This was based on the twin premises that the needs of depressed patients exceeded what could be offered in a group and that the group process would contribute to a negative spiral of unfavorable self-comparisons, and displays of pessimism and hopelessness about the possibility for change. During their initial explorations of a group CBT approach, Hollon and Shaw suggested that these factors would be less of an issue in a homogeneous group of depressed patients than in a heterogeneous group that included only some depressed patients; that is, previous accounts of group process tended to consider the impact of only one or two very depressed individuals within a group of higher functioning, less impaired individuals. However, the more compelling question was what would happen in a setting in which patients all suffered from depression? Would depression in a group setting cause a spiraling depressive process?

The ensuing years and experience with CBT groups for depression suggest that, in the main, group process does not result in patients becoming worse, nor do depressed group members typically "act" in a stereotypically depressed way. Indeed, the efficacy of group CBT approaches is testimony that the dire predictions of increasing pessimism and hopelessness are unfounded. At the same time, when process problems do occur in depression, hopelessness, pessimism, and social comparison are often the culprits.

For example, one of the most common process problems in a CBT group is when one patient considers him- or herself, perhaps accurately, as more depressed and impaired than some others in the group. Such a patient may not participate as actively in the group, and may evidence pessimism about the homework, for example, by predicting that a pleasant activity exercise will not be at all enjoyable and is not worth doing. Both the group leaders and the group itself play a key role in resolving this kind of process problem. Ideally, the response to pessimism and hopelessness is a combination of empathy, encouragement, and also persistence. Indeed, this happens almost naturally in most groups. Earlier writers may well have underestimated the capacity for empathy and understanding that most depressed people have for others, especially fellow sufferers. In the preceding example, pessimism about the usefulness of pleasant activities, an ideal and quite typical response is for other group members to empathize with the patient who is pessimistic, possibly by relating times when they have been pessimistic themselves. If this does not occur spontaneously, empathy, support, and encouragement can also be modeled by group leaders, possibly drawing out other members' examples of low points through which they have battled. To conclude the example, group leaders would then need to carefully leverage this empathy and support with gentle persistence about at least attempting the pleasant event before drawing conclusions about whether it is worhwhile. This fairly simple approach—empathy, understanding, and support, followed by a change strategy—is a critical tool for dealing with other "depressogenic" group processes, including social comparison, rejection of help, and even suicidal or self-harm ideation. In each instance, the group must acknowledge the validity of the person's feelings and thoughts, yet also communicate that change, even from this difficult position, is not only possible but also has happened for others.

There are few, but not insignificant, instances in which specific members of a group do have needs that exceed the capacity of the group. Patients with very serious suicidal ideation and intent, and those whose concentration and ability to understand the material falls well below the group average, may need to seen individually. At the same time, one instance of a group member not understanding or being very pessimistic should be tolerated within the group. Many times these behaviors change over the course of sessions, and such progress can provide important examples of overcoming obstacles and typically end up increasing cohesion. Only if group members consistently demonstrate a lack of understanding or interest in the group process should other treatment options be considered. A rigorous screening process, described earlier in this chapter, also contributes to minimizing the number of patients who might need an alternative approach.

Just as depressed individuals' capacity to support one another is often underestimated, so too is the ability of depressed patients to note "depressive" cognitive distortions and biased thinking in others. In a number of ways, this notable capacity is not surprising. In individual CBT, a common approach in having people question their thoughts is the general strategy of "perspective shift," in which a therapist asks the patient to consider how he or she would respond to a friend who had negative thoughts, or what friends would say if he or she shared these thoughts. In group treatment, having other people offer fresh perspectives is integral to nearly all cognitive interventions, and it is an important form of sharing and mutual support for members to ask questions about one another's thoughts and even point out alternative perspectives. At the same time, some group members may tend to focus on offering others new perspectives or to note others' distortions without recognizing their own! Thus, an important part of group process in depression is, ironically, to ensure that participants focus on the ability to question their own thoughts as incisively as they help others to question theirs. Whenever one patient uses a questioning strategy to help someone else, it can be useful for therapists to reflect those questions back, to determine whether the group member is learning to question his or her own negative thoughts and assumptions.

CONCLUSIONS

The group CBT format was pioneered in the area of depression, and evidence for the effectiveness of the approach has accumulated for over 20 years. The techniques used in depression represent almost all of the basic cognitive strategies, and for this reason, CBT depression groups are a very effective introduction for therapists who are new to the group format. Mastering these techniques in a depression group is an important building block for treating more complex disorders such as bipolar disorder and Axis II conditions in a group. Finally, although a reasonable volume of efficacy data has accumulated for CBT groups in depression, much remains to be discovered about process factors and effective ingredients. We anticipate that the next challenge in the field will be to document which factors are associated with individual and group change. This could in turn lead to further specification and optimization of techniques and process to achieve the best possible outcomes.

APPENDIX 10.1. OUTCOME MEASURES
FOR CBT DEPRESSION GROUP

Self-Report Symptom Scales

Beck Depression Inventory, Second Edition (BDI-II; Beck, Steer, & Brown, 1996)

This 21-item measure is perhaps the most frequently used measure of severity of depressive symptoms. The items are based on criteria from DSM-IV, including sadness, guilt, suicidal thoughts, loss of interest, and physical manifestations such as sleep, appetite, and energy difficulties. The measure takes only 5–10 minutes to complete, and cutoff scores are available to characterize the ranges of depression symptoms, though the instrument does not make a diagnosis per se (Beck et al., 1996). A score of 0–13 reflects minimal depression, 14–19 reflects mild depression, 20–28 reflects moderate depression, and a score of 29 or more reflects severe depression. Reliability of the scale is excellent and validity is also high. For example, the correlation with the best known interviewer-administered scale for depression, the Hamilton Rating Scale for Depression (HRSD), is .71 (Beck et al., 1996).

Depression Anxiety Stress Scales (DASS; Lovibond & Lovibond, 1995a, 1995b)

This scale, available either in a 42-item version or a 21-item short form, has the advantage of assessing both depression and anxiety symptoms, as well as a more general stress dimension. Indeed, the scale was expressly designed to discriminate between anxiety and depression, which typically correlate highly. The factor structure and reliability of the scale have been established in clinical populations (Antony, Bieling, Cox, Enns, & Swinson, 1998). The DASS does indeed distinguish between features of depression, physical hyperarousal, and psychological tension and agitation, and has good-to-excellent concurrent validity. Moreover, various diagnostic groups have different DASS profiles that are consistent with their clinical presentation (Antony et al., 1998).

Zung Self-Rating Depression Scale (Zung SDS; Zung, 1965)

The Zung SDS, a 20-item self-report measure designed for individuals with a primary diagnosis of depression, asks the participant to rate what proportion of time a symptom is experienced (*a little time* to *most of the time*). The scale is based on a factor analysis of the common symptoms of depression and appears to have good reliability. The Zung SDS correlates highly with other measures of depression (.80 with the HRSD, and .54 with the first edition of the BDI; Nezu, Ronan, Meadows, & McClure, 2000).

Quality-of-Life Measures

Quality of Life Enjoyment and Satisfaction Questionnaire (Q-LES-Q; Endicott et al., 1993)

The Q-LES-Q was developed as a self-report instrument (60 items) to assess the enjoyment and satisfaction experienced in numerous areas of daily life. The measure has five subscales: physical health, subjective feelings, leisure time activities, social relationships, and general activities. The Q-LES-Q has quite high internal consistency and test–retest stability (Rabkin, Wagner, & Griffin, 2000), and is associated in expected ways with measures of symptoms and impairment. The Q-LES-Q has been shown to detect clinical changes in response to treatment (Rabkin et al., 2000).

Quality of Life Index (QLI; Ferrans & Powers, 1985)

The QLI is a self-report measure (70 items) developed to measure satisfaction with various life domains. The scale has two sections: One assesses satisfaction with each of 35 items; the other assesses the importance of these 35 specific items. The four domains covered by these items are health and functioning, socioeconomic, psychological or spiritual, and family. Internal consistency has been established for both the total scores and subscales, and test–retest stability over 2 weeks and 1 month was quite high. The QLI is correlated with other life satisfaction measures and is associated with levels of symptoms and coping in expected ways (Rabkin et al., 2000).

Functioning Measures

Illness Intrusiveness Rating Scale (IIRS; Devins, 1994)

Illness intrusions refer to lifestyle and activity disruptions that arise as a result of an illness and/or its treatment (Devins, 1994). The construct of illness intrusiveness, and the scale to assess it, has been used in a variety of both medical and psychiatric illnesses (Bieling, Rowa, Antony, Summerfeldt, & Swinson, 2001). The IIRS measure assesses the extent to which a particular problem causes impairment in 13 different life domains, including health, diet, work, active recreation (e.g., playing sports), passive recreation, finances, relationship with partner, sex life, family relations, other social relations, self-expression/improvement, religious expression, and community and civic involvement. The IIRS has shown good reliability (alphas ranging in the .80s and .90s) in both medical and psychiatric settings, and appears to be associated with symptom severity in anxiety disorders (Bieling et al., 2001).

Sheehan Disability Scale (SDS; Sheehan, 1983)

The SDS is a composite of three self-rated items designed to measure the extent to which three major sectors in the patient's life—work, social life, and family life—are impaired by psychiatric symptoms. Despite its brevity, the scale does display high internal consistency and substantial correlations among its three items (Williams, 2000). SDS scores are higher in patient groups compared to those who do not have psychiatric disorders; importantly, the sensitivity (.83), specificity (.69), positive predictive value (.47), and negative predictive value (.92) have been established for this scale (Williams, 2000). The scale is also sensitive to changes with treatment.

Social Adjustment Scale (SAS; Weissman & Bothwell, 1976)

The SAS is both an interview and a self-report used to assess social functioning over a 2-month (interview) or 2-week period (self-report). The SAS assess six areas: work, social and leisure activities, relationships with extended family, marital role as a spouse, role as a parent, and role as a member of the family unit. The questions in instrument center around the person's ability to complete tasks, degree of conflict, interpersonal behavior, and subjective sense of satisfaction (Weissman, 2000). The scale has adequate internal consistency and test–retest stability (over 2 weeks; Weissman, 2000). The SAS has been found to discriminate between groups with and without psychiatric illness, and is somewhat sensitive to changes due to treatment (Weissman, 2000).

Measures of Vulnerability to Depression

Attributional Style Questionnaire (ASQ; Peterson et al., 1982)

The ASQ is a self-report measure designed to assess perceptions of causality for negative and positive events, specifically, whether an event was due to external or internal factors, whether the cause is stable or fleeting, and whether the cause is global or specific. These attributions, or explanatory styles, are described as specific vulnerabilities to depression. For example, when negative events are interpreted as being due to internal, stable, and global causes, and positive events are seen as being due to external, fleeting, and specific causes, the individual is vulnerable to depression. The measure uses six vignettes and asks the respondent to make four ratings for each vignette. Reliability of this measure is adequate both in terms of internal consistency (Cronbach's alpha) and test–retest reliability. The validity of this instrument has previously been shown, and the ASQ has been utilized in the multisite Temple–Wisconsin Vulnerability to Depression Project (Alloy & Abramson, 1999). Importantly, high ASQ scores do seem to predict development of depressive disorder and symptoms in individuals who are asymptomatic (Alloy et al., 2000).

Dysfunctional Attitude Scales (DAS; Weissman & Beck, 1978)

The DAS was designed to assess maladaptive beliefs associated with depression. Many of the DAS items are explicitly written as "if . . . then" statements, that, if held in an extreme way, are rigid, maladaptive, and likely to lead to the experience of difficult emotions, including depression. The DAS is actually available in three forms, a 100-item version, and two more commonly used 40-item versions (Forms A and B). The factor structure of the DAS is determined by which version is at issue, and the two forms (A & B) appear to have different factors structures. Form A factors consist of need for approval, perfectionism, and avoidance of risk. Form B factors are need for success, need to impress others, need for approval, and need to control feelings (Oliver & Baumgert, 1985). The most comprehensive analysis of the DAS items, using the entire 100-item pool as a starting point, suggests that nine types of beliefs are reliably measured by the DAS: vulnerability, need for approval, success–perfectionism, need to please others, imperatives, need to impress, avoidance of appearing weak, control over emotions, and disapproval–dependence (Beck, Brown, Steer, & Weissman, 1991).

Bipolar Disorder

DESCRIPTION OF BIPOLAR DISORDER

Bipolar disorder is a frequently occurring, often severe psychiatric illness with a tremendous impact on individuals over the course of their lifespan (Cooke, Robb, Young, & Joffe, 1996; Harrow, Goldberg, Grossman, & Meltzer, 1990; Robb, Cooke, Devins, Young, & Joffe, 1997). On the World Health Organization's rankings of disease burden, using disability-adjusted life years (DALYs) as a common metric, bipolar disorder ranked number six in countries with developed market economies even though the prevalence rate for the disorder is just above 1% of the population. With its often unpredictable cycles of deep depressions followed by periods of mania, the disorder can wreak havoc on patients' lives. Bipolar disorder is a frequent cause of inpatient hospitalizations and places sufferers at increased risk of suicide. Both ends of the bipolar continuum lead to problems in functioning; the depressive episodes are characterized by the same symptoms as unipolar depression and undermine the individual's functional capacities. In addition, the manias/ hypomanias often generate their own unique set of problems and stressors in occupational, interpersonal, and financial domains. Bipolar disorder is also, for most, an illness that impacts individuals over their entire adult lifespan, with symptoms waxing and waning in potentially unpredictable ways.

For decades, bipolar disorder has been understood and treated through an exclusively biological lens. Indeed, based on heritability and the necessity of mood-stabilizing medications to achieve even a modicum of recovery, psychosocial interventions have tended to be overlooked, or at the very least understudied, in bipolar disorder. Nonetheless, the past decade has seen a number of developments in psychosocial therapies for this disorder, including a growing body of work advocating CBT as an important and effective adjunct to pharmacotherapy (Basco & Rush, 1996; Newman, Leahy, Beck, Reilly-Harrington, & Gyulai, 2002). This chapter describes bipolar disorder and its key clinical features, followed by a description of recent evidence for CBT, and a group approach to treatment of bipolar disorder.

Diagnostic Features

Fundamentally, bipolar disorder involves a combination of major depressive episodes and shorter, marked elevations in mood and energy called manias and hypomanias. The criteria for depression in bipolar disorder are identical to those for the major depressive episode that characterizes major depressive disorder. A major depressive episode involves at least 2 weeks of depressed mood or loss of interest; accompanied by four or more other symptoms (American Psychiatric Association [APA], 2000), including changes in weight or appetite, dysregulated sleep, physical agitation or retardation, loss of energy, feelings of worthlessness or excessive guilt, difficulty concentrating or making decisions, and suicidal ideation, plans, or attempt. Manic or hypomanic episodes can be seen as the opposite pole (hence, the term "bipolar") of mood, energy, and behavior. However, such episodes go beyond feeling "good." There may be elation and positive affect, certainly; however, often there is also irritability and an admixture of depressive symptoms superimposed on a higher level of driven energy that the affected person cannot control. To meet the criteria for mania, the person must experience 7 days of at least three of the following symptoms: inflated self-esteem or grandiosity; decrease in need for sleep, without loss of energy or fatigue; more talkative or pressured in speech and thought; readily distracted from thoughts or activities; more goal directed, seemingly productive activity; and excessive involvement in pleasurable or impulsive hedonic activities, without recognizing the potential negative consequences (APA, 2000). If such symptoms do not last 7 days but the symptoms are severe enough to warrant hospitalization, criteria for mania have also been met. On the other hand, hypomanias are less severe mood-related experiences, lasting at least 4 days. To meet criteria for a hypomania, the same general criteria are used, except these episodes are shorter and not sufficient to warrant hospitalization (APA, 2000).

This definition of hypomania often leads to considerable confusion for clinicians, because it can be difficult to distinguish "normal" levels of energy and positive affect from a potential hypomania, especially in individuals recovering from depression. Most critically, hypomania applies when the person's "good" mood is clearly different from his or her normal self, and there are behavioral indicators (i.e., greater productivity, decreased need for sleep, talkativeness, and distractibility) that go well beyond a normal euthymic state.

When episodes of depression exist in conjunction with current mania or history of mania, the affected individual is diagnosed with bipolar disorder, type I. When depressions exist in the presence of current or past hypomanias only, the individual is diagnosed with bipolar disorder, type II. There is also increasing recognition that bipolar disorders may exist on a kind of continuum, often referred to as a bipolar spectrum that may reflect both temperament and disease processes (Bieling & MacQueen, 2004). Although this notion is not without controversy, it does seem that more broadly defined cycles of elevated mood followed by dysphoria characterize many patients, with a variety of diagnostic labels, who seem to benefit from mood-stabilizing medications (Perugi & Akiskal, 2002). This has led to argument that the definition of "bipolar" should be expanded and that the spectrum diagnosis more accurately reflects phenomenology and underlying pathophysiology (Akiskal & Pinto, 1999).

CBT FOR BIPOLAR DISORDER

The application of CBT to bipolar disorder is actually relatively recent when compared to treatments for depression and anxiety disorders. This is understandable when considering the centrality of biological treatments, mainly mood stabilizers, for the management of bipolar disorder. Thus, management of bipolar disorder was largely left within psychiatric settings using a completely medical model that called for somatic treatments only. However, it is clear now that supplying a prescription and clinical management of mood stabilizers is simply not sufficient to meet criteria for the best possible care. Indeed, other factors, including patient and family education about the nature and treatment of the illness and formation of a strong collaborative alliance between the patient and the treatment team, are now viewed as critical ingredients in effective treatment (Basco & Rush, 1996). These developments helped to kindle further interest in dedicated, specific treatments that could serve as a useful adjunct not only to control symptoms but also to help patients to live more satisfying and productive lives.

A number of specific issues are a priority in treatment of bipolar disorder. Perhaps the most vexing problem is noncompliance with medication; about 15–46% of patients do not comply with their pharmacological regimen (Basco & Rush, 1996). This has a tremendous impact, because taking this medication not only reduces symptoms during episodes but also has a prophylactic effect (Basco & Rush, 1996). Patients who stay on mood stabilizers are less likely to have repeated mood and mania/hypomania episodes. Thus, management of bipolar disorders and CBT for bipolar disorders explicitly include interventions designed to educate the patient and address, very directly, the notion of medication compliance and obstacles to compliance. There is perhaps no other disorder in which CBT strategies work in such an interconnected way with medications, and in which therapists advocate a true biopsychosocial model.

A second area that is distinctive and unique to bipolar disorder is use of CBT to help orient the patient, early in the cycle, to any shifting between depression and manic mood states. Transitions from the depressed phase of the illness to the manic phase can sometimes be rapid, and it is important for patients to bring the shift to the attention of the treatment team so that decisions can be made about how to manage such a shift. For example, the start of a depressive episode might require adjustment of antidepressant medication or mood stabilizer. Similarly, a shift in the direction of mania could trigger treatment decisions that will help to reduce the possibility of self-defeating behaviors. As an example, many bipolar patients with a history of impulsive, excessive spending may want to consider, with the aid of their treatment team, means to curtail their spending ability by surrendering credit cards or access to bank accounts when they are vulnerable to mania. Patients are unlikely to be able to follow such plans during a full-blown manic episode; thus, early detection and management of mood cycles is a priority. CBT protocols teach patients the skills to better manage the early stages of mania and depression, with a view toward modulating the "amplitude" of swings to either extreme.

The cognitive model of bipolar disorder suggests that manic and hypomanic phases of illness are associated with content that is diametrically opposite the cognitive "pole" of major depression along the same content dimension (Schwannauer, 2004). Thus, the same schema, for example "worth," will be activated in both depressions and manias; however, the valence of that schema will be radically different. During normal moods, such a schema may function at a healthy midpoint; in manias, the schema is positively biased, and in depressions, negatively biased. The cognitive model integrates biologically determined activation of these modes, as well as external triggers (Beck, 1996). But consistent with the general cognitive approach, the model for bipolar disorder also suggests that the kinds of external events that trigger mode activation differ between individuals. For example, a promotion at work may initiate a hypomania in one affected individual, whereas in another, such an episode is triggered by a new romantic relationship, an observation consistent with available data (Schwannauer, 2004). Thus, as in unipolar depression, much depends not only on events but also the affected individual's beliefs and idiosyncratic schemas. Once this manic pole of the motivational and affective subsystems is activated, the person sees the triad of self, world, and future in glowing, positive, and very unrealistic terms (Scott, 2001). This extremely positive cognitive processing is believed to be associated with individuals' consequent behavioral choices because of their belief in themselves as omnipotent, and in the future as limitless in the context of a world of infinite opportunities. These unrealistic thoughts and beliefs, especially when identified early in a mood cycle episode, can be subjected to cognitive techniques involving reality testing and consideration of multiple perspectives.

Because external stressors play an important role in episodes of both depression and mania/hypomania (Goodwin & Jamison, 1990), reducing the frequency and intensity of such difficulties is also an important goal. Here, classical CBT strategies can be used in conjunction with problem solving; where stressors and daily hassles can be reduced, detected early, or defused with problem solving, the patient is likely to have a greater overall level of stability. Moreover, there is evidence that during the depressed phase of bipolar disorder, the cognitive "profile" of thoughts is similar to unipolar depression in terms of content and structure (Clark, Beck, et al., 1999; Rose, Abramson, Hodulik, Halberstadt, & Leff, 1994). Cognitive vulnerability to depression appears to be similar in unipolar and bipolar mood disorders as well (Scott, Stanton, Garland, & Ferrier, 2000). Thus, techniques used in unipolar depression that help individuals to monitor and evaluate their thoughts and beliefs have also been adapted to bipolar disorder. Indeed, the sections on treatment protocols in bipolar disorder for the depressive phase of illness are largely identical to those for unipolar depression, with some additions that are described in the subsequent protocol.

Evidence for CBT and Group CBT in Bipolar Disorder

The first formal description of individual CBT for bipolar disorder was published in 1996, preceded by a number of case reports that cited promising outcomes when CBT was used as an adjunct treatment (cf. Scott, 2001). To date, the outcome data for bipolar disorder is still preliminary; there are as yet no large-scale, randomized, controlled trials for group CBT in bipolar disorder. However, three randomized trials are available for individual CBT treatment. In one trial, 68 patients were provided with either a CBT-oriented intervention designed to help recognize early signs of an episode plus routine care or routine care alone (Perry, Tarrier, Morriss, McCarthy, & Limb, 1999). The intervention group had significantly fewer manic episodes, higher levels of functioning, and fewer days in hospital compared to the routine care group. In a second study, 42 patients were randomized to receive either 20 sessions of CBT or be placed on a waitlist (Scott, Garland, & Moorhead, 2001). The active treatment reduced depression and mania symptoms, and benefited 70% of the patients who were treated (Scott et al., 2001). In the largest available trial, 103 patients with bipolar disorder were randomized to a CBT group or a treatment-as-usual control group in a relapse prevention study. During the first available year of data, the patients who received CBT (for an average of 16 sessions) had fewer depression symptoms and less fluctuation in manic symptoms (Lam et al., 2003). The patients in the CBT condition also had better social functioning than the controls. Finally, in an interesting quasi-experimental design, Zaretsky, Segal, and Gemar (1999) found that currently depressed bipolar patients improved as much as matched unipolar depressives on depression symptom measures after 20 sessions of individual CBT.

The efficacy of group CBT has also been studied, though these studies tend to have only a small number of patients and sometimes no control condition. Cochran (1984) compared a cognitive therapy group treatment to increase adherence to lithium and usual care in 28 patients with bipolar disorder. The group receiving the CBT had fewer hospitalizations and was less likely to discontinue medications (21% discontinuation rate in the CBT group and 57% in the control group). A pilot study conducted by Palmer, Williams,

Gorsefield, and Adams (1995) involved six patients offered a group CBT approach that was more comprehensive than Cochran's. Treatment focused on education about the illness, processes of change, and coping strategies. All participants benefited on at least one outcome measure. Finally, Patelis-Siotis and colleagues (2001) investigated a CBT group approach based on a manual influenced by Beck and colleagues' (1979) approach to depression, as well as specific education about bipolar illness, and strategies to reduce and control mood cycles. A total of 49 individuals participated in the study. Even though all patients had well-controlled depression and mania symptoms as a criterion for study entry, Global Assessment of Functioning (GAF) and psychosocial functioning measures increased significantly by the end of treatment, with nearly 80% of patients adherent with treatment (Patelis-Siotis et al., 2001). Thus, overall evidence for a CBT approach in bipolar disorder is clearly emerging and existent evidence about individual and group treatment is positive.

GROUP ASSESSMENT ISSUES

Assessing Eligibility for Group CBT

Because of the significant heterogeneity of bipolar illness and the nature of "spectrum" bipolar disorders, a thorough diagnostic assessment should be carried out prior to considering group CBT. Even with very structured assessment approaches, it may be difficult to distinguish between bipolar and more characterological presentations of mood cycling. Perhaps most important is the differentiation between bipolar disorder and borderline personality disorder, which can also co-occur (Bieling & MacQueen, 2004). Significant and impairing mood fluctuations may be part of both disorders, yet the two disorders have very different interpersonal and psychological implications. A bipolar group that includes patients with borderline personality disorder plus comorbid bipolar disorder and patients with bipolar disorder only will have unpredictable and likely unproductive group dynamics. It is clearly preferable to have a patient's history well characterized and understood before making the decision to place him or her in a CBT group. In our clinical settings, this is standard practice. Treatment of patients with bipolar disorder begins with planning a pharmacotherapy regimen aimed at achieving some stability in mood. This is then followed by considering the patient's other psychosocial treatment needs and any need to improve functioning and quality of life. It is at this point, when diagnosis is well known, that placement in a CBT group should be considered.

Patients with bipolar type I and type II disorder appear, given extant data, to have equally good potential as candidates for CBT. More challenging decisions occur when a given patient also meets criteria for another disorder, whether an Axis I or Axis II condition. Reviews suggest that comorbidity rates for bipolar and Axis II disorders are in the range of 30–50%, with the most frequent diagnoses being obsessive–compulsive, histrionic, and borderline personality disorder (Bieling & MacQueen, 2004). In a recent pooled analysis of seven studies described by Brieger, Ehrt, and Maneros (2003), the overall Axis II disorders prevalence rate was 45.6% in data for 393 patients; obsessive–compulsive, histrionic, and borderline personality disorder each had a prevalence rate of approximately 15% in that pooled data. Anxiety comorbidity rates in bipolar disorder are between 30 and 50% (Boylan et al., 2004; Cassano, Pini, Saettoni, & Dell'Osso, 1999; Pini et al., 1997; McElroy et al., 2001). In day-to-day clinical practice it is therefore likely that any group of patients with bipolar disorder will contain considerable heterogeneity; however, when another condition may be considered the primary diagnosis, individual treatment might be the preferred choice. For example, for a patient with bipolar disorder that has been well controlled with medications, with no recent history of manias but a notable presentation and impairment due to paranoid personality disorder, a bipolar CBT group is not indicated and individual, schema-based cognitive therapy is likely to be the preferred option. On the other hand, an individual recovering from a manic episode that resulted in a recent hospitalization, who also meets criteria for social phobia at the assessment, may well benefit from a group, even if at a later stage it also becomes necessary to address the social phobia with additional treatment. Thus, the presence of comorbidity should not be an automatic exclusion factor for a group, and clinicians need to decide to what extent each disorder predominates and leads to impairment, and whether the comorbidity could undermine positive group process.

In addition to basic Axis I and II diagnostic screens, a group suitability interview (described in Chapter 5, this volume) can be an important tool to ascertain fit with a group CBT approach. However, there are also important features that make suitability assessment a somewhat unique process in bipolar disorder. First, a stated aim of CBT for bipolar disorder is education about the nature of the illness. This recognizes the fact that individuals with bipolar disorder tend to have misconceptions about the disorder and may even deny they have it, despite considerable proof (Basco & Rush, 1996). Although exact mechanisms for this are not well understood, it is not uncommon for patients to have inaccurate recall of their symptoms and levels of impairment, especially within their manias. Whether this is state-dependent memory or, as previously considered, lack of insight, these factors have traditionally been thought to make therapy difficult in bipolar disorder (Schwannauer, 2004). Nonetheless, prior to treatment patients with bipolar disorder are unlikely to acknowledge triggers to depressive or manic episodes, or to describe their negative thoughts and feelings. Denial of illness may also be part of the picture. This is not necessarily a predictor of poor outcome, because the treatment explicitly addresses readiness to address cognitive and behavioral domains. A second factor that must be acknowledged in suitability interviewing is that patients with bipolar disorder are not likely to have a biopsychosocial view of their illness; thus, they may not recognize what role they may play in helping themselves. Instead, patients with bipolar disorder more typically have a strong biological view, which is not surprising given the centrality of medications in their illness and the exclusively biological model of the disorder that is propagated in some psychiatric circles. Thus, what is important to explore in suitability interviewing is openness to a model that includes external triggers and that offers opportunities for affected individuals to take some responsibility and control for the disorder and for their lives.

A final issue that is of central concern in selecting patients for a bipolar group is state of illness. Clearly, assessed patients who are found to be at one of the two extreme ends of the spectrum of the illness are poor candidates. Patients who are on a hypomanic or manic upswing will likely be a challenge for group process and are unlikely, in many instances, to be able to attend a 2-hour group session and follow group rules and norms. Similarly, patients in a very extreme depression may struggle to follow the concepts or to participate in the group process. Such patients are also often undergoing dramatic and sometimes difficult-to-predict changes in their medication regimen. In any case, it is critical to consider a CBT group only when patients have been offered a pharmacotherapy treatment plan with known efficacy and side effects, and have achieved some modicum of stability.

What is less clear is at what level of illness below these extremes a group would be useful to a patient. For example, a group in an inpatient context may allow quite depressed patients to enter in for the sake of activation, if not long-term change or prevention. In some settings, writers have proposed that the maximum benefit of a group is most likely to occur when both depression and mania/hypomania are nearly to the point of remission (Patelis-Siotis et al., 2001). Indeed, selecting patients who are relatively stable is more likely to maximize the relapse prevention aspects of CBT, which in this chronic disorder are seen to be as important as acute reductions in symptoms (Lam et al., 2003). However, because many patients with bipolar disorder spend a considerable period of time with syndromal or subsyndromal depression symptoms, we suggest that patients with mild-to-moderate level of depression, as well as patients who are presently euthymic but motivated to prevent relapses, be included in group treatment.

Assessing Treatment Outcome

The focus of CBT treatment in bipolar disorder, and by extension, measures of outcome, go well beyond symptoms. Nonetheless, it is very useful for clinicians to track current depression and mania/hypomania symptoms during the course of treatment. This clearly favors the efficient self-report scales described in Appendix 11.1. The Beck Depression Inventory (BDI), also described in Chapter 10, this volume, is an excellent choice for tracking severity of depression symptoms. Self-report scales that measure the other "pole" of the disorder are less developed; thus, we have also included a description of the "gold-standard" interviewer-based measure that is used in most treatment studies of bipolar disorder, the Young Mania Scale. A promising and efficient self-report scale that assesses mania/hypomania in addition to depression is the Internal State Scale. Like the BDI, it is short enough (15 items) that it can be completed at each group session. The scale uses a visual analogue scale that must be measured to be scored; however, subscales allow the user to classify the state of the respondent as depressed, manic/hypomanic, mixed, or euthymic, using carefully constructed algorithms (Bauer, Vojta, Kinosian, Altschuler, & Glick, 2000).

Other outcome domains of interest beyond symptoms are quality of life and functioning; and measures that address these domains are also described in Appendix 11.1. These measures are particularly meaningful for patients who are relatively stable in terms of their mood symptoms and for whom a major goal of group therapy is to decrease the impact of bipolar disorder on functional impairment. A focus on functioning is also consistent with a recovery-based perspective on serious mental illness, in which the focus is living as well as possible even when an underlying illness is not "cured." A number of factors can also be assessed over time that may not involve standardized measures but are important indicators. For example, number of hospitalizations and compliance with pharmacotherapy are two outcomes that may be assessed from chart review.

STRUCTURING GROUP TREATMENT

Number of Participants

As in unipolar depression, data-driven conclusions about the optimal number of participants are not readily available. Given the complexity of this disorder, the number of participants should be somewhat smaller than that for unipolar depression, perhaps between 7 and 10 individuals. Because of the inherent heterogeneity with regard to stage of illness, comorbidity, and lability of mood states, therapists need to have an opportunity to work with and monitor each participant at each group meeting. This is unlikely to be realistic for two therapists if group size is in the double digits.

Structure of Group Sessions

The protocol and general group structure described here is for a closed group format, similar to that for unipolar depression. Two coleaders are likely to be necessary, and the preferred length is 2 hours. One notable difference between unipolar and bipolar groups is that there are two formal psychoeducation sessions; family members are invited to hear the information and participate in a question and answer period. This is not intended to be "family therapy" but rather to provide necessary basic information about a disorder that is complicated and difficult to understand to those close to the affected individual. These two sessions, because they involve larger numbers and a large flow of information, have a very different process and format from subsequent sessions. Aside from questions and facts, there is little emphasis on disclosure or group process per se. Subsequent sessions follow the elements of within-session structure laid out in Chapter 5.

Therapists

There is general agreement that the level of therapist expertise required for CBT in bipolar disorder is higher than that for unipolar depression (Scott et al., 2001). There are several reasons for this. First, from a content perspective, the treatment for bipolar disorder uses almost the entire protocol for unipolar depression, while adding more material devoted specifically to adherence, mania/hypomania, and problem solving. Second, bipolar disorder is inherently more complex as a clinical entity; therapists must be carefully attuned to potential cycling in patients, and the impact of this on group process. Third, therapists are required to have a command of biological theories and pharmacotherapy approaches, whether they are prescribers of medications or not. To accurately represent the biopsychosocial approach in bipolar disorders, therapists in these groups need to be able to consider all aspects of the patients' difficulties and answer critical questions when needed. We recommend that, prior to leading a CBT group for patients with bipolar disorder, therapists first become adept in leading CBT groups for unipolar depression and also have considerable exposure to the clinical management of bipolar disorder.

OVERVIEW OF CBT STRATEGIES IN BIPOLAR DISORDER

The 20-session group protocol described here (see Table 11.1) was derived from a combination of sources, including Basco and Rush (1996), Newman and colleagues (2002), and a group protocol developed for an outcome study (Patelis-Siotis et al., 2001). The first 17 sessions occur weekly, followed by three monthly booster sessions for follow-up, although such boosters could be continued at increasing intervals. The weekly sessions are carefully structured to cover the critical content areas, including psychoeducation, behavioral strategies for depression and mania/hypomania, cognitive strategies for depression and mania/hypomania, problem solving, and core belief work related to bipolar disorder. The booster sessions are relatively less structured and are likely to reflect each group's needs for certain strategies or content areas. In the next section, we describe the major components of treatment and the session-by-session flow of the protocol outlined in Table 11.1.

**TABLE 11.1. Sample Outline of Treatment Protocol for Group CBT
for Bipolar Disorder**

Session	Strategies covered
Session 1	• Psychoeducation I: Family present. • Introduction of therapists. • Overview of the protocol, including psychoeducation plan and brief description of sessions. • Description of bipolar disorder. 1. Signs and symptoms, using examples. 2. Biopsychosocial model, including what is known about genetics, stressors, and psychological factors. 3. Course of illness. 4. Treatments, including medication and therapy. • Impact of bipolar disorder. 1. Impact on affected individual. 2. Impact on family and loved ones.
Session 2	• Psychoeducation II: Family present. • Review of medications used in bipolar disorder. 1. Mood stabilizers: types, therapeutic effects, side effects. 2. Antidepressants: types, therapeutic effects, side effects. • Psychological treatments. 1. Adherence with medications. 2. Early intervention in cycling. 3. Behavioral and cognitive strategies. • Question-and answer period.
Session 3	• Group CBT "rules." 1. Confidentiality. 2. Check-in and rating scales. 3. Homework. 4. Missing appointments. • Group members' narratives concerning their illness. • Goal setting. 1. Elicit goals around treatment adherence. 2. Elicit goals around early prevention of episodes. 3. Elicit goals for problem solving/stress reduction.
Session 4	• Outline relationship between mood state and behavior in depression. • Introduce mood/emotion rating system. • Demonstrate relationship between activities and mood (i.e., what activities improve mood, what activities worsen mood). • Homework: Complete activity schedule with activities and mood ratings.
Session 5	• Behavioral interventions: Modifying activities to improve mood in depression. • Introduce the concepts of mastery (sense of accomplishment) and pleasure, using examples from past to illustrate these types of activities. • Focus on adding mastery and pleasure activities to establish balance of reinforcement. • Homework: Complete activity schedule with new activities added in and rate mood.

(continued)

TABLE 11.1. *(continued)*

Session	Strategies covered

Session 6	• Examine outcome of behavioral modifications for depression.
	• Behavioral signs of mania/hypomania.
	  1. Activity levels.
	  2. Productivity increases.
	  3. Physical signs of mania/hypomania.
	• Behavioral strategies for reducing mania/hypomania.
	  1. Simulation control.
	  2. Strategies for normalizing sleep.
	  3. Relaxation strategies.
	  4. Contacting treatment team.
	• Homework: Patient reviews own early behavioral signs of mania/hypomania and lists alternatives.

Session 7	• Identify negative "mood shifts" to target with cognitive interventions. • Label and rate emotion(s) experienced in difficult situations from examples. • Describe interpretation and "self-talk" as the link between situation and emotion, using patient examples. • Automatic and "hot thoughts": Focusing on the thought most related to the emotion. • Homework: First three columns of dysfunctional thought record (DTR; situation and emotion) to be completed.
Session 8	• Review examples of thought records. • Describe relationships between positive thoughts and early signs of mania/hypomania. • Historical review of "activating" situations and associated positive automatic thoughts. • First three columns of DTR using positive automatic thoughts. • Homework: First three columns of the DTR, and identifying hot thoughts.
Session 9	• Review examples from thought records: Situation, mood, and thoughts. • Identify hot thoughts in the examples. • Introduce the evidence technique, finding evidence "for" and "against" the hot thought and distortions. • Evaluate evidence and distortions for "depression" thoughts examples. • Homework: DTR, including evidence gathering.
Session 10	• Review examples from thought records: Situation, mood, thoughts, evidence, and distortions. • Introduce evidence gathering and distortions for positive automatic thoughts in early signs of mania/hypomania. • Review examples to illustrate elicit evidence for and against positive automatic thoughts. • Homework: Complete sample DTR for positive automatic thoughts.
Session 11	• Introduction of "alternative thoughts" for depression and mania/hypomania. • Troubleshooting Alternative Thoughts and thought records, including ignoring evidence, misspecification of hot thought, activation of deeper beliefs. • Homework: Complete DTRs as needed.

(continued)

TABLE 11.1. *(continued)*

Session	Strategies covered
Session 12	• Review thought record examples where insufficient information exists to draw a conclusion. • Introduce experiments: When there is insufficient evidence to draw a conclusion and more information is needed, devise a way to collect that information. • Create an experiment that is consistent with a patient example. • Homework: Execute an experiment and monitor the outcome.
Session 13	• Review thought records that identified a problem that needed to be solved. • Review problems related to goals around adherence to medication regimen, and stressors from goal setting. • Examine connection between stressors and onset of episodes. • Interpersonal relationships stressors. • Intrapersonal stressors. • Homework: Construct list of stressors to be resolved.

Session 14	• Introduce problem-solving strategies.
	  1. Problem definition.
	  2. Brainstorming solutions.
	  3. Evaluating alternatives.
	  4. Implementation and feedback loop.
	• Introduce coping strategies.
	  1. Emotion-focused.
	  2. Distraction coping.
	  3. Action coping.
	• Balancing coping and problem solving.
	• Homework: Complete a problem-solving exercise.

Session 15	• Introduce "deep cognition"; concepts of conditional assumptions and core beliefs. • Illustrate deep cognition using "downward arrow" technique. • Describe downward arrow as used for conditional assumptions about self, others, and the world. • Homework: Complete a downward arrow exercise.
Session 16	• Explain connection between conditional assumptions and core beliefs. • Illustrate "continuum" model of core beliefs and emphasize prospective techniques to change core beliefs. • Describe evidence-gathering, experiment, and problem-solving plans for changing typical patterns of coping, and collect information to support alternative core beliefs. • Homework: Generate a continuum of core beliefs and keep track of evidence concerning alternative core beliefs.
Session 17	• Core beliefs associated with bipolar disorder. • Defectiveness and shame beliefs. • Interventions for coping with illness based beliefs. • Responsibility and biological "determinism" of illness. • Homework: Implement CBT strategies as needed.

(continued)

TABLE 11.1. (continued)

Session	Strategies covered
Session 18	• Monthly booster session to integrate and implement skills learned, as directed by patients.
Session 19	• Monthly booster session to integrate and implement skills learned, as directed by patients.
Session 20	• Monthly booster session to integrate and implement skills learned, as directed by patients.

Psychoeducation

The first two sessions of this protocol are largely didactic, but it is important to leave time for discussion and questions. Given that patients in the group, and their family members, may have variable understanding of this disorder, many questions are likely to arise. A significant theme in these sessions is related to moving patients from one stage of change to another, based broadly on the transtheoretical model of change pioneered by Prochaska and DiClemente (1983). Not all patients accept that bipolar disorder is "real" or an "illness," and such individuals often do not fully acknowledge that a problem exists at all. As in the substance abuse literature, it is important to emphasize that the individual's problem has a name, diagnostic features, and very important treatment implications, and that the problem is real and needs to be addressed. Including family members is another avenue to communicate fully the nature and seriousness of the problem and its implications. Family members are also included so that they better learn to recognize and, as much as possible, help manage emerging symptoms of depression or mania/hypomania.

At the same time, therapists should be prepared to discuss both the centrality and limitations of medication treatment in this disorder. Many patients will have experienced variable benefits from medications, considerable side effects, difficulties accessing proper treatment, or significant negative experiences during hospitalizations. The implications of these experiences for process are described more fully in a subsequent section.

During these psychoeducational sessions, provision of empathy and understanding is critical, but negative treatment-related experiences can also be reframed to point out the benefits of active management of the illness through proper medical and psychosocial treatment. Moreover, such difficult questions can often be used to set the stage for viewing the disorder in broader psychosocial terms, thus helping the sufferer to wrest back some degree of control over this difficult illness. Around the issue of medication, it is important to combat "all-or-none" thinking in both the affected person and his or her loved ones. Medications may have side effects and other limitations, but the option of not taking medications at all will undoubtedly leave the affected person much worse off.

Therapists are encouraged to use a resource list, both for themselves and for patients to peruse in the group and for homework. A number of audiovisual materials, mainly illness education videos, are also available form a variety of sources. Prepackaged educational materials are available, though therapists can also construct brochures, pamphlets, or a frequently asked questions (FAQ) list that covers the points described in this protocol. For further detail, Basco and Rush (1996) list a number of educational resources, materials, and distribution channels in a very useful appendix in their monograph.

Behavioral Techniques

As in the depression protocol, behavioral strategies begin with increasing reinforcement during episodes of depression or low mood (Sessions 4 and 5), and readers should consult Chapter 10 for details on how to conduct these sessions. Session 6 is clearly unique, in that therapists review the behavioral indicators of mania and hypomania. As described earlier, a key feature of CBT for bipolar disorder is early detection of cycling, and subtle behavioral changes are likely the first sign for most patients that mania/hypomania episodes are starting (Basco & Rush, 1996).

Before such episodes are "clinically" problematic, patients may notice themselves feeling more energetic, productive, or rested on a minimum of sleep. As a response, patients are taught the basics of good sleep hygiene and a variety of strategies to reduce stimulation. Depending on the specific triggers, reduction of stimulation is likely to be desirable. Patients are encouraged to eliminate use of any stimulating substances, including caffeine or sugar. Practical limitations are discussed to prevent physical overstimulation (e.g., overexercising), and plans are drawn up to reduce environmental stimulation by having patients avoid overly social situations or too much sensory input. Patients on an upswing are likely to actively seek out situations that reinforce mania in a positive feedback loop. For example, they may seek out exciting and stimulating environments that speak to their particular triggers; persons for whom overspending is a reliable indicator of mania are likely to seek out their favorite store for "bargains." Of course, such behavior simply provides a kind of incubation for mania and, unfortunately, sets the stage for a situation that is likely to cause further damage. This cycle should be illustrated to patients, and several group members can be encouraged to offer their own unique examples. What can be emphasized is the extent to which different decisions may mitigate or in some cases enable patients to avoid self-defeating outcomes, so long as such plans are carefully made and followed.

Relaxation strategies may also be useful but involve more than progressive muscle relaxation. Indeed, in early mania/hypomania, patients may be unlikely to be able to follow up on an approach that involves sitting for long periods. Stretching exercises, yoga, walking, and other slow physical move-ment, with an emphasis on limited stimulation, are more likely to be feasible. Also, practical "brakes" on manic behavior should be discussed. For example, patients can be encouraged to surrender their credit cards, methods of identifi-cation, or even car keys, so that they cannot spend excessively or travel impul-sively. Early in a manic cycle, patients may well still understand the wisdom of giving up some of their freedoms and autonomy. However, once an episode has peaked, they are unlikely to see a need to curtail their behavior. The ear-lier the patient, family, and care providers are aware of a potential episode, the more management strategies can be planned, and the greater the effective-ness of prevention efforts.

For some patients who have had numerous manic episodes, this portion of treatment is particularly useful. Those who have not had a manic episode for some time, months or years, may have more difficulty recalling exactly their triggers and early behavioral signs. These patients should be encouraged to participate as much as they can, but the group's attention is likely to focus more on those with recent manic episodes. Moreover, the ability to apply behavioral techniques may be limited by the speed and severity of a manic cycle in any given individual. Some patients may be able to apply the strategies well; for others, these strategies will have limited utility when they are most needed. It is important to emphasize that these are strategies that ought to be attempted and refined, not that they are a panacea for mood cycling. Patients who struggle to use these strategies can experience considerable shame and guilt when they are unable to prevent a mood cycle. What should be empha-sized in the group process is that these strategies have promise and should be given an opportunity to work.

An Overview of Cognitive Techniques in Bipolar Disorder

As described earlier, during the depressive phase of bipolar disorder, thinking reflects the negative "cognitive triad" that is also typical of unipolar depres-sion. Thus, the procedures for introducing the connection between situations, negative emotions, and automatic thoughts, as well as evidence gathering in Sessions 7 and 9, are largely identical to the approach in Chapter 10, this vol-ume. Sessions 8, 10, and 11, however, are clearly distinct, in that they describe the centrality of thoughts and their relevance to the "pole" of the disorder that is associated with mania/hypomania. A similar pattern occurs around deeper beliefs and cognitive processes. The strategies and processes used in a unipolar group are similar to those used for bipolar groups. However, at the "deep cog-nition" level, this protocol also explores beliefs uniquely related to bipolar dis-order and that do not arise in unipolar depression. In the sections that follow we focus on the unique strategies used in bipolar disorder. We refer the reader to Chapter 10, this volume, for details on working with the depressive end of cognitive spectrum.

Specific Cognitive Strategies for "Manic Thinking"

In Session 8, the group is introduced to the connection between positive thoughts and the emergence of a potential mania or hypomania. In addition to working on evidence gathering to help counteract the impact of these thoughts on the behavioral and affective domains, this aspect of the treatment maintains the theme of treatment compliance. Changes in thoughts in a positive direction should cue the individual to seek the advice of his or her treatment team and inform loved ones, so that more careful monitoring can be put in place.

Patients in the group will already have learned skills to monitor negative and pessimistic thoughts. Indeed, because most patients are likely to have spent far more time with symptoms of depression as opposed to mania, they are likely to have more facility recording and sharing negative automatic thoughts. Monitoring the positive thoughts associated with the relatively rare manic and hypomanic states may well involve a more historical perspective. Such thoughts are also heterogeneous, given the various kinds of phenomenology of mania. Some patients may have experienced early signs of mania in the form of expansive well-being and positive evaluations of themselves and their abilities. Others may notice a sense of irritation and being "driven" toward some goal, along with thoughts that are in line with those states. By revisiting, with each member, if possible, their thoughts during the most recent manic/ hypomanic episode group members will undoubtedly learn to recognize the many guises in which such episodes appear.

Basco and Rush (1996) list nine types of positive thinking associated with mania, and their examples can be useful to round out the group's experiences and examples. Adapting this list for the group may be especially useful when patients have forgotten, or are unaware of, past manic thoughts. Each type of thought is listed below:

1. Increased sexual thoughts as libido rises. This can often involve misinterpretation of normal positive social cues as indicative of sexual interest.
2. Concern that other people and events are moving too slowly. Because emergent mania may result in increased energy, the affected person may experience others as slowing down, when it is the affected person that is speeding up.
3. A need to go to the highest level to accomplish some goal, for example, having a complaint about a product and asking to speak to the CEO of the company. This grandiose thought, which may also be evident in narcissistic personality disorder, does not place the needs of the affected person in the proper context.
4. Thoughts and impulses involving the need to insert humor when it is inappropriate. The affected person may see a serious situation (a

meeting at work) as being in need of "lightening up" to reflect his or her expansive mood.

5. A sense that others believe that the affected person is very smart and has excellent ideas. This usually involves misinterpretation of some signs of general approval and seeing these as very strong support for novel ideas or plans the manic person may have.

6. Thoughts about other people being humorless, slow, or dull. These also are based on not recognizing that it is the self that has become different.

7. Thoughts related to the medication as a brake on the current good feeling, or as being unnecessary.

8. A set of beliefs that the affected person knows more than anyone else about him- or herself or situations; thus, he or she does not accept feedback from others.

9. A focus on the present as the only thing that counts, and possibly losing sight of learning from the past or the consequences of actions for the future.

It is easy to appreciate how each type of thought can readily lead to more dysfunction by supporting self-defeating behavioral choices, for example, pursuing an inappropriate relationship or acting on some other immediate or grandiose impulse. Each type of thought can be written on a whiteboard in Session 8, and the group can discuss the relationship of the thought to bipolar symptoms, as well as the problems and dysfunction that arise from the thought. Group members can then be taught to use evidence-gathering strategies, as they did with depressive thoughts, so that these thoughts, too, can be subjected to "reality" testing.

Equally important is to emphasize first that these thoughts matter for prevention, and that cognitive strategies can be integrated with behavioral "calming" strategies. To achieve prevention, patients should be taught that the first step is simply to notice and to have "meta-awareness" that these kinds of thoughts are occurring. Second is to emphasize slowing those thoughts with rational thinking and evidence strategies, and third, informing loved ones or the treatment team that these thoughts have occurred. If not checked early, at some point in a manic cycle these thoughts can reach a level of intensity that is beyond the reach of these standard thought change techniques (Basco & Rush, 1996). Describing this phenomenon to patients is itself tricky; on the one hand, it is important for patients to try to change their own thoughts; on the other hand, the nature of the changes they experience may make such thoughts hard to derail. As with behavioral control strategies, it is important for participants to understand that cognitive strategies can work, but they may not always be able to stop a manic cycle.

By Session 10, the group is working on and discussing thought records that involve both positive and negative thoughts. To illustrate questioning strategies and evidence gathering for both poles of the bipolar spectrum, therapists may wish to include examples of thoughts that are overly positive and overly negative. Thus, over the course of Sessions 7 to 11, all participants gain familiarity with examining both kinds of distorted thinking, because skills for examining both kinds of thoughts are necessary for their current needs and any future prevention efforts.

Problem-Solving and Coping Strategies

Session 13 introduces action plans in response to thought records, and Session 14 introduces coping and advanced problem-solving strategies. As described earlier, the main reason for including these topics explicitly is the resolution and prevention of stressors and problems that might set the stage for a depressive or manic/hypomanic episode. The topics introduced here are also revisited in subsequent sessions; there are often intimate links between the stresses and problems associated with bipolar disorder and the formation of core beliefs about the self as flawed or damaged. Indeed, it is difficult to conceive of an illness that would be a better catalyst for producing stressors and lasting problems; by the time a patient has reached a bipolar group for CBT, the illness is likely to have caused any number of interpersonal problems: loss of jobs or ability to function in expected roles, difficulties associated with psychiatric hospitalization, and economic hardships. Thus, it is necessary to introduce both problem-solving strategies to assist with major difficulties and to resolve smaller problems, and coping strategies to help patients manage already entrenched problems that may be difficult to eliminate entirely.

By Sessions 13 and 14, group members and therapists are likely to have had many opportunities to obtain a good understanding of each person's current life situation, past episodes of illness, and goals. Therapists may also have a strong sense of what issues are most useful for each group member to address, and can assist in the selection of problem-solving areas by using Socratic dialogue. The exact domains considered vary considerably and may involve interpersonal relationships, work, or important life goals, such as financial security. Such goals are unlikely to be attained during the group; the intent is to launch a process of working toward long-term goals and heading off problems.

Session 13 uses the action plan approach to dealing with thought records that point out the existence of a problem; this session is very similar to teaching action planning to patients with unipolar depression. However, in the protocol for bipolar disorder, problem solving similar to the strategies described in Chapter 4, this volume, is carried on more extensively than in unipolar depression. Group members select broader areas, beyond those identified by thought records, that they would like to work on with concerted problem solving. Patients are then taught a series of steps to work toward a solution to one problem area they wish to work on during the group (D'Zurilla & Goldfried, 1971; Hawton & Kirk, 1989; Mueser, 1998).

The steps described to the group are problem definition and assessment, brainstorming solutions, evaluating the possible plans for their advantages and disadvantages, and implementing and evaluating the solution. In Step 1, "Defining the problem," group members are encouraged to contemplate the nature of the problem, their feelings about it, and the specific issues that need to be concretely resolved. In Step 2, "Brainstorming," the participant with a problem and the other group members are encouraged to come up with ideas for resolving a problem, with the only instruction being that there are no instructions; open-minded thinking and creativity are encouraged. In Step 3, "Evaluating options," the focus changes to the practical advantages and disadvantages of the options generated by brainstorming. Step 4, "Action and feedback," involves implementing, in step-by-step fashion, the best of the options and assessing how well that action achieves the goal. Working through a complete example with the group is likely to take considerable time; thus, therapists should take care to select an area that is relevant to as many group members as possible.

The second component of Session 14 is to present coping strategies that are introduced as another set of tools to deal with ongoing stressors. Group members are introduced to three different types of coping: emotion-focused, distraction–avoidance, and action-oriented. Therapists emphasize the need to choose a balance of strategies depending on the type of stress, and help to identify when coping strategies may fail. For example, distraction–avoidance coping may actually be useful when someone is facing a transient stressor that he or she can neither prepare for nor put off. On the other hand, the patient who opts for distraction coping to deal with a financial crisis is highly likely to make the problem worse rather than better. It is useful for the group to discuss a number of different problems and chronic stressors, and how to balance the different coping strategies to adapt to those circumstances.

Working with Beliefs in Bipolar Disorder

This component of therapy, Sessions 15, 16, and 17 has considerable technique overlap with belief work in unipolar depression. For example, use of prototypical thought themes to identify underlying cognitive "rules," or of a downward arrow to uncover conditional assumptions and core beliefs are applicable techniques to both bipolar and unipolar depression groups. Processwise, higher levels of affect are common during these sessions, and therapists should be prepared to use the techniques in a less structured but no less directive manner to help participants confront their long-standing beliefs and schemas. However, the design of the sessions in this portion of the protocol also reflects a number of unique challenges to belief work in bipolar disorder.

First, it is not unusual for patients with bipolar disorder to be struggling with issues of "self" and identity (Patelis-Siotis et al., 2001). Indeed, the nature of the illness—tremendous swings in energy levels and affect, and wide variations in levels of productivity and functional capacity—often lead to a profound sense of confusion about "who I am." Moreover, patients with early-onset (child or adolescent) bipolar disorder may have been delayed in reaching certain developmental milestones (Patelis-Siotis et al., 2001). The disorder may have interfered significantly with family relationships, forming and maintaining romantic attachments, and attaining achievement goals, such as graduation from high school or college. Even in patients who did not have an early onset, repeated episodes that result in hospitalization, loss of a job, or other role losses often result in difficulties with shame and guilt. Because of these factors, core belief work in bipolar disorder often focuses on a deeply felt sense of "defectiveness." Participants may describe confusion between "me" and "the illness", and be uncertain of what they control in their lives through their own volition and what is caused by symptoms of the disorder. Even more complex is when hypomania or mania at some point lead to increased functioning, for example, in academic or vocational contexts, and the affected individual is uncertain whether he or she deserves credit for those achievements.

During these three "beliefs" sessions in the protocol, therapists should focus the discussion on these defectiveness beliefs. For positive adjustment to occur, participants need first to understand that these beliefs do exist and are important in governing their emotions, where such beliefs originate, and what consequences they have. An important exercise during these sessions is working with participants to delineate carefully what they are responsible for in their lives and what is not under their control because of the disorder. Time should be spent on helping participants feel more empowered by making choices about their identities, values, and goals. Once a proper equilibrium is established, and affected individuals have a better sense of self versus symptoms, there is a much higher probability that patients will accept having an illness that needs to be treated medically and at the same time engage in psychological strategies to cope and limit the impact of the illness on their lives.

The shame and defectiveness beliefs so common in this disorder are unlikely to shift completely in these three sessions, and often this topic area is revisited in the booster groups. It is important to emphasize that changing such beliefs requires more time and attention, and that doing so reflects a process of recovery and acceptance that may involve occasional setbacks. The final sessions of the group also typically represent a subtle but important shift from an emphasis on management of symptoms to broader questions concerning changes to enhance quality of life and long-term adjustment to what is, for almost all sufferers, likely to be a chronic illness.

GROUP PROCESS FACTORS IN CBT FOR BIPOLAR DISORDER

Although there are a number of notable similarities in process factors in depression groups and bipolar groups, there are also unique challenges associated with bipolar disorder that make leading such groups more challenging.

Bipolar disorder depressive mood states are often much more entrenched, and therapists should expect a less robust response to specific depression-relieving interventions compared to unipolar depression. Nonetheless, group members currently in a depressed phase of the illness will, in most respects, react to interventions and other members in manner that is often indistinguishable from that of individuals with unipolar depression. Thus, a thorough understanding of process factors described in Chapter 10, this volume, is prerequisite for therapists interested in treating patients with bipolar disorder. However, three other process areas are relatively unique to bipolar disorder: the patient's model of the illness, mood cycling over the course of treatment, and difficult past treatment experiences. Each area and its impact on process is described.

Because one of the stated goals of a CBT group for bipolar disorder is illness education, patients enter the group with various levels of understanding and often wildly varying views of the disorder. Some group members may be skeptical about "talking" therapy for what they regard, and have often been told, is an entirely biological illness. Patients with a biological view have different expectations and level of commitment to the group experience than those who have sought out CBT expressly because it offers important psychological skills to assist them with their illness. Still other group members may be at a stage in which they are not yet convinced they have an illness at all. Clearly, people with such varied views will have to come to some shared understanding and acceptance of one another's position. Therapists are advised to allow time for such discussions to take place, and to be ready to revisit the biopsychosocial model when needed to help group members find common ground, especially in the early psychoeducation sessions.

Patients skeptical of therapy, who may also be reluctant to disclose or participate actively, should be encouraged to allow the experience of treatment to unfold. Therapists may need to be patient, allowing time and opportunity for these group members to participate fully. Relative to other kinds of CBT groups, therapists may wish to place less demands on group members who do not participate equally. It may also be necessary sometimes to discuss this issue directly by making the group aware that each member comes to the experience with different expectations and may participate in a variety of ways. Participants who are not yet ready to change actively may still gain valuable information and motivation despite their reluctance to be fully engaged in all components of treatment. Even if group members start the group at different stages, by the time the group ends, it is not unusual for all members to be full participants, because they have been allowed the time and opportunity to resolve their skepticism and denial through the experiences of the group itself.

The second issue that not only affects process but also has important clinical implications is when a patient moves into a manic/hypomanic phase. Often the first knowledge the clinical care team has about a patient starting such a cycle is when he or she arrives at group demonstrating signs of mania.

A patient may act, talk, and dress differently than the week before, in ways that are likely to be quite obvious to the group and the therapists. This can be a challenging situation, especially when the patient attributes the change to a "cure" or improvement in the illness rather than recognizing that he or she is having a manic upswing. In the group sessions, such a patient may be overly talkative, wish to dominate the agenda, or even ignore group rules entirely. At a certain point of severity, therapists may have little choice but to work with the person one-on-one and arrange for a more detailed mood and mental status assessment. In those rare instances, one of the coleaders can carry on with the rest of the group. In any case, when such signs begin to emerge in group, it is often very useful for group members to discuss what they are seeing, if possible by questioning the affected person directly. This can be a very useful demonstration of the early signs of an upswing for all group members, and may give the affected patient insight into his or her emerging mania/hypomania as well.

Finally, a significant proportion of patients with bipolar disorder are likely to have had unsatisfying experiences with mental health treatment settings and practitioners. The kinds of difficulties experienced vary widely but may include misdiagnosis (or a very delayed correct diagnosis), problematic treatment procedures, upsetting experiences with involuntary hospitalization or being treated against one's will, and medications with serious side effects but no impact on symptoms. Not surprisingly these experiences may inform the person's view of treatment more generally; some patients undoubtedly express considerable anger, especially as the group explores illness experiences, shame, and guilt. Trust in the therapists and the group process in general can also be affected. It is important for therapists to appear neither defensive nor nihilistic about treatment in particular and the mental health system more generally. Therapists should acknowledge that the mental health care system has flaws, especially when it comes to understanding and treating bipolar disorder. Moreover, it is useful to discuss that there are "no right answers" when it comes to knowing, for example, exactly when hospitalization is required (or not required), or when people should be treated, even against their will. This acknowledgment of difficulties must also be balanced with provision of hope that good care is possible, and that one negative set of experiences is not sufficient to conclude that the entire system is fatally flawed. Fortunately, too, this is an issue in which the presence of multiple group members can be very helpful; others who have had similar difficulties can "model" positive coping strategies they have used. Other group participants who have experienced similar events can be asked to share their experiences in coming to terms with such difficult experiences. Therapists above all need to be sure to position themselves as advocates of the patient's best interests, not as defenders or apologists for past injustices of the health care system. These issues may arise at almost any time during treatment, and therapists need to be sure to allow time to discuss and explore these issues, even if doing so means falling a step behind in the expected time line of the protocol.

CONCLUSIONS

The recent addition of CBT-based strategies, alongside standard medication treatments, has been an important step forward in the management of bipolar disorder. In a condition with such dramatic consequences for emotions, functioning, and quality of life, treatments that go beyond mood-stabilizing medications have been much awaited and needed. The group CBT approach offers a number of useful ingredients, treating not only the symptoms of the condition but also patients in the context of their lives and the desire for recovery. For many patients, this biopsychosocial view is breath of fresh air and welcome news that there is something they can do aside from taking medications. Evidence for the approach is still growing, and it will be useful to evaluate more directly group versus individual CBT for this disorder. Bipolar disorder is an illness that often leads to a sense of isolation and hopelessness. A CBT group provides an important antidote to the view, "I am alone" and it offers patients a host of strategies to help them take back control over their lives and futures.

APPENDIX 11.1. OUTCOME MEASURES
FOR CBT BIPOLAR GROUP

Depression and Mania Symptom Scales

Beck Depression Inventory, Second Edition (BDI-II; Beck, Steer, & Brown, 1996)

This 21-item measure is perhaps the most frequently used measure of severity of depressive symptoms. The items are based on criteria from DSM-IV, including sadness, guilt, suicidal thoughts, loss of interest, and physical manifestations such as sleep, appetite, and energy difficulties. The measure takes only 5–10 minutes to complete and cutoff scores are available to characterize the ranges of depressive symptoms, though the instrument does not make a diagnosis per se (Beck et al., 1996). A score of 0–13 reflects minimal depression, 14–19 reflects mild depression, 20–28 reflects moderate depression, and a score of 29 or more reflects severe depression. Reliability of the scale is excellent and validity is also high. For example, the correlation with the best known interviewer-administered scale for depression, the Hamilton Rating Scale for Depression (HRSD), is .71 (Beck et al., 1996).

Internal State Scale (ISS; Bauer et al., 1991)

The ISS is a 15-item self-report scale using a visual analogue scale approach. The scale seems to work well even when patients are manic or hypomanic. Patients respond to various items (e.g., "Today I feel irritable," "Today I feel 'sped up' inside") by placing an "X" along a 100 mm line, anchored by *not at all, rarely* and *very much so, much of the time*. The instrument takes 5–10 minutes to complete and produces four subscales: Activation (ACT), Well-Being (WB), Perceived Conflict (PC), and Depression Index (DI). The scores for each subscale are calculated by measuring the distance along the line where the X is made for each item of a subscale and summing these distances. Because of the nature of the various subscales, it is also possible to combine subscales to classify patients as depressed, manic/hypomanic, euthymic, or mixed (Bauer et al., 2000), though the algorithm for doing this is complex and may not need to be performed to monitor changes in group members. In terms of validity, the scale has moderate agreement with physician-rated mood state (Bauer et al., 2000) and is able to correctly classify individuals in various mood states with good accuracy (Bauer et al., 1991). It also demonstrates a factor structure consistent with the various proposed subscales, and those scales demonstrate good-to-excellent alpha reliability (Bauer et al., 1991).

Young Mania Rating Scale (YMRS; Young, Biggs, Ziegler, & Meyer, 1978)

The YMRS is the most frequently used measure of mania/hypomania, although it does require an interview-based assessment. However, because mania symptoms can sometimes involve a loss of insight or an inability to complete self-report measures, this scale is based on more objective observation and is typically considered the gold standard in bipolar disorder. The authors of the YMRS intended to develop an efficient (17 items, taking 15 minutes to administer) measure of the severity of mania, and the scale was intended to parallel the well-established HRSD. Trained interviewers rate the items, and reliability ratings have been high in multiple studies (Yonkers & Samson,

2000). The scale has also been shown to correlate with more elaborate measures of mania and is sensitive to changes as a result of treatment (Yonkers & Samson, 2000).

Quality-of-Life Measures

Quality of Life Enjoyment and Satisfaction Questionnaire (Q-LES-Q; Endicott et al., 1993)

The Q-LES-Q was developed as a self-report instrument (60 items) to assess the enjoyment and satisfaction experienced in numerous areas of daily life. The measure has five subscales: physical health, subjective feelings, leisure time activities, social relationships, and general activities. The Q-LES-Q has quite high internal consistency and test–retest stability (Rabkin et al., 2000). The Q-LES-Q is associated in expected ways with measures of symptoms and impairment, and has been shown to detect clinical changes in response to treatment (Rabkin et al., 2000).

Quality of Life Index (QLI; Ferrans & Powers, 1985)

The QLI is a self-report measure (70 items) developed to measure satisfaction with various life domains. The scale has two sections: One assesses satisfaction with each of 35 items; the other assesses the importance of these 35 specific items. The four domains covered by these items are health and functioning, socioeconomic, psychological or spiritual, and family. Internal consistency has been established for both the total scores and subscales, and test–retest stability over 2 weeks and 1 month was quite high. The scale is correlated with other life satisfaction measures, and the QLI is associated with levels of symptoms and coping in expected ways (Rabkin et al., 2000).

Functioning Measures

Illness Intrusiveness Rating Scale (IIRS; Devins, 1994)

Illness intrusions refer to lifestyle and activity disruptions that arise as a result of an illness and/or its treatment (Devins, 1994). The construct of illness intrusiveness, and the scale to assess it, has been used in a variety of both medical and psychiatric illnesses (Bieling et al., 2001). The IIRS measure assesses the extent to which a particular problem causes impairment in 13 different life domains, including health, diet, work, active recreation (e.g., playing sports), passive recreation, finances, relationship with partner, sex life, family relations, other social relations, self-expression/improvement, religious expression, and community and civic involvement. The IIRS has shown good reliability (alphas ranging in the .80s and .90s) in both medical and psychiatric settings, and appears to be associated with symptom severity in anxiety disorders (Bieling et al., 2001).

Sheehan Disability Scale (SDS; Sheehan, 1983)

The SDS is a composite of three self-rated items designed to measure the extent to which three major sectors in the patient's life, work, social life, and family life are impaired by psychiatric symptoms. Despite its brevity, the scale does display high internal consistency and substantial correlations among its three items (Williams, 2000). SDS scores are higher in patient groups compared to those who do not have

psychiatric disorders; importantly, the sensitivity (.83), specificity (.69), positive predictive value (.47), and negative predictive value (.92) have been established for this
scale (Williams, 2000). The scale is also sensitive to changes with treatment.

Social Adjustment Scale (SAS; Weissman & Bothwell, 1976)

The SAS is both an interview and a self-report used to assess social functioning over a
2-month (interview) or 2-week period (self-report). The SAS assess six areas: work,
social and leisure activities, relationships with extended family, marital role as a
spouse, role as a parent, and role as a member of the family unit. The questions in
instrument center around the person's ability to complete tasks, degree of conflict,
interpersonal behavior, and subjective sense of satisfaction (Weissman, 2000). The
scale has adequate internal consistency and test–retest stability (over 2 weeks;
Weissman, 2000). The SAS has been found to discriminate between groups with and
without psychiatric illness, and is somewhat sensitive to changes due to treatment
(Weissman, 2000).

CHAPTER 12

Eating Disorders

DESCRIPTION OF EATING DISORDERS

Diagnostic Features

Currently, the official eating disorder category according to the text revision to the fourth edition of the *Diagnostic and Statistical Manual of Mental Disorders* (DSM-IV-TR; American Psychiatric Association [APA], 2000) includes anorexia nervosa (AN), bulimia nervosa (BN), and eating disorder not otherwise specified (EDNOS). However, these categories do not adequately reflect the most common clinical presentations of eating disorders. Although binge eating disorder is widely studied, it is currently classified as EDNOS. In addition, patients presenting with partial syndromes (e.g., subthreshold AN or BN) are also common and are typically assigned a diagnosis of EDNOS. Evidence suggests that the presence of partial syndromes is clinically significant given the high degree of similarity in patients presenting with full and partial syndromes (Crow, Agras, Halmi, Mitchell, & Kraemer, 2002).

AN is characterized by the following features: (1) refusal to maintain a minimum normal body weight for the individual's age and height (i.e., less than 85% of expected or a body mass index [BMI] equal to or less than 17.5); (2) intense fear of weight gain that is magnified with weight loss; (3) distortion of the significance and importance of weight and shape, such that self-esteem is largely dependent on weight and body shape, and lack of recognition of the serious health consequences of being underweight; and (4) the loss of at least three consecutive menstrual cycles (amenorrhea) in postmenarcheal females (APA, 2000). The two types of AN, distinguished by the absence or presence of regular binge eating and/or purging (self-induced vomiting, misuse of laxatives, etc.) behavior, are restricting type and binge-eating/purging type.

BN is characterized by the presence of recurrent episodes of binge-eating and compensatory behaviors to prevent weight gain (vomiting; misuse of laxatives, diuretics, or other medications; fasting; excessive exercise; etc.) that occur at a minimum of twice per week for at least a 3-month period (APA, 2000). Similar to AN, BN is also characterized by self-evaluation that is largely influenced by body shape and weight. However, unlike individuals with AN, individuals with BN are generally normal weight or above. A "binge" is defined as consumption of an objectively large amount of food within a discrete period of time, accompanied by a sense of lack of control over one's eating (APA, 2000). The two types of BN, distinguished by the presence or absence of purging behaviors described earlier, are purging type and nonpurging type.

EDNOS is the category reserved for eating disorders that do not meet the full criteria for AN and BN but have clinically significant symptoms (e.g., an individual who meets all of the criteria for BN but only binges and purges once per week). EDNOS also includes individuals who report symptoms of binge-eating disorder (BED), currently classified as a disorder for further study in DSM-IV-TR (APA, 2000). BED is characterized by recurrent episodes of binge eating in the absence of any inappropriate compensatory behaviors.

Descriptive Features

Although the prevalence rates of eating disorders are low, their associated psychiatric and medical morbidity are high. Based on a recent review of epidemiological studies and eating disorders, average prevalence rates were found to be 1% for BN in young females, 0.1% for BN in young males, 0.3% for AN in young women, and 1% for BED (Hoek & van Hoeken, 2003). However, these prevalence rates reflect only those meeting strict diagnostic criteria and do not take into account the significant number of individuals presenting with partial syndromes. Evidence shows that both full and partial syndrome eating disorder cases are associated with significant comorbid psychopathology, particularly depression (Lewinsohn, Striegel-Moore, & Seeley, 2000).

Although there are many similarities between AN and BN, individuals with AN typically require more intensive treatment within a multidisciplinary team environment to facilitate the necessary weight gain required for recovery, as well as to manage medical complications. BN is the most researched eating disorder, likely due to the higher prevalence rate than AN. Individuals with BED are quite similar to individuals with BN with regard to maladaptive concerns regarding shape and weight. However, BED is characterized by considerably reduced dietary restriction compared to BN; thus, it is not surprising that BED is significantly related to obesity (Wilfley, Schwartz, Spurrell, & Fairburn, 2000). There are few differences between individuals with BED and individuals with BN nonpurging type, although compared to BN, BED is associated with greater age of onset, increased BMI, and a less pronounced gender difference (e.g., Rammacciotti et al., 2005; Striegel-Moore & Franko, 2003).

BED is also associated with comorbid psychiatric disorders, particularly depression (Wilfley, Friedman, et al., 2000).

Eating disorders are much more prevalent in females than in males. Sociocultural emphasis on thinness as the female beauty ideal exerts pressure on women to try and achieve an unrealistic standard (Striegel-Moore, Silberstein, & Rodin, 1986). Not surprisingly, this sociocultural factor plays a role in the etiology of eating disorders, because both across and within different ethnic groups, there is a correlation between the prevalence of eating disorders and societal pressures to be thin (Hsu, 1990).

COGNITIVE-BEHAVIORAL APPROACHES TO UNDERSTANDING EATING DISORDERS

CBT models of eating disorders place central emphasis on the role of cognitive factors in the development and maintenance of the core eating disorder features of dietary restraint, binge eating, and behaviors aimed at weight control (Garner & Bemis, 1982, 1985). These cognitive factors include abnormal attitudes about weight and shape, information-processing biases, and beliefs about the self (Vitousek & Hollon, 1990; Vitousek & Ewald, 1993). CBT for eating disorders targets negative thoughts and schemas, and core eating disorder psychopathology, as well as maladaptive eating disorder behaviors, with an emphasis on both cognitive and behavioral change (for review, see Bowers, 2001; Shafran & de Silva, 2003).

CBT for BN was developed by Fairburn and colleagues (Fairburn, 1981, 1985; Fairburn, Marcus, & Wilson, 1993) and emphasizes the key role of both cognitive and behavioral processes in the development and maintenance of the disorder. In their model, Fairburn et al. (1993) detail a causal sequence of factors involved in the development and maintenance of the disorder as follows: Low self-esteem in the context of extreme personal value placed on an idealized body shape and low body weight leads to the development of strict dieting. Lapses in dietary restraint lead to episodes of binge eating that are followed by compensatory behaviors, such as vomiting, resulting in a perpetuating cycle of symptoms. Bingeing may serve to reduce negative affect in the short term, and is maintained in part by purging behaviors that reduce anxiety about possible weight gain. In the long term, binge eating and purging cause further distress and lower self-esteem, thus contributing to further dieting and consequent binge eating. For a detailed manual on conducting CBT for BN, see Fairburn et al. (1993). CBT for BN typically lasts 20 sessions. Fairburn et al. structure treatment in three phases. In the first phase, treatment strategies include self-monitoring, weekly weighing, psychoeducation about weight and eating, prescription of regular eating patterns, and self-control strategies. The second phase of treatment focuses on eliminating dieting, teaching problem-solving skills, implementation of cognitive restructuring, and behavioral strategies. The third stage of treatment focuses on relapse prevention strategies.

In CBT for AN (Garner, Vitousek, & Pike, 1997), abnormal concerns about shape and weight are conceptualized as the core feature. Greater emphasis is placed on interpersonal factors in CBT for AN than in CBT for BN. CBT for AN, developed by Garner and Bemis (1982, 1985), emphasizes three treatment phases: (1) development of trust and establishment of treatment parameters (e.g., minimal body weight threshold, target body weight range, meal planning); (2) modification of beliefs related to food and weight, and associated symptoms (e.g., behaviors aimed at weight control), followed by broadening to other relevant issues (e.g., self-esteem, self-control, impulse regulation, interpersonal functioning, emotional expression); and (3) relapse prevention.

Fairburn, Shafran, and Cooper (1999) presented a new conceptualization of the maintenance of AN based on the work of Slade (1982), in which extreme need to control eating is the central maintaining feature of the disorder. A general need for self-control is driven by a general sense of ineffectiveness and perfectionistic tendencies, combined with low self-esteem. According to Fairburn et al. (1999), difficulties controlling various life aspects lead to a specific focus on control over eating for a number of powerful reasons. Restriction of eating provides evidence of successful control that is immediate; it has a strong effect on the individual's social environment, and eating is a salient behavior in families. In addition, control over eating allows the interruption or reversal of puberty, and it is reinforced by Western values emphasizing dieting as a means to control shape and weight. Fairburn et al. specify three mechanisms through which control over eating is maintained: enhanced sense of personal control, starvation sequelae (e.g., intense hunger) that drive further caloric restriction, and extreme concerns about shape and weight. CBT for AN typically lasts much longer than CBT for BN, from 1 to 2 years. A longer duration of treatment is necessitated by motivational obstacles, the degree of weight gain needed to achieve a minimal healthy weight, and the necessity for occasional hospitalization or partial hospitalization (Garner et al., 1997).

Empirical Support for CBT

In clinical practice, CBT interventions are often used with a mixed group of patients with eating disorders, although there are very few studies examining CBT in such samples. In one study, CBT was found to be well-received by a mixed group of patients on an inpatient eating disorder unit, with patients preferring a brief CBT intervention over a psychoeducation group (Wiseman, Sunday, Klapper, Klein, & Halmi, 2002). Another study found that a 13-week group CBT intervention was efficacious in producing symptom reduction in an adolescent sample with mixed eating disorders (Charpentier, Marttunen, Fadjukov, & Huttunen, 2003).

In the research literature, CBT interventions for eating disorders have been developed specifically for BN, AN, and BED. Overall, there is greater evidence for the efficacy of CBT in BN and BED, and preliminary evidence that it may also be helpful in the treatment of AN.

CBT is considered the first-line treatment for BN (Wilson, 1999; Wilson & Fairburn, 2002). Approximately 50% of individuals receiving manual-based CBT for BN cease binge eating and purging (Wilson & Fairburn, 2002). In addition to improvement in the core clinical features of the eating disorder (binge eating, purging, caloric restriction, and maladaptive thoughts and beliefs about weight and body shape), improvement in concurrent psychological symptoms is also observed (e.g., low self-esteem and depression; Wilson & Fairburn, 2002). CBT for BN has been associated with good treatment efficacy and maintenance of gains (Jacobi, Dahme, & Dittmann, 2002). In one study, 69% of patients had no current eating disorder diagnosis and 85% no longer met criteria for BN at a 3-year follow-up post-CBT (Carter, McIntosh, Joyce, Sullivan, & Bulik, 2003). At 10-year follow-up, CBT was associated with improved social adjustment compared to the control group (Keel, Mitchell, Davis, & Crow, 2002). For CBT nonresponders, the success of secondary sequential treatments, such as interpersonal psychotherapy (IPT) and pharmacotherapy, appears to have little added benefit (Mitchell et al., 2002). In addition, there is some evidence that combining CBT with pharmacotherapy (fluoxetine) does not lead to better outcome than CBT alone (Jacobi et al., 2002). CBT for BED is based on CBT for BN and has been shown to have good efficacy for reducing binge eating (for review, see Wilson & Fairburn, 2002).

Application of CBT to AN has been understudied for a number of reasons: The low prevalence of the disorder hinders recruitment to ensure adequate power for detection of statistically significant effects; treatment is lengthy, averaging at least 1 year; study recruitment is hampered by difficulties with motivation; and the presence of serious medical illness due to complications does not allow for participation in a randomized, controlled trial (Wilson & Fairburn, 2002). However, preliminary evidence indicates that CBT for AN shows promise. There is some indication that CBT is preferred over standard behavioral treatment and is associated with significant symptom reduction in AN (Channon, de Silva, Hemsley, & Perkins, 1989; Serfaty, Turkington, Heap, Ledsham, & Jolley, 1999). Based on the utility of CBT in BN, there is good reason to believe that it may be beneficial for treatment of AN (Wilson & Fairburn, 2002).

However, the clinical efficacy of CBT in the treatment of eating disorders is not ideal. Although CBT is clearly a beneficial treatment for BN, the degree of symptom improvement is limited, with about 50% of patients achieving symptom remission (Wilson, 1999). The remaining half of patients achieve partial improvement or exhibit no response to treatment (Wilson, 1999). Given this reality, Wilson has proposed that current CBT be improved either through expansion of clinical focus to broader issues (self-esteem, emotion regulation, interpersonal issues, etc.) or through increased emphasis on the core features of BN, especially weight-and shape-related cognition. Fairburn,

Cooper, and Shafran (2003) have proposed a transdiagnostic theory of eating disorders that extends the focus of standard CBT to encompass additional mechanisms that serve to maintain an eating disorder, including low self-esteem, perfectionism, mood intolerance, and interpersonal difficulties. CBT based on transdiagnostic theory encompasses a broader range of mechanisms that serve to maintain the eating disorder and may be applied across diagnostic categories (AN, BN, EDNOS) due to the emphasis on shared clinical features across eating disorders (Fairburn et al., 2003). Research currently under way is examining the efficacy of this new and expanded CBT for eating disorders.

Evidence for Group Treatments for Eating Disorders

This section focuses solely on CBT. For a review of other types of group treatments, see Polivy and Federoff (1997). Many studies demonstrate the effectiveness of group CBT, with significant reductions in bulimic symptoms (e.g., Leung, Waller, & Thomas, 2000). One study directly comparing individual and group CBT for BN found that both modalities were equivalent on the majority of outcome variables and in attrition rates; however, patients receiving individual CBT had a greater degree of abstinence from bulimic behaviors than did those in group CBT. However, this difference was not evident at follow-up (Chen et al., 2003). Although there is some evidence that group treatment may be associated with a higher dropout rate than individual treatment (Garner, Fairburn, & Davis, 1987), other research, including a meta-analysis (Hartmann, Herzog, & Drinkmann, 1992), suggests that the two modalities are essentially equivalent. In one study, group CBT was associated with higher abstinence rates than pharmacotherapy (fluoxetine) only, or CBT combined with pharmacotherapy (Jacobi et al., 2002).

There has been limited research on group CBT for AN, with mixed results. One study provided evidence that group CBT leads to symptom reduction (Aranda et al., 1997). However, in another study, a 10-week CBT group was not associated with any significant symptom reduction, likely due to the short-term nature of the intervention, as well as process factors important for symptom change, such as motivation, insight, and ambivalence toward treatment (Leung, Waller, & Thomas, 1999). Given the lack of controlled trials examining CBT in AN, it is premature to come to any conclusions at this time.

Few studies have examined group CBT for BED. There is some evidence that CBT is equivalent to IPT (with 79% and 73% recovery rates, respectively) in a study comparing 20 weekly sessions of group CBT or group IPT for overweight patients with BED (Wilfley et al., 2002). In addition, evidence suggests that extending the course of CBT treatment may be beneficial for those who do not cease binge eating after a 12-session group treatment, with treatment gains observed through an additional 12-week course of treatment (Eldredge et al., 1997).

ASSESSMENT ISSUES

Before treatment begins, assessment is conducted one-on-one, typically beginning with a diagnostic interview to confirm that an eating disorder is present
and is the primary disorder, and to identify any comorbid disorders present. A
thorough clinical interview is necessary to assess the important features of the
eating disorder and to determine eligibility for group treatment. Issues for
determining eligibility for group treatment are discussed in later sections in
this chapter.

The clinical interview should cover the following topics: demographic
features, current body weight and weight history, weight-controlling behaviors, food and liquid consumed on a typical day, binge-eating and eating
behavior (e.g., food intake on a typical day), attitudes toward weight and
shape, activity level, family history, medical history, social supports, history of
self-harm, trauma and abuse, comorbid conditions, motivation, and treatment
goals. A useful assessment tool for providing a detailed assessment of the
intensity and frequency of eating disorder symptoms is the Eating Disorder
Examination (EDE; Cooper & Fairburn, 1987; Fairburn & Cooper, 1993), a
semistructured interview consisting of 62 questions that provide five subscale
scores based on symptoms over the past month: dietary restraint, bulimia, eating concern, weight concern, and shape concern.

To supplement the clinical interview, self-report measures are recommended to assess initial symptom severity and treatment response in the following areas: eating disorder symptoms and associated features, self-esteem,
depression, anxiety, and personality functioning. Some of the most popular
measures for eating disorders are described here. For a more comprehensive
review of a range of assessment tools for eating disorders, the reader is
referred to Allison (1995) and Peterson and Miller (2005).

To assess eating disorder features, the Eating Disorder Inventory (EDI;
Garner, Olmsted, & Polivy, 1983) and the Eating Disorder Inventory–2 (EDI-
2; Garner, 1991) are excellent measures to capture symptoms across eating
disorder diagnoses. Norms are available for both eating disorder patient and
nonpatient samples. The original EDI is a 64-item measure with three subscales assessing specific eating disorder attitudes and behaviors (Drive for
Thinness, Bulimia, and Body Dissatisfaction), and five subscales assessing general features associated with an eating disorder (Maturity Fears, Ineffectiveness, Perfectionism, Interoceptive Awareness, and Interpersonal Distrust). The
EDI-2 includes an additional 27 items that form three additional subscales
(Asceticism, Impulse Regulation, and Social Insecurity). The EDI-3 (Garner,
2005) has recently been released; however, to our knowledge, there are no
published studies using this version of the EDI as of yet. There is also a self-
report version of the EDE, the Eating Disorder Examination Questionnaire
(EDE-Q; Fairburn & Beglin, 1994), although data are inconsistent on the
degree of agreement between the EDE and the EDE-Q (for review, see Peterson & Miller, 2005). Furthermore, a number of studies suggest that the reliability and validity of the EDE-Q may be enhanced by providing definitions of

the concepts (e.g., "binge") asked about prior to administration of the EDE-Q (Peterson & Miller, 2005). In addition, there are measures specific to eating disorder diagnosis, such as the Eating Attitudes Test (EAT; Garner & Garfinkel, 1979) for assessment of AN, and the Binge Scale (Hawkins & Clement, 1980) and Bulimia Test—Revised (BULIT-R; Thelen, Farmer, Wonderlich, & Smith, 1991) for assessment of BN.

STRUCTURING GROUP TREATMENT AND PROCESS ISSUES

Table 12.1 provides details of group composition and treatment format from a number of studies on group treatment for BN and BED. In this section, we make specific recommendations based on the research literature and our own clinical experience with regard to group context, composition, group inclusion considerations, the structure of group sessions, and treatment considerations, paying attention to how various aspects may affect group process. In addition, challenges to group process are discussed.

Context

Group CBT for eating disorders may be conducted in an outpatient, day hospital, or inpatient setting. Given that each CBT session builds on previous sessions, with an emphasis on skills development, a closed group is required, with group members remaining together from the outset until completion of the group. This format works well in an outpatient setting but will likely present a challenge to the day hospital or inpatient context, where open groups tend to be utilized as patients enter and leave the program at varying times due to differing lengths of stay and treatment needs. Incorporation of small, brief modules (cognitive strategies, behavioral strategies, etc.) that are closed may provide one format that is suitable for a day hospital or inpatient setting.

Composition and Format

Composition of Groups

It is generally recommended that the group be run by two therapists. Based on efficacy studies of CBT, the average number of group members ranges from 6 to 12 in studies of BN and BED (see Table 12.1). There is a lack of studies on group CBT for AN, but it is has been speculated that patients with AN may do better in a smaller group (from four to five participants), which allows more group time for each member and maximizes patient interaction (Hall, 1985). It is advisable to allow a few extra members in the group to balance group attrition rates, which may range from 11% for BED (Wilfley et al., 2002) to over 30% for AN (Chen et al., 2003) and BN (Leung et al., 1999, 2000).

TABLE 12.1. Format and Composition for a Sample of Group Eating Disorder Treatments

Study	No. of sessions	Group composition	Session length	Strategies
BN				
Bailer et al. (2004)	18 weekly sessions	8 to 12 patients 2 therapists	1.5 hours	Psychoeducation Self-monitoring CBT model of BN Cognitive and behavioral strategies for symptom control Cognitive restructuring, behavioral experiments Relapse prevention
Chen et al. (2003)	19 weekly sessions	6 patients 1 therapist	1.5 hours	CBT based on Fairburn, Marcus, & Wilson (1993)
Jacobi, Dahme, & Dittmann (2002)	20 sessions over 16 weeks (twice weekly for first month and weekly for remaining 3 months)	Number of patients not specified 2 therapists	2 hours	CBT based on Fairburn (1985), Agras (1987), and Jacobi et al. (1996)
BED				
Wilfley et al. (2002)	20 weekly sessions	9 patients 2 therapists	1.5 hours	Behavioral strategies and self-monitoring, with a focus on normalizing eating, cognitive restructuring, and relapse prevention techniques
Gorin, Le Grange, & Stone (2003)	12 weekly sessions	6 to 11 patients 2 therapists	1.5 hours	Cognitive and behavioral strategies to promote symptom reduction and normalization of eating based on Telch and Agras (1992), including self-monitoring, examination of triggers for binges, development of exercise program, and relapse prevention

Number and Frequency of Sessions

The few existing studies of group CBT for BN and BED have typically consisted of 18 to 20 sessions of 1½ to 2 hours' duration, with sessions held on a weekly basis (see Table 12.1). In the protocol presented in this chapter, we recommend 20 weekly 2-hour sessions. Further research is needed to determine the optimal number of group CBT sessions for BN, BED, AN, and mixed disorders.

Inclusion Guidelines

The suggestions in this section describe ideal conditions under which eating disorders are treated in groups. In clinical practice, it is unlikely that such conditions will be met in assembling an ideal group, although it may be useful to consider these guidelines.

Diagnosis and Clinical Severity

Although research studies examining treatment efficacy using randomized, controlled trials have focused on a homogenous composition of group members (e.g., only patients with BN), in clinical practice, this may not always be feasible or practical. It is common for groups in clinical settings to comprise patients with a range of eating disorder diagnoses. However, there is very little research on which to base this decision. There is some evidence that mixed groups of AN, BN, and groups including males do not have a negative impact on outcome (e.g., Inbody & Ellis, 1985); however, this work was not specific to CBT group therapy.

If resources allow, we recommend separating groups by diagnosis for a number of reasons, both process and practical. Mixed groups include differences in symptom presentation and treatment goals that may detract from cohesiveness (e.g., weight gain for AN vs. no weight goal for BN). Variation in symptom severity is a factor that may detract from treatment gains when individuals with less severe symptoms develop greater symptom severity when exposed to individuals with more severe disorders (Frommer, Ames, Gibson, & Davis, 1987). In addition, a mixed group may contribute to a group culture of envy (e.g., individuals with BN and BED admiring the low weight of those with AN) and competition (MacKenzie & Harper-Guiffre, 1992), although competition can exist in a homogeneous group as well. Differences in disorders may also contribute to a reduction in safety and comfort of self-disclosure in the group. For example, BN is associated with shame, guilt, and embarrassment that is not present to the same degree with AN. Individuals with BN may be more comfortable revealing their feelings in a group of individuals sharing their concerns (Roy-Byrne, Lee-Benner, & Yager, 1984). There is evidence that individuals with BN report feeling intimidated by individuals with AN; thus, a mixed group may contribute to an individual with

BN feeling self-disgust and shame (Enright, Butterfield, & Berkowitz, 1985). Individuals with BED tend to be older, with a greater proportion of males; thus, they may not relate to younger, predominately female patients with AN and BN in terms of stage of life and life issues. Finally, patients with AN require a longer course of treatment than do individuals with BN or BED.

Given the practical necessity of running a mixed group composed of patients with varying symptom presentations in most clinical settings, it is worth noting that there are also benefits to a heterogeneous group composition. Patients may benefit from being exposed to group members of varying body sizes, all of whom share common concerns and fears. Patients with more severe symptoms may gain hope and possible strategies from interacting with group members who have less severe symptoms and have achieved greater symptom control. In patients with AN, a mixed group may lessen competition among group members and challenge weight stereotypes and prejudice. The potential difficulties that may arise with a heterogeneous group (noted earlier) can be managed within the group by acknowledging individual differences at the outset of the group, then emphasizing commonalities and shared concerns.

Ideally, when treating eating disorder in a group, the eating disorder should be the primary diagnosis. Given the significant comorbidity with other Axis I disorders, the presence of additional disorders should be considered when determining an individual's suitability for group inclusion. For example, the presence of severe social phobia may interfere with an individual's ability to participate fully in a group format. Alternatively, the presence of a substance use disorder may compromise an individual's ability to benefit from a group treatment.

If group members have mixed diagnoses, it is ideal to have a balance of the disorders represented, as well as symptom severity (e.g., including at least two individuals with the same diagnosis). For example, a group consisting primarily of individuals with BN and BED and only one individual with AN symptoms may not function well, because the individual with AN may view herself as not fitting in or may feel that her needs are not being met. Individuals with very severe symptoms may benefit more from individual treatment tailored to meet treatment needs. Feeling that a group is not addressing one's needs has been shown to be significantly related to dropout in a CBT group for BN (McKisack & Waller, 1996).

Comorbidity

Comorbidity is not a rule out for group membership, although there is little research examining the impact of comorbidity on treatment outcome. Given the high degree of comorbidity in a population with eating disorders, comorbidity is more the norm than the exception. Generally speaking, when comorbidity is present, the therapists should consider whether the individual's treatment needs would be better met with individualized treatment. In addition, the impact of comorbidity on the treatment experience of other group members should be considered when determining eligibility for group treatment. For example, an individual with comorbid borderline personality disorder who engages in frequent self-harm and suicidal behaviors may not be best served in a group format. If an individual presents with comorbid symptoms that would interfere with participation in the group, negatively impact other group members, or interfere with the ability to follow through with treatment, then it is best to have that person treated on an individual basis. Examples of comorbid diagnoses that may warrant exclusion from the group include psychotic disorders and substance use disorders.

Motivation and Commitment

CBT is an active treatment intervention requiring a great deal of effort on the part of the patient through extensive between-session homework exercises. If an individual is not ready to engage in a change intervention, then group CBT is not a good match. Such an individual would benefit more from a treatment focused on enhancing motivation for change. An important part of the assessment is determining an individual's motivation for change and commitment to therapy. Dropout rates for a CBT group for BN were as high as 42% in a study by Jacobi et al. (2002). Thus, therapists need to prepare group participants for involvement and try to boost commitment. Establishing a contract with group members regarding attendance, participation, and expectations may be useful (Lacey, 1983). It is important for group members to be able to commit to all the group sessions to minimize disruption to their own treatment, as well as that of the rest of the group. It may also be useful to provide educational sessions that clearly outline what the treatment process involves to address potential concerns and to correct misinformation.

Treatment ambivalence and ego syntonicity of some symptoms may require more direction from therapists to address aspects that patients do not see as being problematic (i.e., low weight in AN). There is some evidence that readiness for change is associated with better treatment outcome in BN (Franko, 1997). In addition, reduced symptom severity has been related to group dropout in a CBT group for BN (McKisack & Waller, 1996), most likely due to impact on treatment motivation. A useful exercise in the initial stage of treatment is to have group members examine personal costs and benefits of living with an eating disorder versus recovery, then share their experiences in the group. This motivational interviewing intervention helps to increase awareness and boost motivation for treatment.

Therapist Training

Attention should be given to the training and background of the cotherapists. Therapists should be trained in application of CBT to a population with eating disorders. It can be beneficial to have a dietician with training in CBT for eating disorders as one of the cotherapists. This is especially important in a group for AN, where emphasis is placed on increasing food intake for weight gain, but it may also be helpful in groups for BN and BED given the major role that normalized eating plays in treatment. A dietician serves as a credible resource for education regarding issues related to food intake and caloric needs, thus engendering trust in patients to make behavioral changes to their eating.

Structure of Group Sessions

Sessions should be scheduled to last 2 hours (see Table 12.1). Each session begins with setting an agenda, in which therapists give a brief overview of the topics to be covered. Patients may be given the opportunity to add items to the agenda (e.g., questions, issues arising from the last session). Material and homework from the previous week are then reviewed. Once self-monitoring begins, group members are asked to refer to their monitoring forms to discuss how their homework went. It can be helpful for therapists to collect the monitoring forms, so that feedback can be provided. This is especially important in the initial weeks of normalized eating, because patients benefit from specific feedback and clarification regarding food servings and classification of food. Collection of homework also underscores for patients the importance of homework completion. Homework review often takes half the session; concepts are highlighted and reviewed, group members' experiences are linked, and obstacles and challenges are identified and problem-solved within the group. The remainder of the group session focuses on new material. The last part of the session involves assigning homework for the next week, such as cognitive restructuring, assertiveness, nutrition skills, activity guidelines, and so forth.

KEY TREATMENT COMPONENTS

This section provides an overview of the main CBT components for treating eating disorders. For a more detailed description of treatment, see Wilson, Fairburn, and Agras (1997) for AN, and Garner et al. (1997) and McCabe, McFarlane, and Olmsted (2003) for BN. Table 12.2 provides a summary of what is covered in each session. This outline is based on a group treatment for mixed eating disorders developed by Laliberté and McKenzie (2003).

Psychoeducation

Psychoeducation is a critical component in CBT for eating disorders. In one study, a brief psychoeducation group treatment was found to be as effective as individual CBT with the least symptomatic patients with BN (Olmsted et al., 1991). Many of the maladaptive compensatory behaviors are based on misinformation (e.g., that vomiting and laxatives are effective ways of controlling weight). Thus, provision of corrective information assists individuals in giving

TABLE 12.2. Sample Outline of Treatment Protocol for Group CBT for Eating Disorders

Session	Strategies covered
Pretreatment individual meeting	• Explain how the group will work and what to expect. • Introduce norms and rules for group and provide practical information (e.g., location). • Answer any questions and address concerns.
Session 1	• Introduction to group members (group members share personal experiences of what brought them to group). • What to expect from treatment. • Psychoeducation: Physical and psychological consequences of eating disorders. • Discussion of reasons for change, and the benefits and costs. • Homework: Exercise to determine the pros and cons for giving up eating disorder and working on recovery.
Session 2	• Homework review. • Psychoeducation: Set point theory and normalized eating. • Discussion of what this means for group members and what they need to work on. • Homework: Readings.
Session 3	• Homework review. • Psychoeducation: CBT model for understanding an eating disorder. • Group members discuss how the model is personalized for them, based on their experiences.
Session 4	• Homework review. • Introduce role of self-monitoring. • Each group member develops a personalized plan for working toward normalized eating and sets an eating goal to work toward over for the next session. • Homework: Daily monitoring of food intake.
Session 5	• Homework review. • Group members discuss progress make toward working on eating goals. • Obstacles and challenges are identified and problem-solved within the group. • Behavioral strategies for normalizing eating are reviewed. • Homework: Daily monitoring of food intake and situational context; each group member sets new behavioral goal related to normalizing eating.
Session 6	• Homework review. • Discussion of the connection between situational context and eating. • Exploration of social, interpersonal, and emotional triggers for eating disorder symptoms. • Behavioral strategies for managing symptoms are reviewed. • Homework: Daily monitoring of eating, eating disorder symptoms, and triggers; each group member sets new behavioral goal related to normalized eating.
Session 7	• Homework review. • Group members discuss connections between triggers and symptoms, and identify patterns; high-risk situations are identified for each group member.

(continued)

TABLE 12.2. (*continued*)

Session	Strategies covered
Session 7 (*cont.*)	• Group problem solving is used to manage triggers and risky situations. • Homework: Daily monitoring (eating and symptoms, triggers); behavioral goals are set for normalizing eating and managing risky situations.
Session 8	• Homework review. • Check-in on progress toward normalized eating. • Discussion of common challenges to normalized eating (e.g., restaurants, buffets, parties, illness, holiday meals). • Strategies for managing these challenges are discussed. • Individualized goals are set. • Homework: Daily monitoring (eating and symptoms, triggers); working toward behavioral goals.
Session 9	• Homework review. • Discussion of exercise as an eating disorder symptom. • Group members share their current level of activity and how it may play a role in their eating disorder. • Discussion of reasons to exercise other than weight control (e.g., health, stress relief, fun). • Homework: Daily monitoring (eating and symptoms, triggers); working toward behavioral goals; development of a healthy exercise plan. (*Note.* For an individual with AN, this would mean no exercise until a minimum healthy weight is achieved.)
Session 10	• Homework review. • Discussion of emotional triggers and introduction of techniques to manage strong emotions and anxiety (e.g., tolerating discomfort, self-soothing, relaxation, mindfulness). • Identification of obstacles and challenges, problem solving, and goal setting. • Homework: Daily monitoring (eating and symptoms, triggers); working toward behavioral goals.
Session 11	• Homework review. • Psychoeducation: Role that thoughts play in the eating disorder. • Introduction of cognitive strategies (e.g., identifying thoughts, cognitive distortions). • Homework: Daily monitoring (eating and symptoms, triggers); working toward behavioral goals; completion of monitoring form; recording situation, thoughts, and feelings.
Session 12	• Homework review. • Introduction to cognitive strategies for challenging thoughts using group examples from the homework. • Setting of behavioral goals. • Homework: Daily monitoring (eating and symptoms, triggers); working toward behavioral goals; completion of a thought record.
Session 13	• Homework review. • Review of group examples from thought records to identify common challenges or difficulties. • Further discussion of application of cognitive strategies. • Setting behavioral goals. • Homework: Daily monitoring (eating and symptoms, triggers); working toward behavioral goals; completion of a thought record.

TABLE 12.2. *(continued)*

Session	Strategies covered
Session 14	• Homework review. • Review of group examples from thought records to identify common challenges or difficulties. • Introduction to core beliefs, underlying rules and assumptions and strategies for shifting core beliefs. • Setting behavioral goals. • Homework: Daily monitoring (eating and symptoms, triggers); working toward behavioral goals; using a thought record to identify core beliefs.
Session 15	• Homework review. • Review of group examples from thought records to identify common challenges or difficulties. • Group discussion of core beliefs and exploration of their origins. • Introduction to the connection between core beliefs and compensatory strategies (perfectionism, need to please others, etc.). • Introduction to behavioral experiments. • Setting behavioral goals. • Homework: Daily monitoring (eating and symptoms, triggers); working toward behavioral goals; using a thought record to identify core beliefs, explore origins and related compensatory strategies; plan behavioral experiment.
Session 16	• Homework review. • Psychoeducation: Review of the basic building blocks of nutrition. • Review of progress toward normalized eating for each group member. • Discussion of challenges and problem solving. • Homework: Daily monitoring (eating and symptoms, triggers); working toward behavioral goals; completion of thought record.
Session 17	• Homework review. • Discussion of challenges and problem solving. • Discussion of strategies for managing interpersonal triggers and conflicts (e.g., assertiveness, communication, problem solving). • Homework: Daily monitoring (eating and symptoms, triggers); working toward behavioral goals; completion of thought record.
Session 18	• Homework review. • Discussion of challenges and problem solving. • Body image. • Homework: Daily monitoring (eating and symptoms, triggers); working toward behavioral goals; completion of thought records.
Session 19	• Homework review. • Discussion of challenges and problem solving. • Discussion of issues and problems that may underlie the eating disorder and strategies for dealing with these issues (e.g., problem solving, further therapy needs). • Homework: Completion of exercise to review progress made in group and identify continued goals and areas of vulnerability.
Session 20	• Homework review. • Identification of potential triggers for relapse. • Relapse prevention strategies.

up purging behaviors and provides a basis to buy into the treatment rationale (e.g., that normalized eating will reduce binging urges caused by caloric restriction). Psychoeducation may be provided in a separate group, before the CBT group begins, or it may be fully integrated into the CBT group.

It is important to cover a number of topics in the psychoeducational material:

- A CBT model for understanding how eating disorders develop, and the biological and psychological processes that maintain the disorder (e.g., eating disorder symptoms play a role in maintaining the eating disorder: caloric restriction leads to a binge, which then leads to steps to eliminate the calories consumed in the binge, such as vomiting, overexercising, use of laxatives, and further caloric restriction, thus leading to a vicious cycle of symptoms).
- The connection between eating disorder symptoms (dietary restriction, binge eating, purging, etc.) and self-esteem and related problems, and the many functions that the eating disorder may serve in the individual's life (self-protection, distraction from overwhelming problems, a way of taking control, getting attention, etc.).
- The process of weight regulation and set-point theory of body weight (e.g., the idea that body weight physiologically regulates around a "set point" that the body tries to "defend" to prevent significant changes in weight [Keesey, 1993]) and more recent findings on the role that biological factors play in stable body weight.
- The link between strict dieting (eating too little, avoiding pleasurable foods) and binge eating.
- The physical, psychological, and social consequences of an eating disorder and the health risks associated with starvation, low body weight, vomiting, laxative and diuretic abuse, and excessive exercise.
- Guidelines for normalized eating (restoration of regular eating patterns) and activity level, and their role in recovery.
- The idea of a healthy weight range (vs. an "ideal" number) or a personalized "natural" weight associated with a healthy lifestyle (vs. a prescribed "ideal" weight).

Across treatment sessions, the therapists serve as sources of education. It is also helpful for all patients to be given a list of self-help treatment manuals to read as they go through treatment, such as *The Overcoming Bulimia Workbook* (McCabe et al., 2003). For more detailed information on the psychoeducational topics described the reader is referred to Garner (1997).

Weekly Weighing

Regular weighing is essential for AN, in which work toward establishing a healthy weight is a central goal of treatment. In the case of BN, weighing is optional. Patients may be instructed to weigh themselves on their own once per week, then discuss their thoughts and feelings about their weight in the group. The rationale for weekly weighing should be presented. Weighing is a behavioral strategy for assessing concerns about weight and shape, as well as a source of feedback on changes related to eliminating symptoms (e.g., binges, overexercising) and efforts toward normalizing eating. Emphasis is placed on accepting a weight range rather than a specific number. In addition, education is given regarding natural fluctuations in weight. For individuals who weigh themselves frequently, reducing this behavior to once per week is a form of response prevention. Excessive weighing is a checking behavior typically used to reduce anxiety about what the number on the scale might be, as well as a source of information that guides behavior and increases symptoms (e.g., if one's weight has increased, more caloric restriction or exercising is indicated). Weighing is also useful once patients have normalized their eating and activity, because it demonstrates the stability of weight even after exposure to "forbidden" foods or eating a large meal. This information helps to reduce anxiety about normalized eating.

Self-Monitoring

Self-monitoring is an integral tool in CBT. When working with eating disorders, self-monitoring is used to detect triggers of symptoms, patterns of symptoms and urges for symptoms, and to identify goals. Self-monitoring also increases awareness of the links among thoughts, feelings, and behaviors, and the environmental context. In addition, self-monitoring forms the basis for homework assignments across treatment. Patients should be provided with the treatment rationale for self-monitoring, including the purpose and why it is important, as well as guidelines for how to self-monitor (e.g., recording data specifically and accurately as soon as possible after an event). To monitor eating symptoms, patients typically record patterns of food and liquid intake on a daily basis. In addition, the context (e.g., situation, time, and place) and associated thoughts, feelings, and behaviors are also recorded. Patients are encouraged to record data directly after eating, if possible. Given the labor-intensive nature of self-monitoring, therapists should focus on having the group track only those aspects that will be discussed in the group.

In the group setting, patients review their self-monitoring records in detail. Therapists and other group members may help the patient to identify patterns and gaps, situational triggers, and context. The quantity, as well as the quality and timing of eating is reviewed to establish homework goals. Cognitive and behavioral strategies are then applied in the group to manage triggers and urges for symptoms.

Normalized Eating

One of the main strategies for recovery from an eating disorder is promotion of normalized eating and reduction of dietary restraint. "Normalized eating" refers to a meal plan consisting of three nondieting meals and one to two snacks per day, with meals incorporating variety and including high-energy foods (typically avoided foods) and added fats. Eating typically is planned to start within 1 hour of waking, then every 3 to 4 hours thereafter. Elimination of diet products is an important part of exposure to more normal foods, in addition to allowing the patient to achieve the necessary energy intake. A normalized meal plan is approximately 2,000 to 2,200 calories for females and 2,300 to 2,500 for males, although these totals may vary depending on age, height, and activity level. Ideally, a dietician estimates the exact energy needs for the individual. Individuals work to normalize eating at their own pace, with emphasis on the timing and structure of meals, increased variety, and exposure to feared or "risky" foods. Cognitive-behavioral strategies are used to manage urges, to identify high-risk situations that trigger symptoms, and to develop skills for coping with high-risk situations (e.g., stimulus control, meal planning, introduction of feared foods). It is important to prepare patients to tolerate the physical discomfort that may come from normalized eating and to emphasize that the discomfort will gradually pass. This is especially true for individuals with AN or for patients who frequently purge, both of whom may suffer from delayed gastric emptying. In some cases, when expert medical advice is available, medication may be useful to help manage gastrointestinal symptoms that occur in the early stages of normalized eating.

Behavioral Strategies for Symptom Control

Behavioral strategies are a key component for achieving symptom control. Strategies should be individually tailored, planned, specific, and simple. Patients are encouraged to distinguish between an urge and actually engaging in symptomatic behavior. Once the urge is identified, strategies can be applied until the urge passes or reduces in intensity. Separation of the urge from the symptom itself helps to increase feelings of personal control. It is helpful to remind patients that the strategies they use are not necessarily permanent, but represent a temporary tool used for recovery. Also, patients are encouraged over time and with self-monitoring to anticipate the circumstances commonly associated with urges for symptomatic behavior. In this way, the situation can be managed by problem solving and planning, which is easier than dealing with the symptom once it is activated. It is also helpful to review the benefits and costs for acting on an urge versus not acting on an urge. In terms of not acting on an urge, the cost is short-term distress and the benefit is long-term, permanent change and increased control. We next discuss behavioral strategies to manage symptoms.

Delay and Distraction

Delay involves introducing a waiting period between experiencing an urge and acting on the urge with symptomatic behavior (e.g., vomiting). Delay is typically combined with the use of distraction. For example, in response to an urge to vomit, an individual may decide to delay acting on the urge for 10 minutes, in the hope that the urge will pass. During the 10-minute period, the individual is instructed to engage in activities to distract him- or herself from acting on the urges (leaving the house, calling a friend, etc.).

Mechanical Eating

Mechanical eating involves planning meals in advance (including the time and place, and the food and liquid to be consumed), then following through with the plan no matter what (e.g., despite not feeling hungry or being busy). The goal of this strategy is to eliminate confusion (e.g., wondering what and when to eat) that may lead to restriction, as well as the anxiety associated with having to make a spontaneous decision regarding what and how much to eat.

Exposure

Exposure-based strategies involve having the individual gradually confront feared and/or avoided situations or foods. Examples include eating an avoided food (e.g., a risky dessert), wearing a bathing suit or a particular item of clothing, or looking in a mirror. Exposure should be combined with response prevention when appropriate, for example, preventing the response of checking weight change on the scale following consumption of an avoided food. Usually, treatment is focused initially on exposure to risky/avoided foods. Exposure to body image situations occurs in the later stages of treatment, once the individual's symptoms have stabilized.

Coping Phrases

Coping phrases are also a helpful strategy for managing an urge to engage in symptomatic behavior. Coping phrases should be individualized and meaningful, and often incorporate goals for recovery (e.g., "Restricting now will only lead to bingeing later," "Vomiting will not help me in my recovery process," "Food is my medicine," "This urge will pass," "Feeling full is not the same as feeling fat"). Coping phrases are useful when it may be too difficult to challenge thoughts associated with the eating disorder and may incorporate education received in earlier sessions.

Environmental Control

Controlling environmental stimuli that are associated with symptoms is another useful strategy. Patients should be encouraged to take an environmental inventory of triggers for symptomatic behavior, then make a plan to eliminate these items (a picture on the fridge as a source of motivation, a measuring cup for food, an item of clothing used to measure size, laxatives in the medicine cabinet, etc.).

Additional behavioral strategies include reduction of checking behaviors (weighing, looking in the mirror, reassurance seeking related to appearance, etc.), planning for high-risk situations (e.g., taking a list when grocery shopping and going with a supportive friend), and activity planning (e.g., activities involving new interests and hobbies).

Cognitive Strategies

Cognitive strategies for eating disorders focus on maladaptive automatic thoughts related to food, weight, and shape. Chapter 3 in this volume provided a detailed discussion on the application of cognitive strategies in a group session. In this section, we describe the use of cognitive strategies in the context of treating individuals with eating disorders within the four categories of strategies described in Chapter 3.

Exploring the Relationship between Thoughts, Situational Triggers, and Affect

Early on in treatment, group members are taught to examine the connections among their feelings, the situational context, and their thoughts. Self-monitoring by using thought records facilitates this process. Examples of common eating disorder thoughts include the following:

"I am a weak person, because I ate that piece of pizza."
"I will only eat one meal today, because my weight is too high."
"If I eat a fattening food, the fat will go directly to my thighs."
"I am a loser. I need to lose weight."
"I am not going to the pool party. I cannot wear a bathing suit. People will think I am disgusting."

Exploring Evidence and Challenging Cognitive Distortions

Individuals with eating disorders engage in a variety of cognitive distortions. Common ones include extreme or black-and-white thinking (e.g., seeing oneself as either thin or fat, strong or weak), harsh self-judgment (e.g., "I am a pig," "I am disgusting," "I am a freak"), emotional reasoning ("I felt like I gained 5 pounds from eating that piece of chocolate; therefore, I did"), and using "feeling fat" to mask true feelings about real-life situations and problems. Patients also engage in frequent social comparison, typically in the upward direction (others are more successful, thinner, more attractive, etc.).

These distortions may be challenged by examining evidence that supports or does not support the thought, and by considering alternate perspectives (e.g., "What would someone without an eating disorder think about this situation?"). Consider the following example:

Situation:	I was at a party with friends and they ordered pizza. I hadn't eaten all day, so I ended up having three pieces.
Feelings:	Disgust—90 out of 100 Anxiety—95 out of 100 Out of control—98 out of 100
Thoughts:	I shouldn't have had that pizza. I am a weak pig. I feel like I binged. I need to go vomit.
Supporting evidence:	I broke all of my rules. I don't eat after 6 P.M., and pizza is a forbidden food.
Disconfirming evidence:	Even though I feel like that was a binge, it is normal to eat three pieces of pizza. People without an eating disorder would think nothing of it. Given that I hadn't eaten all day, the pizza was really like my dinner. I know that I need to start incorporating forbidden foods in my recovery. Just because I feel out of control doesn't mean I should vomit. Vomiting won't really solve things, and I will just feel worse about it later. Not eating after 6 P.M. is one of my eating disorder rules, and breaking it is going to be a part of my recovery.
Balanced thought:	It is okay to have had the pizza. Everyone else was having it. It was really like my dinner. Not eating all day set me up for feeling out of control. If I tolerate this discomfort, my urge to vomit will pass.
Revised feeling levels:	Disgust—40 out of 100 Anxiety—60 out of 100 Out of control—50 out of 100

Exploring Underlying Beliefs and Assumptions

In addition to examination of core beliefs, rules, and assumptions that underlie thoughts associated with eating disorders, it is also very important to focus on schema-level cognitions (core beliefs) unrelated to eating disorder themes (e.g., self-worth). The central feature across AN and BN is that weight is an important determinant of self worth. Core beliefs unrelated to food, shape, and weight have been associated with treatment outcome (Leung et al., 2000). Core beliefs often focus on themes in which individuals believe that they are worthless, ineffective, defective, or insufficient. Interpersonal and competency themes are common as well. Individuals who have a history of being teased or abused may have core beliefs associated with rejection and likability. Behaviors aimed at weight control serve as compensatory strategies for these underlying beliefs. Perfectionism may also serve as a compensation strategy for a core belief of incompetency.

It is also important to explore what "thin" and "fat" mean to the individual. Thinness is typically related to positive themes (e.g., success, control, power, beauty), whereas "feeling fat" is typically related to negative themes (e.g., failure, weakness, unattractiveness). Once these connections are identified, individuals are encouraged to examine these connections and their validity, as well as how these beliefs fit with personal values and goals (e.g., "Do you want to be remembered for being 'thin' or for being a good person?"; "Do you judge other people based on their weight? If not, why?"). In the process of shifting core beliefs, it is important to examine how these beliefs may have developed (family factors, past experiences, traumatic events, episodes of teasing, etc.).

Behavioral Experiments

Behavioral experiments are an excellent strategy for targeting both automatic thoughts, and underlying assumptions and beliefs. In a behavioral experiment, group members are encouraged to test the validity of their beliefs, the way a scientist might test a hypothesis. Examples of behavioral experiments that may be useful for people with eating disorders include the following:

- Wearing a bathing suit to the pool to see what happens. Focusing attention on what other people are doing, to see whether they are repelled or repulsed.
- Purposely trying not to do something perfectly.
- Going to a party or social event when "feeling fat" to see what the outcome might be.
- Engaging in an activity that has been put on hold until a certain weight has been achieved (getting a massage, buying a new outfit, etc.).
- Letting go of weight control measures.
- Trying normalized eating and activity.

Relapse Prevention Strategies

In the final phase of treatment, it is important to incorporate relapse prevention strategies for maintenance of change and continued recovery. These strategies include identifying and preparing for high-risk situations, development of coping and problem-solving skills to manage stress, and using past relapses as learning opportunities. Resources should be facilitated so that group members can continue work on underlying issues (e.g., self-esteem, body image, abuse, relationships, anger and stress management) after the group has finished. Exploring what has led to past relapses provides important information that can be used in dealing with similar situations in the future. It is also beneficial to examine group members' expectations about recovery, so that the therapists may ensure that expectations are realistic and conducive to continuing and maintaining the gains patients made during treatment.

Lapses are highly likely, so it is important for the therapists to help group members prepare for such instances and use them as a opportunities to learn, as well as to practice the skills they have developed. Establishing a concrete plan of what to do in case of a slip is a useful exercise for the last group session.

SAMPLE CBT GROUP PROTOCOL FOR EATING DISORDERS

Although research has focused on the development of separate treatment protocols for individuals with AN and BN, it is more common in clinical practice to treat individuals with a variety of eating disorder symptoms, due to often limited resources and the variety of symptoms in individuals presenting for treatment. Thus, the following 20-session protocol is outlined for a mixed group and is based on CBT treatments described by Laliberté and McKenzie (2003), Garner et al. (1997), McCabe et al. (2003), and Wilson et al. (1997). Treatment begins with an individual pretreatment session, followed by 20 group treatment sessions. A brief description of what occurs in each session (elaborating on the summary provided in Table 12.2) follows.

Pretreatment Individual Meetings with Group Members

Before the group begins, we recommend that each group participant meet with at least one of the therapists. The purpose of this meeting is twofold: to ensure that the individual is ready and that group treatment is appropriate for him or her and to allow each group member to know at least one person before the group starts (thus increasing his or her comfort level). During the meeting, the therapist explains how the group will run and what to expect. Group norms and rules are briefly reviewed and practical information (location, time, etc.) is provided. This is also an opportunity to address any concerns or questions that an individual has in relation to the group treatment.

Session 1: Treatment Rationale and Commitment to Change

In the first session, group members are oriented to each other and to the group treatment. They are provided with an understanding of what to expect from treatment, as well as psychoeducation on the nature of an eating disorder, and its physical and psychological consequences. The various functions of an eating disorder are explored within the group, with discussion of group members' reasons for wanting to change. The costs and benefits of recovery (giving up the eating disorder) versus keeping the eating disorder are discussed. For homework, group members conduct a cost–benefit analysis for giving up the eating disorder and working on recovery versus keeping the eating disorder.

The purpose of this exercise is to build motivation and provide a realistic appraisal of the challenges of recovery (i.e., overcoming the costs of giving up the eating disorder).

Session 2: Introduction to Normalized Eating

Session 2 and all sessions following it begin with setting an agenda, addressing any questions from the previous week, and homework review. During homework review, a whiteboard is often used to illustrate common themes within the group. Therapists make an effort to involve the group as each group member provides a review, using questions such as "Did anyone else have difficulty with _____?" and "Can other people relate to _____?" In addition, group members are encouraged to help each other through problem-solving obstacles and challenges. In Session 2, psychoeducation on set-point theory and weight regulation, the link between dieting and eating disorders, and the concept of normalized eating is provided. Concerns and issues raised by this information are the focus of group discussion. Group members discuss their reactions to set-point theory and how they may start to work toward normalizing their eating. For homework, group members are given material to read on the topics raised in group.

Session 3: The CBT Model of Eating Disorders

Following a review of the homework and discussion of issues raised, the CBT model for understanding an eating disorder is presented. Group members discuss how the model is personalized for them, based on their own experiences. The role that self-monitoring will play in recovery is introduced. For homework, group members complete daily monitoring of food intake.

Session 4: Working toward Normalized Eating

Following a review of homework and discussion of issues raised, group members develop personalized plans for working toward normalized eating. Each group member sets an eating goal to work toward for the next session. The role of coping statements to aid normalized eating is discussed. Homework is daily monitoring of food intake.

Session 5: Behavioral Strategies and Planning for Normalizing Eating

Following a review of self-monitoring homework and progress on eating goals, CBT strategies for eating/restricting are introduced (mechanical eating, meal planning, coping strategies, etc.). The connection between the situational context and eating symptoms is discussed. For homework, group members continue monitoring of food intake and also note the situational context. Each group member sets a new behavioral goal related to normalizing eating (e.g., increasing quantity, improving quality/variety, working on structure/timing).

Session 6: Behavioral Strategies for Managing Symptoms

During the homework review, the connection between situational context and eating is highlighted. Group discussion focuses on an exploration of the social, interpersonal, and emotional triggers for eating disorder symptoms. Psychoeducation on the difference between an urge and a symptom is presented. CBT strategies for managing the range of eating disorder urges and symptoms (bingeing, vomiting, laxative/diuretic abuse, overexercising, etc.) are reviewed (e.g., delay, distraction, coping statements). For homework, group members complete daily monitoring of eating, eating disorder symptoms, and triggers. Each group member sets a behavioral goal related to normalized eating.

Session 7: Managing Risky Situations

Following homework review, group members discuss connections between their eating disorder symptoms and triggers, and identify patterns (e.g., risky situations/mood states that typically lead to symptoms). Group problem solving is used to generate strategies and plans for managing triggers and risky situations. For homework, group members continue daily monitoring of eating, symptoms, and triggers. Behavioral goals are set for normalizing eating and controlling symptoms.

Session 8: Managing Challenges to Normalized Eating

Following homework review, each member checks in regarding progress toward normalized eating (e.g., what changes they have made, what goals they will continue to work on). Group discussion focuses on the common challenges to normalized eating, such as eating in restaurants, dealing with a buffet situation, coping with eating at parties, how to eat during illness, and managing eating at holiday meals and family gatherings. Strategies for managing these situations are reviewed. For homework, group members continue daily monitoring of eating, symptoms, and triggers, as well as working toward behavioral goals.

Session 9: The Role of Exercise in an Eating Disorder

Following homework review, group discussion focuses on exercise as an eating disorder symptom. Group members share their current level of activity and how it may play a role in their eating disorder. Reasons for exercising, other than weight control, such as health, stress relief, and fun, are brainstormed. Types of exercise that tend to be associated with the eating disorder are identified (e.g., solitary exercise), as well as "safer" types of exercise that are not typically used for weight control (e.g., team sports, yoga). For homework, group members develop a healthy exercise plan, taking into consideration their eating disorder symptoms and recovery. For an individual with AN symptoms, this may mean planning not to exercise until a minimum healthy weight is achieved, then selecting activities that were not part of the eating disorder. For an individual with symptoms of BED or BN, where exercise did not play a role, this may mean planning to incorporate new activities. In addition, group members continue daily monitoring of eating, symptoms, and triggers, as well as working toward behavioral eating goals.

Session 10: Identifying and Managing Emotions

Homework is reviewed, and the role of emotional triggers is highlighted. Emotions are discussed, with emphasis on identifying emotions that may be masked by other states (e.g., feeling fat, feeling numb). Strategies for managing strong emotions and anxiety are introduced (e.g., tolerating discomfort, self-soothing, relaxation, and mindfulness). The remainder of the session is spent on identifying and problem-solving obstacles and challenges thus far, and goal setting related to eating and symptoms. For homework, group members continue daily monitoring of eating, symptoms, and triggers, and working toward behavioral goals.

Session 11: Introduction to Cognitive Strategies

Homework is reviewed, with emphasis on problem-solving obstacles identified through self-monitoring, as well as detailed discussion of each group member's exercise plan. The remainder of the session focuses on the introduction of cognitive strategies. Topics covered include the role of automatic thoughts in eating disorder symptoms; the connection among thoughts, feelings, and behavior; identification of automatic thoughts; and cognitive distortions. For homework, group members continue monitoring of daily eating, symptoms, and triggers, as well as working toward behavioral eating goals. In addition, group members complete a new monitoring form whenever they experience an urge to engage in symptomatic behavior, and record the situation, their thoughts, and their feelings.

Session 12: Challenging Automatic Thoughts

Homework is reviewed, with an emphasis on the connection among thoughts, situations, feelings, and urges to engage in symptomatic behavior. Cognitive strategies for challenging eating disorder thoughts are introduced (e.g., exploring the evidence, cost–benefit analysis, shifting perspective), and exemplified using group members' examples from the homework. Working with a thought record is illustrated. For homework, group members complete thought records and continue daily monitoring of eating and symptoms, as well as progress toward behavioral eating goals.

Session 13: Applying Cognitive Strategies

Homework is reviewed. The group problem-solves challenges or obstacles identified as individual group members practice challenging their eating disorder thoughts. The remainder of the session focuses on mastering the application of cognitive techniques for challenging eating disorder thoughts using group members' experiences. For homework, group members complete thought records and continue daily monitoring of eating and symptoms, as well as progress toward behavioral eating goals.

Session 14: Examining Underlying Rules, Assumptions, and Core Beliefs

Following homework review, the concepts of underlying rules, assumptions, and core beliefs are introduced. Topics discussed include their origins and how they develop, how they differ from automatic thoughts, and methods for identification (e.g., the downward arrow technique). Strategies for shifting rules and challenging core beliefs, as well as establishing new core beliefs, are reviewed. For homework, group members complete thought records, with a focus on identifying and working with the rules, assumptions, and core beliefs underlying their initial automatic thoughts. In addition, group members continue daily monitoring of eating and symptoms as well as working toward behavioral eating goals.

Session 15: Origins of Core Beliefs and Compensatory Strategies (e.g., Perfectionism)

Homework is reviewed, with an emphasis on working with group members' examples from their thought records to identify common challenges or difficulties. Group discussion focuses on core beliefs that were identified and their origins. The connection between core beliefs and compensatory strategies, such as perfectionism and efforts to please others all the time, is discussed, with group members identifying possible compensatory strategies that they may use. Homework focuses on using thought records to identify core beliefs, to explore their origins, and to identify related compensatory strategies. In addition, group members continue monitoring of eating and symptoms, and working on goals for normalized eating.

Session 16: Progress toward Normalized Eating

Homework is reviewed, with a focus on the origins of core beliefs and identification of compensatory behaviors. Strategies for changing compensatory strategies are discussed, with an emphasis on behavioral experiments, such as purposely making a mistake (perfectionism) and saying no to a request (pleasing others). The remainder of the session focuses on reviewing individualized progress toward normalized eating. Information on the nutritional building blocks is presented. Common challenges and obstacles are discussed. Group problem solving is used to identify strategies to overcome obstacles. For homework, group members continue to complete thought records, monitor eating and symptoms, and work toward goals for normalized eating. Group members also set goals for behavioral experiments, if relevant.

Session 17: Managing Interpersonal Triggers

Homework is reviewed and feedback regarding group members' activity plans is given. The role of interpersonal triggers and conflicts in the eating disorder is discussed. The remainder of the session is spent on practicing social skills techniques (e.g., assertiveness, communication styles) and reviewing strategies for managing interpersonal situations (e.g., problem solving). The group practices different forms of communication (passive, assertive, and aggressive), then group members engage in role plays of various conflict scenarios. For homework, group members continue self-monitoring of eating and symptoms, completion of thought records, and work on behavioral eating goals.

Session 18: Body Image

Homework is reviewed, with a focus on the learning gained from completion of behavioral experiments related to group members' compensatory strategies. The group focus then shifts to body image. Topics dealing with body image include the longer-term work of recovery, individualized meaning of fat versus thin, triggers of negative body image, the role of the scale, CBT strategies for dealing with negative body image, coping with sociocultural influences and weight prejudice, and strategies for developing a healthier body image. For homework, group members continue self-monitoring of eating and symptoms, completion of thought records, and work on behavioral eating goals.

Session 19: Dealing with Underlying Issues

Following the homework review, group discussion focuses on the issues and problems that may underlie the eating disorder for each group member. Strategies for dealing with these issues are discussed, such as problem-solving or seeking further treatment for secondary disorders (social phobia, post traumatic stress disorder, etc.). For homework, group members complete an exercise designed to review progress made in group and to identify continued goals and areas of vulnerability.

Session 20: Relapse Prevention

Homework is reviewed, with emphasis on reinforcing progress made in the group and plans for continued recovery work. The remainder of the session is spent on relapse prevention issues, including common triggers for relapse (e.g., stress) and strategies for dealing with slips. Finally, termination issues are discussed (feelings about the group coming to an end, saying good-bye to the group, etc.).

Follow-Up

It is important to plan scheduled follow-up sessions or booster sessions to check progress. Research suggests that patients with BN who have difficulty following successful treatment are unlikely to seek additional visits of their own accord to help manage relapse (Mitchell et al., 2004). Planned sessions or phone calls are recommended as a relapse prevention strategy. This is especially important in the first 6 months posttreatment, when risk of relapse is high (Olmsted, Kaplan, & Rockert, 1994). It is also useful to have an individual meeting with each group member following the end of the group to identify further treatment needs and to offer direction to appropriate resources. Many day hospital and outpatient eating disorder programs have groups that would be of great benefit following this 20-session CBT group, such as a body image group or a monthly relapse prevention group.

TREATMENT CONSIDERATIONS FOR ADOLESCENTS

Group CBT in adolescents with eating disorders requires family involvement to enhance motivation, to provide a supportive environment for change, and to buffer stress that could trigger relapse (Lock, 2002). It is recommended that family therapy sessions be held in conjunction with CBT sessions for younger patients (Garner et al., 1997). A model for involving parents in CBT for adolescents with BN is described by Lock (2002). Adult patients may also benefit from family sessions, where family members receive education and have the opportunity to ask questions about the treatment process.

GROUP PROCESS ISSUES THAT MAY CHALLENGE GROUP THERAPISTS

Running a group for eating disorders is particularly challenging to group therapists compared to running groups for other disorders (e.g., panic disorder, depression) due the ego-syntonic nature of eating disorders. Even when individuals are motivated to change, letting go of the eating disorder is a challenging process punctuated by periods of ambivalence. One study comparing an eating disorder group to a mixed psychiatric control group found that the eating disorder group reported not only greater engagement in treatment but also greater avoidance of treatment content (Tasca, Flynn, & Bissada, 2002).

A major concern for any eating disorder group, but particularly for a homogeneous group, is that members will teach each other techniques and encourage symptoms that contribute to increased pathology (e.g., Hall, 1985). It is important for group leaders to be aware of this possibility and be prepared to manage its occurrence within the group. This issue should also be addressed in the pregroup individual meeting and in Session 1, where group members are encouraged to support each other in trying to achieve recovery and make every effort to avoid teaching one another new behaviors that worsen their eating disorder. At the outset, it is helpful to provide specific guidelines to group members regarding limiting discussion of symptoms, such that they describe a difficult symptom week without mentioning specific strategies used to engage in symptoms (e.g., methods of purging). This guideline also applies to discussions that may occur between group members outside of the group, because it is common for group members to form relationships with each other that take on a life of their own, separate from the group. Despite the therapists' intention to discourage relationships outside the group, this common occurrence is beyond the therapists' control. Another potential issue that the group therapists should be aware of is group members' formation of a strong eating disorder identity through overidentification with other group members (Polivy & Garfinkel, 1984). This may be addressed to some extent by encouraging group members to expand their awareness beyond others' eating disorders and to develop attachment opportunities that diversify their sense of self.

Group leaders need to examine their own beliefs and personal issues related to body image and weight (MacKenzie & Harper-Guiffre, 1992). Group leaders can also benefit from clinical supervision given that patients with eating disorders are well known for focusing on therapists' weight and shape. Such scrutiny may be difficult for some therapists to manage; thus, an outlet for debriefing and discussing such issues is valuable for facilitating the therapeutic experience. In addition, given the role of modeling in CBT, we would recommend that the therapists be nondieters who are able to model a nondieting, normalized eating approach, and that they be fairly comfortable with their weight and shape, and the scrutiny they may receive from group members. For these reasons, therapists who have recently recovered from an eating disorder or who have active weight and shape issues should reconsider their appropriateness as therapists in an eating disorder group.

Another issue that may affect group process is ambivalence regarding recovery. Given that ambivalence is expected at various points throughout treatment, it is important for group leaders to be prepared for and to manage the impact of a group member's ambivalence on the rest of the group. Treatment ambivalence may manifest itself in a variety of ways, both passive (e.g., homework incompletion, absenteeism) and explicit (e.g., stating in group that "recovery is impossible"). Failure to manage ambivalence may have a negative impact on other group members' level of motivation. Normalizing ambivalence, processing feelings, and validating the challenges group members face in their recovery are all useful therapeutic strategies for maintaining the group environment.

CONCLUSIONS

Eating disorders include AN, BN, and EDNOS. The presence of partial syndromes is also clinically significant and warrants intervention. Following an overview of the diagnostic and descriptive features of eating disorders, this chapter focuses on reviewing the cognitive-behavioral approach to eating disorder treatment, with an emphasis on group intervention. Despite greater evidence for the efficacy of CBT for BN, preliminary data suggest that CBT may also be helpful in the treatment of AN. This chapter provides an overview of various issues in structuring a group treatment for eating disorders. In addition, particular attention is paid to the issues involved in group process with an eating disorder group. The essential treatment components for a CBT group are presented, along with a 20-session sample protocol geared to a mixed patient group. In clinical practice, groups are more likely to be run with mixed groups of patients rather than groups tailored to specific eating disorders, largely due to resources and practical constraints. However, research has tended to focus on "pure" diagnostic groups. Further research is needed to examine the efficacy of group CBT for mixed groups of patients with eating disorders.

CHAPTER 13

Substance Abuse

Frederick Rotgers
Trinh An Nguyen

DESCRIPTION OF SUBSTANCE USE DISORDERS

The misuse of psychoactive substances poses the most significant health threat to Americans in the 21st Century (Robert Wood Johnson Foundation, 2001). A sizable majority of Americans will experience some significant negative consequences as a result of substance use at some time in their lives. Nonetheless, most substance use does not result in significant problems for the user, unless use is chronic. Despite the fact that most substance users avoid lasting significant negative consequences associated with use, epidemiological data suggest that substance use disorders (SUDs) are the among most prevalent psychiatric disorders in the wider population, second only to depressive spectrum disorders in their frequency of occurrence (Regier et al., 1990).

Diagnostic Features

Although there are many terms used in the vernacular to denote these disorders ("alcoholism" and "addiction" being the most commonly used), the text revision of the fourth edition of the *Diagnostic and Statistical Manual* (DSM-IV-TR; American Psychiatric Association, 2000) specifies two types of substance use–related disorders: substance-induced disorders and substance-related disorders. Substance-induced disorders typically consist of problems that appear to be the direct result of substance use, such as intoxication, withdrawal symptoms, substance-induced psychosis, and so forth. These disorders are generally treated medically, and they do not play a role in the discussion that follows.

More prevalent and directly pertinent to our discussion are the substance-related disorders, of which DSM-IV-TR specifies two types: substance abuse and substance dependence.

Substance abuse, presumed to be less severe than substance dependence, is marked by repeated use of a substance in situations in which such use is potentially harmful to oneself or others, or despite knowledge that such use causes or is associated with significant social or psychological problems. Table 13.1 presents a synopsis of the criteria for substance abuse.

Substance dependence is more serious in its implications, and closer in meaning to what most laypeople consider to be "addiction." Substance dependence requires substance use to have created three or more of a list of negative consequences in a person's life over the course of time. Criteria for substance dependence are summarized in Table 13.2.

There are several important implications of the DSM-IV-TR approach to diagnosing substance-related disorders. First, these disorders are not unitary entities, nor are all persons who meet criteria for these diagnoses alike in the particular symptom picture they present. Second, it is important to note that substance use per se is not part of the diagnostic criteria for either substance abuse or substance dependence except as a baseline requirement (e.g., one cannot be alcohol-dependent if one does not drink!). Third, once a person has been diagnosed as substance dependent, he or she never completely loses that diagnosis. At best, the disorder, successfully resolved, is considered to be in sustained full remission. Finally, resolution of substance abuse and dependence does not necessarily require a cessation of substance use. It only requires that the person's substance use no longer result in the symptoms considered to constitute the disorders. Thus, lifelong total abstinence from substance use is not a prerequisite for resolution of substance-related disorders, although, pragmatically, it is a certain way to ensure that the person will no longer experience problems related to substance use.

As well as variability across individuals in the ways in which substance abuse and dependence are manifested, there is variability among psychoactive substance in the extent to which users are likely to develop either of these substance-related disorders. Thus, it is not clear, for example, whether and to

TABLE 13.1. Criteria for Substance Abuse

1. One or more of the following criteria for over 1 year:
   a. Role *impairment* (e.g., failed work or home obligations)
   b. Hazardous use (e.g., driving while intoxicated)
   c. Legal problems related to substancel use
   d. Social or interpersonal problems due to substance use
2. Has never met criteria for substance dependence

TABLE 13.2. Criteria for Substance Dependence

1. Three or more of the following occurring at any time in the same 12-month period:
   a. Tolerance to the effects of substance as defined by either:
      • Need for markedly increased amounts of substance to achieve desired effect.
      • Markedly diminished effect with continued use of the same amount of substance.
   b. Withdrawal symptoms or use of a substance to avoid withdrawal.
   c. Substance is consumed in larger amounts or over longer time periods than was intended.
   d. Presence of a persistent desire or unsuccessful attempts to cut down or control substance use.
   e. A great deal of time is spent using, obtaining the substance, or recovering from the effects of substance use.
   f. The person gives up important social, work, or recreational activities in order to use the substance or as a result of substance use.
   g. Substance use continues despite the person's knowledge that he or she has a persistent or recurring physical or psychological problem that is likely to be due, to or made worse by, substance use.

what extent hallucinogens produce a dependence syndrome similar to that of other substances for which dependence syndromes are well established (e.g., alcohol, opioids, stimulants). The nature of the dependence syndrome for a particular drug can also vary from individual to individual, as can patterns of use leading to abuse or dependence. For these reasons, individualized assessment and treatment planning is a critical part of any cognitive-behavioral treatment for SUDs. We discuss assessment in greater detail in a subsequent section.

COGNITIVE-BEHAVIORAL APPROACHES TO UNDERSTANDING SUDS

CBT approaches to understanding SUDs are based solidly in social learning theory (SLT; Rotgers, 2003). According to SLT, SUDs develop initially as a result of an interaction between biological predispositions toward a positive experience with a particular substance, availability of that substance for initial experimentation, and conditioning and modeling factors that result in learning how to use and appreciate the effects of the substance. Temperament and personality factors also appear to play a role in determining who among the vast majority of people who experiment with psychoactive substances will likely abuse or become dependent upon them (Rotgers, 2003).

Initial use of a substance, according to SLT, occurs when an individual has models who demonstrate a positive expectancy for the use of a substance; that is, initial substance use is prompted by an expectation of reinforcement for use behavior. This reinforcement can take a variety of forms, not all of which are directly due to the pharmacological effects of the substance. For example, researchers have demonstrated that children as young as 5 and 6 years old have strong expectancies regarding the effect of drinking alcoholic beverages (Leigh & Stacy, 2004). These expectancies, coupled with social reinforcement (often termed "peer pressure"), trigger initial use in most young people.

Most young people experiment with psychoactive substances (with tobacco and alcohol being the most commonly tried "first" drugs; Kandel, 2002), but only a minority go on to develop problems related to substance use. Although it is clear that, for some individuals, there is a innate tendency to respond to the pharmacological effects of particular substances in ways that increase the risk of future problematic use (Schuckit, Smith, & Tipp, 1997), biological variables play only a small role in the continuation of substance use and occasional development of SUDs following a period of use.

Continuation of use, according to SLT, results from the reinforcing properties of the substance for the individual. These, in turn, lead to the strengthening of positive outcome expectancies for use of the substance, which in turn feed back to produce increased use. With repeated use over time, biological changes begin to occur (in the form of development of tolerance to the substance's effects) and use begins to be driven, at least in part, by consequent changes in the reinforcing properties of the substance for the individual. Thus, as the individual uses the substance repeatedly, and develops tolerance to the substance's effects but maintains strong positive outcome expectancies for substance use, there is a tendency to use more of the substance more often to achieve the expected effects. This process then begins a "vicious cycle" in which the person uses more of a substance, or uses more frequently, both to achieve expected positive outcomes and, as dependence begins to develop, to reduce the negative effects of substance withdrawal following an episode of use.

Although much of the process of development of SUDs occurs outside of awareness, through a combination of both classical and operant learning processes, coupled with biological changes that occur as part of the body's adaptation to the presence or absence of the substance, changes are occurring on a cognitive level as well. Expectancies often manifest themselves as cognitions coupled with both physical sensations and affect. Depending on the nature of the specific reinforcement contingencies for substance use experienced by a particular individual, cognitions often develop that, themselves, serve as stimuli to continued use. These cognitions are often experienced as "urges" to use or "cravings" for the substance, and can serve as proximal stimuli for behavior aimed at obtaining the substance (Tiffany, 1990).

Thus, an individual who is alcohol-dependent may develop cognitive distortions related to alcohol use. For example, the individual may make implicit self-statements such as "I can't function without a drink" or "I need a few drinks in order to relax." It is clear that substance use serves a variety of intrapersonal and interpersonal functions that vary from individual to individual, with consequent variations in the types of self-statements/cognitions regarding substance use that develop (Khantzian, 1985). Identification of these functions and the stimuli associated with them form a critical part of CBT approaches to helping people overcome SUDs.

To the extent that substance use has become a focal point of the individual's daily activities, cognitions may develop in which the individual exaggerates the positive outcome expectancies for substance use, and minimizes the negative outcome possibilities. Despite this, however, the individual is typically fully aware of both the positive and negative aspects of substance use. Assistance in changing substance use often depends upon working with these outcome expectancies in the form of a "decisional balance" self-assessment in which the individual is guided through weighing the pros and cons of substance use and change.

Once a person has developed an SUD, there are several possible outcomes. The SUD may exacerbate over time (traditional lore suggests, incorrectly, that this is the most common outcome); it may be resolved by the person without assistance (according to research, the most common outcome; Dawson, 1996); or the person may seek assistance to alleviate the negative effects of substance use. CBT approaches to the treatment of SUDs postulate that for change to occur, several factors must be in place. These have been summarized as the person being "ready, willing, and able" (Rollnick, Mason, & Butler, 1999). In more technical language, the individual must be prepared to make changes in his or her life and behavior that support a reduction or cessation of substance use ("ready"). He or she must also be willing to sustain effort and commitment to changing substance use behavior ("willing"). Finally, he or she must have the requisite skills to implement planning changes in behavior, thinking, and lifestyle ("able").

The process by which the individual moves from problematic use of a substance (abuse or dependence) toward a healthier relationship with that substance (either moderate use or abstinence) has been described DiClemente and Prochaska (1998) in their transtheoretical model of motivation (TMM), which proposes that change occurs as the individual progresses through a series of stages (outlined in Figure 13.1).

The stages are presumed to be sequentially invariant, in that the individual must pass through them in order during each change-attempt episode. Each of the stages in the TMM involves different cognitive, behavioral, and affective processes that serve either to facilitate or to inhibit movement toward change. For example, in the Precontemplation stage, characterized by minimal problem recognition, consciousness-raising activities, such as information provision, are particularly important in moving the individual into the next stage of change. CBT approaches have a significant advantage within the TMM framework, in that they are consistent with the change processes that are presumed to operate in a variety of the early stages, and certainly are applicable in the Action stage, when the individual is clearly engaged directly in changing behavior.

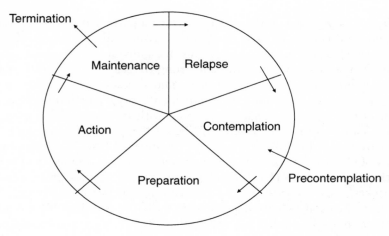

FIGURE 13.1. Stages of change.

For many substance-abusing clients, specific thinking patterns perpetuate the disorders and may block change. Beck, Wright, Newman, and Liese (1993) identified these thinking patters with addictive beliefs that fall into two general categories: expectation beliefs and permission-giving beliefs. Expectation beliefs are those that relate to what the client feels are, or will be, the benefits of use. These beliefs involve ideas of pleasure seeking, problem solving, relief, and escape, and as discussed earlier, may be formed quite early in the person's life (Beck et al., 1993). Permission-giving beliefs relate to justification, risk taking, and entitlement, and serve as the energizers of substance seeking and use (Beck et al., 1993). Additional research by Freeman (1992) further classify permission-giving beliefs into (1) denial-related beliefs—those that the client uses to tell him- or herself that the problem or behavior does not exist or to minimize it, and (2) rationalizing beliefs—those beliefs that admit, at least partially, to the behavior but justify, explain, entitle, attribute, or deny the connection between behavior and consequences.

The beliefs associated with SUDs are often closely connected to particular states or contexts, often referred to as "triggers." Triggers elicit both expectation beliefs and permission-giving beliefs, and serve as the proximal stimulus to the initiation of substance-seeking behavior. Triggers may also elicit the complex constellation of thoughts and behaviors associated with substance craving. Triggers can be either internal (affective states such as anxiety, depression, anger, or happiness; Marlatt & Gordon, 1985) or contextual (involving events and circumstances outside the individual). Such contextual triggers are often associated with internal states. Situations that involve conflict, peer pressure, or celebration often evoke particular emotions that become conditioned cues to initiate substance use. The particular triggers that are most salient for a particular individual are highly idiosyncratic; that is, individuals vary greatly in the extent to which a particular emotional state or environmental context is associated with craving and substance-seeking behavior. Thus, anger may be a trigger for one individual but not for another. One individual may find bars to be a strong trigger to use, whereas another may be indifferent to this context. This idiosyncratic patterning of triggers makes it necessary to identify each individual's trigger patterns to assist the person in developing strategies for coping with triggers without using substances. This process is the essence of the CBT approach to treating SUDs.

In overview, the CBT approach to treatment of SUDs focuses on two aspects of client behavior and cognition: motivation to change, and skills to facilitate and maintain changes (relapse prevention). Although motivational approaches, such as motivational interviewing (Miller & Rollnick, 2002), have developed somewhat independently of CBT approaches, there is a natural compatibility between these approaches. Research on motivational interviewing has found that addressing client motivation and stage-of-change issues at the beginning of treatment enhances outcomes regardless of the specific content of the treatment that follows. For this reason, we have incorporated motivational components into our sample CBT group protocol.

CBT approaches to the treatment of SUDs have been extensively manualized. Early manuals (Monti, Kadden, Rohsenow, Cooney, & Abrams, 2002) focused primarily on treatment of alcohol problems. Later manuals using a CBT approach have focused on treatment of other drug problems, primarily cocaine and stimulant use (Carroll, 1998). Carroll's manual for treatment of cocaine dependence is an individually delivered program that could easily be adapted for group delivery. The other manualized approaches are specifically designed for group delivery.

A manual has also been published that incorporates the TMM into a group treatment format that focuses on conjoining motivational and CBT approaches (Velasquez, Maurer, Crouch, & DiClemente, 2001). There have also been efforts to manualize motivational interventions, such as motivational interviewing, for group delivery (Ingersoll, Wagner, & Gharib, 1997; Rotgers & Graves, 2004). These manualized treatments both attempt to capture the spirit of motivational interviewing in group format.

Efficacy of CBT

Numerous evaluations of CBT interventions for SUDs have been conducted, and support for the effectiveness of this approach is strong. It has been compared with alternative and control treatments (e.g., Miller, Willbourne, & Hettema, 2003). Both individual and group versions of CBT have been evaluated, with data supporting efficacy in either delivery format. In fact, until recently, the research literature on outcomes of treatments for SUDs generally favored CBT over other approaches. However, it has become clear in recent years that CBT may be differentially effective for some clients (Maude-Griffin et al., 1998). As with most other treatment approaches, the best question to ask may not be "Is CBT treatment effective?" but rather "With what patients is CBT effective, and with what patients is it more effective than other approaches?" This mirror's Paul's classic question about psychotherapy research from the 1960s: "What works, with whom, under what circumstances?" (Paul, 1969).

We have chosen to adopt the "Paulian" perspective on efficacy in this brief review of the efficacy of CBT approaches and focus our brief review on client variables that appear to be associated with outcome of CBT treatments. Research suggests that the following client variables are associated with treatment outcomes using CBT approaches: psychopathology, abstract reasoning ability, religious beliefs, and belief in the "disease model" of addiction.

Psychopathology, Abstract Reasoning, and Outcome of CBT

Research has shown that relapse occurred significantly more slowly when patients with high psychopathology received coping skills treatment, and when patients with low psychopathology received interactional group therapy. Relapse rates were also slower when subjects with high sociopathology were treated with interactional therapy. Patients classified as cognitively impaired, however, had better outcomes in interact ional therapy and worse outcomes in coping skills treatment (Kadden, Cooney, Getter, & Litt, 1989).

Kadden et al. (1989) suggested that patients with more psychopathology may be expected to do better in coping skills treatment because of its structure, and because its goals are limited to relapse prevention. The relative lack of structure and broader goals of traditional therapy may be threatening to patients who have more psychopathology. Patients higher in sociopathy may do better with coping skills treatment, because it does not require strong interpersonal relationships among group members, and because it provides specific anger management skills. On the other hand, patients low in sociopathy may be receptive to the interpersonal focus of more traditional group therapy.

A study of treatment of cocaine users by Hall and associates suggests that CBT approaches may be more effective with patients who have better abstract reasoning ability (Maude-Griffin et al., 1998). When data comparing outcomes of a group CBT and a traditional 12-step approach were analyzed with respect to abstracting ability, CBT clearly produced better outcomes with patients whose abstracting abilities were better.

On the face of it, these two sets of findings (that patients higher in psychopathology and higher in abstracting ability do better in CBT) seem to be in conflict, because it seems logical to assume that co-occurring psychopathology would reduce abstracting ability. It seems likely that the content of the CBT approaches, which focus on enhancing commitment to abstinence and supporting such a commitment systematically through teaching of coping skills, can provide structure and motivation that may be helpful for patients who are initially attempting to overcome co-occurring disorders, but who can then make use of (due to higher abstracting abilities) the technical aspects of CBT treatment.

Beliefs and CBT Outcome

Patients who hold strong religious beliefs tend to do less well in CBT than in a traditional 12-step approach, whereas patients who subscribe to the view that addiction is more like a disease than like a bad habit also do less well with CBT approaches (Logan & Tonigan, 2003). This is not surprising given the strong emphasis in traditional treatments on a philosophy (the 12 steps) that, although not directly affiliated with any religion, incorporates many concepts and ideas from Judeo-Christian thinking (e.g., the notion of a "higher power" and frequent references to turning one's life over to God). This sort of philosophy has often been off-putting for many patients, to the extent that legal actions have been brought in some instances to ensure that non-12-step alternatives are available in some settings on the ground that offering only a 12-step approach violates constitutional guarantees of freedom of religion (Apanovitch, 1998).

Likewise, research suggests that patients who subscribe less strongly to a disease concept of addiction do better with CBT approaches. Again, this is not surprising, because a central tenet of traditional 12-step-based treatments is the notion that one's addiction is a result of a disease that can only be managed, never cured—hence, the emphasis on lifelong abstinence as the only viable approach to resolving addictions. When treatment approaches or support groups are available that allow for moderation or harm reduction goals, researchers have found that they tend to attract people who are both less religious and less committed to the view that their problems with substances are the result of a disease (Humphreys & Klaw, 2001).

Despite the findings we have just reviewed, it is clear that CBT approaches work well with a variety of clients. Whereas the attempt to identify specific matching variables that can be used to prescribe treatments differentially has been ongoing, the results have been less than overwhelmingly positive. In our view, the extensive research evidence for the efficacy of CBT approaches makes them a good initial treatment choice for virtually any client, with the possible exception of those whose abstract reasoning and thinking skills are so poor that they cannot learn effective coping skills or engage in cognitive restructuring on a systematic basis.

ASSESSMENT ISSUES IN CBT OF SUDs

The CBT view of SUDs and the variables associated with change and maintenance of change suggest that five important areas need to be addressed in client assessment: (1) motivation for change, (2) skills assets and deficits, (3) cognitive distortions and expectancies, (4) environmental and internal factors associated with substance use ("triggers"/high-risk situations), and (5) treatment goals and commitment. We briefly address each of these important areas for assessment.

Motivation for Change

As indicated in our brief discussion of the TMM, client motivation and readiness to change are critical to treatment outcome. Mismatching interventions to clients' stage of change has been thought to be a major factor in treatment failure (Prochaska et al., 1994). Therefore, assessing motivation and stage of change become critical to ensuring that interventions are appropriate for particular clients.

A number of instruments have been developed to assess stage of change or readiness to change (Carey, Purnine, Maisto, & Carey, 1999). These include the University of Rhode Island Change Assessment (URICA; DiClemente & Hughes, 1990), the Stages of Change Readiness and Treatment Eagerness Scale (SOCRATES; Miller & Tonigan, 1996), and the Readiness to Change-Treatment Questionnaire (RTCQ, Rollnick, Heather, Gold, & Hall, 1992). All of these instruments have good psychometric properties and have been shown to be at least moderately predictive of treatment outcomes. All are available in the published research literature. With the exception of the RTCQ, which takes only 5 minutes, these instruments take the typical client 10–20 minutes to complete.

Although scores on the URICA, the SOCRATES, and the RTCQ have been shown to predict outcomes such as treatment engagement and retention, they have not done a good job specifying clients' stage of change within the TMM (Carey et al., 1999). They also are somewhat cumbersome to score and interpret. A briefer, more intuitive assessment procedure is the Readiness Ruler technique developed by Rollnick et al. (1999). Using the clinical heuristic of "ready, willing, and able" as a guide to understanding client motivation, the Readiness Ruler technique asks the client to rate him- or herself on three dimensions: importance of changing the target behavior, readiness to change the behavior now, and confidence in one's ability to actually effect changes.

From a clinical perspective, any of these assessment instruments is a useful way of tapping into the change-related factors outlined in the TMM.

Skills Assets and Deficits

Delineating client skills that have been brought to bear on prior change efforts with success, as well as skills deficits that both maintain target behaviors and stand in the way of successful change, is an important aspect of initial assessment. Although space prohibits extensive discussion of skills assessment, suffice it to say that a number of instruments and procedures have been developed that, along with structured behavioral interviewing, can be used to assess levels of client skills (Donovan & Marlatt, 2005). Having a baseline sense of how skillful a client is in relation to behavior change, as well as areas of skills weakness, can allow clinicians to monitor progress through periodic reassessments. It can also alert clinicians to client skills that may have been discounted by the client (e.g., successful smoking cessation in a client seeking help with cocaine dependence), but that may be generalized to the current change effort.

Cognitive Distortions and Expectancies

Assessing cognitive distortions and expectancies provides a baseline from which to measure changes in clients' views of both the costs and benefits of substance use. Both positive outcome expectancies (and cognitive distortions that accompany them) and negative outcome expectancies for substance use have been found to correlate with outcome. Specifically, as positive outcome expectancies are reduced and negative outcome expectancies increase, the likelihood of use (or relapse to previous levels of use once change has occurred) decreases.

A number of instruments are available for measuring positive outcome expectancies (see Allen, 2003). Although these tend to be focused on alcohol use, they can also be used to assess positive outcome expectancies for the use of other drugs. Assessing these positive expectancies also provides an indication of the specific cognitive distortions that clients have with respect to substance use. Given that relapse to previous levels of substance use is often associated with activation of positive outcome expectancies ("I'll feel less angry if I smoke a joint," "A couple of beers would really take the edge off my nervousness"), helping clients identify and develop alternative cognitive and behavioral coping strategies when these expectancies are activated can greatly enhance outcome.

As noted earlier, negative outcome expectancies have also been found to correlate with outcomes (McMahon & Jones, 1993a). Specifically, as negative outcome expectancies for substance use increase ("The hangovers are really bad," "I can't take the paranoia after I smoke crack"), the likelihood of a return to pretreatment levels of use decreases. Periodically assessing negative expectancies using the Negative Alcohol Expectancy Questionnaire (McMahon & Jones, 1993b; reworded if assessing drug-related negative expectancies) can help track a client's progress toward more stable and permanent behavior change.

Environmental and Internal Factors Associated with Use ("High-Risk Situations")

Assessment of so-called "high-risk situations" or "triggers" that are discriminative stimuli for substance use is critical in assisting clients in the development of individualized coping strategies. Although the triggers to substance use are likely as varied and heterogeneous as clients, a number of types of triggering events, situations, and internal states seem to be most frequently associated with relapse to previous use levels across client and drug types (Marlatt & Gordon, 1985). These can be assessed with the Inventory of Drinking Situations (IDS; in Allen, 2003), which not only identifies triggers but also provides information as to the "potency" of the trigger in the form of Likert ratings of the likelihood that the client will use in the context of that particular situation or internal state. Instruments are also available (e.g., the Drug Abuse Self-Efficacy Scale [DASES]; in Allen, 2003) that allow a correlation of triggers with the client's self-efficacy expectation for coping with them effectively without using substances. Again, assessment of these factors allows tailoring of both coping strategies and plans to individual clients, and tracking of progress toward enhanced self-efficacy with respect to coping.

Treatment Goals and Commitment

A number of studies have found that the single best predictor of treatment outcome is the degree of client commitment to a particular change goal (usually abstinence) at treatment entry (Morgenstern, Frey, McCrady, Labouvie, & Neighbors, 1996). Research has also demonstrated that, at least in the context of treatment for alcohol and possibly cannabis problems, allowing the client to select between abstinence and moderate use at treatment entry, then to change that goal as treatment progresses, is associated with better outcomes, regardless of the goal selected (Ojehagen & Berglund, 1989).

The assessment of treatment goals is clearly quite simple. The clinician need only ask the client what goals he or she wishes to pursue. This only becomes problematic for some clinicians when the client appears to be toying with the idea of moderation rather than abstinence. A persistent myth in the treatment community asserts that moderation is impossible for most clients and that, even if it were possible, it is an undesirable outcome. Research, particularly studies focused on alcohol use over the past 30 years, has clearly debunked this myth (e.g., Dawson, 1996). In fact, recent research has found that even clients with relatively severe substance use problems can effectively moderate their use with treatment. That being said, is it responsible and ethical even to allow clients to make their own goal choices?

Research suggests that clinician fears with respect to accepting a client goal of moderation are typically overblown. Clients in treatment rarely choose moderation as their treatment goal, and of those who do, most shift their goal to abstinence as treatment progresses. Of course, it is probably clinical hubris for a clinician to believe that it is the clinician's goal choice that matters at the end of the day. Clearly, what the client chooses is what the client will do! Given the importance of therapeutic alliance in helping clients resolve substance use problems, as well as research suggesting that even minor disagreements between client and clinician at the beginning of treatment are associated with poorer outcomes (Brown & Miller, 1993; Patterson & Forgatch, 1985), it makes sense for clinicians to recognize client autonomy with respect to goals and to work within that limitation to negotiate a treatment goal to which the client can make a strong commitment.

In addition to reducing the likelihood of conflict between clinician and client, some research suggests that imposing a treatment goal (whether it be abstinence or moderation) on a client is associated with poorer outcome (Sanchez-Craig & Lei, 1986). Thus, the broad body of research on client goal choice would seem to point toward a less doctrinaire and prescriptive approach on the part of the clinician as being most likely to bear fruit in terms of positive outcomes. Of course, this does not mean that the clinician should abandon efforts to persuade clients that the safest course (abstinence) is often the best in the long run. Rather, clinicians (and this is certainly in the spirit of CBT) negotiate goals with clients in the context of a thorough examination of the pros and cons of various goal choices.

Once a treatment goal has been agreed upon, assessment of commitment to change relative to that goal is easy. Most research on this topic has used a simple 10-point Likert scale rating, in which the client simply indicates how committed he or she is to the goal selected. The higher the rating, the more committed the client is, and the greater the likelihood of achieving that goal in the long run.

GROUP TREATMENT

The prototype for group CBT for substance abuse is the set of companion manuals by Monti et al. (2002), published in two editions as *Treating Alcohol Dependence*. These manuals are also closely related to the individual treatment manual used in the CBT condition in the multisite study Project MATCH (Matching Alcohol Treatments to Client Heterogeneity). A group treatment manual published by Velasquez et al. (2001) uses CBT in the context of the TMM concept of change. Both these and other manuals contain a core of sessions that we outline here. In addition, we believe that research supports starting off all clients with an initial individual session that consists of a motivational feedback interview based on the assessment data gathered prior to treatment. We have provided an outline of that session as well.

In addition to adding an initial individual motivational feedback session, we also adopt an approach similar to that used in the Project MATCH study. This approach is characterized by what we would term a manual "guided" process in which there is a core set of sessions delivered to every group cohort, with an additional set of "optional" sessions delivered "as needed," or if assessment across clients indicates a dominant group need in that particular area. Thus, for a group of single persons not in relationships, group sessions on couple communication may not be relevant. However, for a group of married clients, such a session may be critical. The ability to tailor the content of some group sessions within the context of providing a systematic core of basic skills for change and relapse prevention seems to us to provide an optimum balance between being strictly manual-driven and nonmanualized, and allows for use of clinical judgment in structuring the curriculum for the specific group of individuals being treated. We call this approach "manual-guided," in that the manual provides specific structured group sessions, with options for changing or augmenting the specific sessions based on clinical judgment and the particular characteristics of the clients in a particular group cohort.

Session Format

Sessions should follow a consistent format from the beginning of treatment. This format has several components, with the length of time devoted to each component determined by the facilitator as the group session unfolds. Thus, for sessions in which there has been no previous homework assignment, this component may be abbreviated or omitted.

We next present the components of a CBT group format.

Welcome and Agenda Setting

After a brief welcome in which the group ground rules are briefly reviewed, the facilitator uses the first 5 or 10 minutes of each session to review the topics to be discussed, and invites participants to submit their own agenda items for consideration. The facilitator leads a brief discussion of how much time the group wants to devote to each participant's agenda items (attempting to consolidate items that are very similar in content), while ensuring that the topic of the day is covered thoroughly. The amount of time devoted to participants' agenda items varies depending on the length of group sessions.

Homework Review

Following agenda setting, the first task is *always* to review and discuss participants' experiences doing the previous session's homework assignment. In this component of the group, there should be particular focus on participant successes and on barriers that participants encountered in attempting to do the homework. Discussion of barriers should include brainstorming of ways to overcome those barriers in the future.

Participant Agenda Items

Although these are often touched upon in the discussion of homework, in this next component, participants may express their own concerns, difficulties, and successes. The facilitator should attempt, as much as possible, to relate participants' agenda items to past or future group session content.

Presentation of the Topic of the Day

Assuming a 90-minute group session, this component should take up at least 45 minutes of the session. Because most topics require not only didactic presentation by the facilitator but also discussion and practice by participants, it is important that sufficient time be allotted for a reasonably thorough presentation of the topic of the day.

Homework Assignment and Wrap-Up

The facilitator presents and explains the homework assignment for the week and invites participant discussion as to the feasibility of the assignment (including potential barriers to completion of the assignment), and questions as to assignment specifics. The session ends with the facilitator's inquiry about participants' view of the session. Was it helpful, not helpful? Was anything unclear, or perhaps offensive to them? Finally, date, time, and place of the next session are presented.

With this structure for delivery in mind, we now briefly outline the content of the core and optional sessions, which are displayed in Table 13.3. The reader should keep in mind that the sessions we suggest have been part of CBT group treatment for some time. These sessions have proven utility with a broad range of clients in a variety of settings, which does not make them sacrosanct, or immutable, but rather suggests that these session topics should have high priority in the design of any particular group program for substance users.

Group Session Summaries

Session 1: Individual Motivational Feedback

In this initial session, the focus is upon exploring the pros and cons of changing substance use. There are several techniques for doing this (e.g., see Miller & Rollnick, 2002; Rollnick et al., 1999; Rotgers & Graves, 2004). We recommend simply putting a decisional balance matrix on a blackboard or in handouts and asking group members to indicate first the pros of continuing unchanged, the cons of changing, then the cons of continuing unchanged, and finally the pros of changing. It is important that clinician remain neutral in this exercise; the point is to encourage group members to develop their own motivational structure for change. The group facilitator should utilize reflective listening techniques (Miller & Rollnick, 2002) to stimulate and facilitate continued participation by the group members.

Session 2: Introduction to High-Risk Situations

In this session, the focus is on helping the client to identify, in as much detail as possible, situations in which he or she is at increased risk for substance use.

TABLE 13.3. Sample Outline of Treatment Protocol for Group CBT of Substance Use

Session	Strategies covered

Session 1	• Individual motivational feedback.
	• Decisional balance matrix.
	  1. Pros of continuing unchanged.
	  2. Cons of changing.
	  3. Cons of continuing unchanged.
	  4. Pros of changing.

Session 2	• Identification of high-risk situations.
	  1. Intrapersonal or interpersonal.
	  2. Triggers: Affect, people, places, things.
	• Action plans for coping with high-risk situations.

Session 3	• Identification of precursors to substance abuse.
	• Planning methods to cope with urges.
	  1. Thought stopping.
	  2. Decisional balance exercise.
	  3. Delaying.

Session 4	• Managing negative thinking. • Relationship of thinking and affect. • Identifying negative thought patterns. • Challenging negative thoughts and cognitive restructuring.
Session 5	• Seemingly irrelevant decisions. • Vigilance for high-risk situations. • Functional analysis to think through risk.
Session 6	• Planning for emergencies. • Emergence of unexpected triggers or high-risk situations. • "If . . . then" action plans. • Hiearchy of coping strategies.
Session 7	• Refusal skills and direct offers. • "No thanks" principle. • Developing personal refusal scripts. • Role-play assertive responses.
Session 8	• Giving and receiving criticism. • Responding assertively to criticism. • Delivering critical comments assertively. • Relaxation skills. • Role plays.
Session 9	• Anger management and substance use. • Identification of signs of anger. • Relaxation skills. • Cognitive restructuring with anger thoughts. • Problem solving in anger scenarios. • Role plays.

(continued)

TABLE 13.3. (continued)

Session	Strategies covered
Session 10	• Pleasurable activites and substance use. • Review of withdrawal from pleasant activities as a result of substance use. • Identify pleasurable activities as a healthy alternative. • Plan for engaging in pleasant activities. • Eliciting a commitment for planful pleasant events.

Session 11	• Stigma and problems related to substance use.
	• Problem-solving skills.
	  1. Problem definition.
	  2. Brainstorming solutions.
	  3. Selecting a solution.
	  4. Implementing a solution.
	  5. Evaluating a solution.
	• In-session examples.

Session 12	• Reinstituting non-substance-focused friendships. • Repairing damaged familial relationships. • Repairing damaged relationships with employers. • Finding a supportive/self-help group to sustain recovery.

Situations are classified as intrapersonal or interpersonal (Marlatt & Gordon 1985), because high-risk situations (often called "triggers") can be affective states, as well as external events (in Alcoholics Anonymous [AA] parlance, "people, places, and things"). Emphasis is also placed on helping the client begin to develop specific, multilevel action plans for coping with high-risk situations without using substances.

Session 3: Managing Urges to Use

The focus of this session is on developing strategies for early identification of precursors to substance use, and planning methods to cope with urges. This session builds upon the notion of high-risk situations (triggers) introduced in Session 2. A variety of methods have been employed to help substance users resist urges to use. Most commonly this involves some version of thought stopping coupled with a brief decisional balance exercise on the pros and cons of using, delaying action on feelings for at least 15 minutes, or what has been called "urge surfing"—simply observing the urge but not acting upon it. In-session practice can often bring home the central point of this session: that urges and cravings typically subside on their own.

Session 4: Managing Negative Thinking

Substance users early in treatment are often subject to a variety of negative thoughts about themselves, their substance use, and their ability to cope with daily living without using substances. Often these negative thought patterns trigger negative affect that, in turn, becomes a high-risk situation for substance use. In this session, participants learn to identify and challenge negative or maladaptive thought patterns. The most frequently used method is to teach Ellis's (Ellis & MacClaren, 2005) A-B-C-D-E approach to cognitive restructuring.

Session 5: Seemingly Irrelevant Decisions

Once substance users have stopped using (perhaps the easiest part of the process of overcoming substance use problems—Mark Twain claims to have done it hundreds of times with smoking!), it is important that they remain vigilant for high-risk situations that may trigger relapse. In this session, participants are taught functional analysis as a means of thinking through the risk potential of various decisions. Often "seemingly irrelevant decisions" can trigger a relapse, so participants are taught to think ahead and evaluate potential courses of action, with an eye toward the degree to which these may lead to high-risk situations that may tax coping skills.

Session 6: Planning for Emergencies

Substance use is associated with a wide variety of discriminative stimuli that serve as triggers. Unfortunately, not all of them are readily apparent to patients, despite their best efforts to identify as many triggers as possible. This session addresses the issue of what to do when an unexpected urge or craving to use occurs outside the context of previously identified high-risk situations or triggers. The focus is on developing specific "if . . . then" action plans that are individualized for each group participant, and involves a hierarchy of coping strategies that can be sequentially implemented. Thus, if a "first-line" strategy fails, the participant has a second (and sometimes even a third) strategy upon which to rely.

Session 7: Refusal Skills

Often one of the most difficult challenges for a substance user to confront without using is a direct offer of alcohol or drugs from another person. Although refusing an offer of substances is quite simple in principle (one need only say "No thanks," repeatedly, if necessary!), this skill is a critical one for many patients in preventing relapse following establishment of abstinence. In this session, participants develop personal "scripts" for substance refusal and role-play practice encounters using assertive responses to increasingly insistent offers of substances from other group members. Emphasis is placed on the basic components of assertive responding: body posture, eye contact, tone of voice, and statement content.

Session 8: Giving and Receiving Criticism

As with assertive refusal of offers of substances, it is frequently the case that substance users are unable to respond assertively and appropriately to criticism from others, and may also be prone to deliver criticisms to others in a way that leads to confrontation and anger rather than problem solution. In this session, the focus is on both what to say and how to say it when responding to critical comments from others, as well as how to deliver critical comments to others without becoming angry or confrontational. This session often includes brief instruction in relaxation techniques used to defuse physiological arousal (either anxiety or anger) in response to or in anticipation of giving criticism. Role-play practice is an important part of this session.

Session 9: Anger Management

Yet another difficult task for many substance users is managing angry responses both to others and to their own perceived inability to organize their lives effectively without substances as a focus. As a follow-up to Session 8, this session teaches a basic anger management strategy that consists of identification of physical indicators of anger, relaxation strategies to reduce arousal, and cognitive restructuring to assist in defusing angry thoughts and implementing a problem-solving approach to anger-inducing encounters. Again, role-play exercises play an important part in this session.

Session 10: Increasing Pleasant Activities

As substance use becomes increasingly the focus of a patient's life (e.g., as substance use shifts into more severe dependence) it is not uncommon for the patient to begin to give up many activities that previously were sources of pleasure and life satisfaction. For patients whose substance use is of long duration, this may mean that they have few, if any, pleasurable activities or outlets left in their lives. Thus, when the patient initiates abstinence from substances (even if only temporarily), there is a psychological and emotional void left in his or her life. In this session, patients are helped to begin to identify and increasingly engage in pleasurable activities that can provide a substitute (albeit, perhaps a less powerful one) for substance use. There is then a process of eliciting commitments from participants to begin to engage in these pleasurable activities in a planful way during the remainder of treatment.

Session 11: Problem Solving

Learning effective problem solving is an essential skill focus for substance users. Despite Herculean efforts by treatment providers and others who advocate for a disability or disease view of SUDs, a substance use diagnosis still carries significant stigma in contemporary American society. Substance users often encounter genuine life problems that, either because their substance use began early and created a developmental lag, or because they have "forgotten" skills they once knew, require active, systematic problem-solving skills to resolve. In this session, participants are introduced to one of the many standardized problem-solving models. For example, the model developed by D'Zurilla and Nezu (1999) consists of a series of steps for effectively identifying a problem, brainstorming possible solutions, selecting a solution to implement, implementing the solution, then evaluating the efficacy of the chosen approach. In-session exercises, in which participants use the problem-solving model to approach standardized problem scenarios, are an important aspect of this session.

Session 12: Developing Support Networks

As with pleasurable activities, it is often the case that as substance users become more and more involved in a substance-using lifestyle and peer group, they begin to lose touch with nonusing friends and become alienated from nonusing relatives. This session addresses strategies for reinstituting old non-substance-focused friendships, repairing damaged family relationships, and establishing new, supportive relationships. Issues such as repairing damaged relationships with employers and spouses/domestic partners are central to this session. In addition, participants (who have been advised to try out self-help support groups early on in the treatment) are encouraged to begin the process of finding a support group in which they feel comfortable. Although there is some clinical controversy about whether persons receiving CBT treatment for substance use disorders should be directed toward 12-step support groups, research clearly shows the advantages of affiliation with these groups for prolonging abstinence (or promoting moderation).

As we indicated at the beginning of this section, this selection of group topics is meant to provide a core set of topics around which a CBT group treatment can be developed. It is important to understand that this outline is neither exhaustive nor prescriptive. Therapists should carefully consider adding or subtracting sessions depending upon group members' needs. For example, in working with coerced clients (such as offenders or persons mandated by an employer to seek treatment), sustaining motivation to change is often an issue that requires more than a single session to address. Therapists working with coerced patients might wish to consider adding periodic motivational enhancement sessions, in which group participants review and revise their personal decisional balance exercises and renew their commitment to goals and change.

Issues in Treatment Implementation and Follow-Up

A variety of issues need to be considered when implementing any treatment for substance users, and CBT group treatment is no exception. In this section we consider some of the issues that are most germane to the treatment of substance users. These include issues regarding the relationship between substance use and other co-occurring disorders (comorbidity), relapse prevention and booster sessions, long-term follow-up of patients, and the issue of support groups and their role in the change process for substance users. We consider each of these in turn.

Comorbidity

Although clinicians have long recognized the close relationship between substance use and other psychiatric disorders, research on this relationship in the last decade of the 20th century began to quantify this issue (Regier et al., 1990). What emerged from research by Regier and colleagues (as well as others) was a picture suggesting that, on average, more than one-third of patients being treated for an SUD suffered from another Axis I or Axis II disorder. In particular, the association between substance use and so-called "severe" mental disorders (schizophrenia, bipolar disorder, etc.) became much clearer.

Until quite recently, it was traditional, perhaps due to the way in which the mental health and substance abuse treatment and reimbursement systems were structured, for patients with both substance misuse and psychiatric disorders to be shuttled back and forth between mental health and substance abuse treatment providers, often being told that one of their disorders (either the psychiatric disorder or the SUD) must be treated before the system with which the patient was currently interacting could treat its particular focus disorders. This frequently led to patients not being treated at all, because neither the mental health nor substance abuse treatment systems would work with patients with co-occurring disorders. This situation began to change in the 1990s, and it is now good practice to treat psychiatric disorders and SUDs concurrently, rather than separately and/or sequentially (Rosenthal & Westreich, 1999).

Contributing to this situation was a belief among many persons with co-occurring disorders (as well as many clinicians), often mistakenly attributed to 12-step philosophies (as opposed to specific 12-step meetings), that psychotropic medications were simply other drugs, analogous to the ones the substance user was trying to stop using; therefore, the substance misuser who suffered from a pharmacologically treatable psychiatric disorder should avoid all "mood altering" substances, including prescribed medications. Efforts by 12-step groups, such as AA, to change this view have largely (but not entirely) been successful, and it is now rare, at least among clinicians, to find opposition to taking prescribed psychotropic medications for co-occurring psychiatric problems.

In the context of this chapter, the question arises as to whether CBT group treatment is appropriate for patients with co-occurring psychiatric disorders, and for which disorders. The research to date on this question is sparse, but it does suggest that patients with significant co-occurring psychopathology can benefit from CBT group treatment (Rosenthal & Westreich, 1999). The main group for whom group treatment may not be indicated, at least at the beginning of treatment, are patients who suffer from severe social anxiety, for whom the group setting itself may become a barrier to treatment.

Also perhaps less likely to benefit from group CBT approaches are patients with neurological deficits that impair learning new skills as complex as some of those taught in group CBT treatments for substance misuse. There is, however, the possibility that many of these patients will find the supportive, problem-focused approach of CBT to be more effective. In the absence of strong research findings on this issue, we recommend that clinicians base the decision whether to refer a particular individual to a CBT group for substance abuse treatment on a thorough assessment.

Relapse Prevention, Booster Sessions, and Long-Term Follow-Up

The question of when treatment is "finished" is important in treating many disorders, but perhaps even more so in substance use disorders. Within both the clinical and "recovering" communities, much debate focuses around whether SUDs are ever "finally and conclusively" resolved, or whether the person who develops an SUD and completes treatment must be considered forever "in recovery," or whether those who have completed treatment, like cancer patients whose cancer has been removed without a return of symptoms for a period of time, can at some point be considered "cured."

It has become a truism in the substance abuse treatment area that longer involvement is associated with better outcomes. Although it is unclear whether this often-cited research finding is due to treatment factors (e.g., a "dose–response" effect) or client motivation (cf. Miller, 2000), the importance of some continuing contact with patients seems clear. The issue of how much contact and how often clients should be provided with booster sessions remains unresolved, at least in terms of research. Although it is speculative at this point, it may be useful for clinicians to schedule a follow-up contact (whether by phone or in person) with clients on a quarterly basis after the end of treatment.

In addition to periodic therapist contact, another means for helping clients maintain treatment gains is to assist them in establishing an affiliation with a free support group such as AA or Self-Management and Recovery Training (SMART). We discuss this option in the next section.

Use of Support Groups

Support groups have been at the core of helping people overcome SUDs for more than 65 years, following the founding of AA in the 1930s. Research has clearly demonstrated an association between support group attendance and long-term positive outcomes after treatment (McKellar, Stewart, & Humphreys, 2003). Although the reason for this association is not clear, it seems likely that either the most motivated patients stick with support group attendance, thus reaping more benefits, or there is something about support groups themselves that facilitate ongoing positive outcomes. The extremely high dropout rates from most support groups (cf. Alcoholics Anonymous, 1999) tend to support the former assumption. Whatever the reason, affiliation with and regular attendance at support group meetings seems to be associated with better posttreatment outcomes.

There are a variety of support groups available for people who are attempting to recover from substance use (McCrady, Horvath, & Delaney, 2002). Most follow the 12-step approach developed by Bill Wilson and Bob Smith, the cofounders of AA. In fact, 12-step-based support groups are available in virtually every metropolitan area in the United States, and in many larger cities abroad. This wide availability makes 12-step groups the first choice for most people who decide to use support groups.

Although 12-step groups espouse a philosophy of life and behavior that is, in some aspects, fundamentally different from the orientation of CBT groups, strong arguments have been made for their inclusion as an option for patients in CBT treatment (McCrady et al., 2002). Certainly, attendance at support groups of any sort provides models for successfully overcoming SUDs, as well as an opportunity to make new friends who are substance-free. The regular reminder of the need for vigilance with respect to triggers and other high-risk situations that 12-step groups provide also facilitates long-term change.

In recent years, a number of non-12-step alternative groups have developed. Two of these, Self-Management and Recovery Training (SMART) and Moderation Management (MM) are based squarely in CBT principles. Both of these groups support the notion (inconsistent with the original writings of the founders of AA) that one can "recover" from SUDs and need not be forever "recovering." These groups also appeal (as does another support group, Secular Organization for Sobriety [SOS]) to patients for whom the spiritual aspects of 12-step groups are inconsistent with personal values and beliefs.

MM has the additional aspect that its program does not establish a predetermined goal of abstinence from substances, as do all other support groups (Rotgers & Kishline, 1999). Rather, MM supports objective, honest examination of the role of substances in the individual's life, and any course that leads to a reduction of negative consequences associated with substance use. Thus, goals of moderation or reduced use are not frowned upon; rather, they are considered an important part of change for individuals who are committed to moderation or who, for whatever reasons, are not yet ready to pursue abstinence. MM espouses the view that any healthy change in behavior should be supported, even if it does not produce perfect abstinence or health. Nonetheless, MM supports members who have chosen abstinence, and the current handbook (Rotgers, Kern, & Hoeltzel, 2002) provides a variety of techniques that members can apply in the pursuit of either reduced use or abstinence.

Advantages and Obstacles in Group CBT for SUDs

Advantages of Group CBT

Group CBT has a number of advantages as an approach to working with substance users. It is highly pragmatic and skills focused, and, despite the group format, is delivered in a fashion that allows a large measure of individualization of treatment. CBT and associated approaches (e.g., group motivational interviewing) have performed quite well with patients with co-occurring disorders. For these patients, the pragmatic, present time, and skills-focused emphasis of group CBT is helpful in reducing the resistance that can often occur in non-CBT approaches. CBT's inherently respectful and collaborative approach to helping patients change is an additional advantage over traditional approaches to group treatment of substance abuse, which are often confrontational and aggressive in their attempts to break through "denial."

Noncompliance with Homework

Homework or assignments to practice new behavioral skills outside of sessions is a cornerstone of CBT, whether delivered in group or individual formats. Persistent noncompliance with homework is a good indicator that some obstacle stands in the way of the patient's progress. It is critical that the group leader inquire into, and help patients deal with, barriers to completion of homework that may exist, both in the patient's environment and in his or her thinking. Typically, these barriers fall into one of several categories that need to be assessed and addressed if treatment is to be fully successful. Typical barriers to homework completion include (1) minimal motivation to change, (2) disorganization and chaotic lifestyle that makes systematic attention to homework difficult, (3) homework assignments that seem overwhelmingly complex or difficult for the patient, and (4) patients' misunderstanding of assignments or the importance of homework in the change process. It is critical that the therapist assess with the patient which obstacle is operative in a particular case (it is important to recognize that more than one may be operative), and begin to develop a plan to help overcome those obstacles and facilitate homework completion.

Motivation issues can be usefully addressed by asking patients to think about the pros and cons of changing by themselves, of changing with treatment, and of following the recommendations that the therapist and group make to help facilitate change. Helping disorganized or chaotic patients learn basic organizational skills is often helpful in reducing that barrier. Incomplete assignments that the patient sees as too difficult or complicated can be dealt with by simplifying the assignments, explaining them in detail to the patient, and requesting that the patient repeat what he or she understands the assignment to be, then clarifying, until the patient understands the assignment accurately. Similarly, a patient's misunderstanding of the assignment or the importance of homework can be addressed by clarifying with the patient the requirements of the assignment and the rationale for asking the patient to do it.

Lack of Spiritual Emphasis

For some patients, especially those who are not particularly religious, lack of spiritual emphasis can be an advantage of CBT. The emphasis on self-efficacy, personal autonomy, and skills is often more compatible with patient views than is the spiritual approach associated with 12-step treatment. However, particularly for patients who have had positive, if temporary, results from following the 12-step philosophy, or for those who are receiving CBT group treatment in the context of a 12-step-oriented program, the lack of a spiritual emphasis can seem to be a disadvantage.

It is important that such concerns be addressed early on in treatment. It is useful for spiritually oriented patients to indicate that nothing in CBT treatment is inherently inconsistent with the 12 steps. Even the wording of Step One, which refers to "powerlessness," focuses on the past (we "were" powerless), and on the use of the substance itself, as well as on the "unmanageable" nature of the user's life. Explaining that CBT directly addresses both of these issues by teaching the skills necessary to navigate through a difficult environment and negative emotional states, without using substances to cope, can often alleviate patient concerns in this regard. Certainly, saying to patients that CBT does not discourage attendance at 12-step groups can also be helpful.

Models of Progress for Slower Members

As with support groups, CBT groups can provide a variety of modeling opportunities for group members who may initially have difficulty in the behavior change process, or who may be slower to pick up and utilize new skills effectively. Group members who rapidly "get" the CBT approach can be helpful to other members, both by example, and in group interactions and role plays. Both group CBT and support groups offer an opportunity for communal problem-solving when a member runs into difficulty. In order to facilitate this process, it is critical that the group facilitator work hard to establish a safe, accepting group atmosphere that is highly tolerant of mistakes and lack of immediate progress.

CONCLUSIONS

Group CBT for SUDs is an approach that has garnered substance research support for its efficacy. The approach is inherently respectful and collaborative, and it fosters client self-efficacy. It is compatible with the most widely available support groups for substance users (e.g., 12-step-based groups). Given its strong skills focus, group CBT is an ideal approach for persons who lack particular coping skills either in direct relation to substance use (e.g., drink/drug refusal skills, emotional coping) or to coping with life circumstances that may trigger substance use. This approach is flexible, able to be tailored to individual needs, and is based solidly on assessment of factors associated with substance use. We believe it is worth considering for virtually any clients except those with extreme social phobia or other disorders that make any group approach problematic.

CHAPTER 14

Personality Disorders

Arthur Freeman
Jessica L. Stewart

DESCRIPTION OF PERSONALITY DISORDERS

Personality disorders (PDs) are long-standing, compulsive, rigid patterns of perceiving, interpreting, and responding to one's environment and to oneself that are characteristic of the individual's functioning and generally present across a wide range of life situations (Freeman, Pretzer, Fleming, & Simon, 2004). PDs consist of pervasive, inflexible, enduring patterns of cognition, poor affective management, and maladaptive behavioral responding (American Psychiatric Association [APA], 1994; Beck, Freeman, & Associates, 1990; Beck, Freeman, Davis, & Associates, 2003; Millon, 1981; Young, 1990). However, the hallmark of individuals with personality disorders are problems relating to others, social skills deficits, and, more generally, interpersonal difficulty (APA, 1994; Beck et al., 1990, 2003). Millon (1981) describes a process by which patients with PD engage in self-defeating sequences that consist of "protective constriction, cognitive distortion, and behavior generalization" (p. 9) that results in the limiting of new learning opportunities, misinterpretation of benign events, and provocation of "reactions from others that reactivate earlier problems" (Millon, 1981, p. 9).

Because of the persistence of patients' underlying beliefs and subsequent cognitive distortions, their often limited motivation for change (or for treatment), the lack of effective pharmacological interventions, and their difficulty in interpersonal relationships, most clinicians commonly perceive individuals with PDs as being among the most difficult and frustrating patients with whom they work.

Patients with PDs have a very high utilization rate of mental health resources (Bender et al., 2001; Hoffman, 2002), but their response to treatment is typically limited or poor (Beck et al., 2003; Freeman, Pretzer, Fleming, & Simon, 1990; Freeman et al., 2004). Patients with PDs are more difficult to treat than those with more episodic (i.e., Axis I) disorders because of the pervasive and rigid nature of the disorders, and because the cognitive, affective, and behavioral style of the individual is generally ego-syntonic, thereby, in the view of the individual, not requiring change or modification (Hoffman, 2002; Millon, 1981; Young, 1990). The empirical data regarding efficacy of treatment indicate that specific symptoms improve more quickly than do the overall social functioning and maladaptive personality traits inherent in PD diagnoses (Leichsenring & Leibing, 2003). Perhaps this relates to the affective and cognitive avoidance evident in most PDs; many patients actively avoid addressing their deep-rooted cognitions and emotions because they are too painful (Young, 1990) or the beliefs related to these emotions are not easily made accessible. Many of their rigid cognitive defenses were developed for this very reason, making the process of therapy potentially difficult, because therapy, by its very focus, aims at gaining access to, creating awareness of, understanding, then restructuring maladaptive thinking–feeling–behaving patterns.

In addition, the issue of patient dropout is an especially unfortunate commonality among patients with PDs that limits the ability of the therapist to work with the patient to access core cognitions and emotions that result in their distress and prove to be impediments to the improvement of their coping—or, phrased differently, to reduce their psychopathology. There is evidence however, that in general, psychotherapy can be an effective treatment for individuals with PDs (Bateman & Fonagy, 2000; Beck et al., 2003; Perry, Banon, & Lanni, 1999). The literature also indicates that the outcome of treatment may differ depending on the form of psychotherapy (Hardy et al., 1995; Libermann & Eckman, 1981) and the specific disorder (Karterud et al., 1992; Stone, 1983).

Clinicians treating patients with PDs must therefore have a clear understanding of the patients and their problems. They must then plan the treatment strategies and the resultant interventions accordingly, based on the conceptualization, and be prepared to continue therapy for a longer period of time than with other populations of patients. In addition, because of the interpersonal difficulties inherent in the disorders, clinicians must pay particular attention to the therapeutic relationship (Beck et al., 1990, 2003; Freeman et al., 1990, 2005; Young, 1990). According to Young (1990), the necessary abilities or characteristics making a patient appropriate for short-term cognitive therapy include (1) access to feelings, with some brief training; (2) access to thoughts and images, with brief instruction; (3) identifiable issues for focus; (4) motivation to do homework assignments and learn self-control strategies; (5) a major problem focus of therapy that is not the therapeutic relationship; and (7) cognitions and behavior problems that can be changed (albeit perhaps gradually) through intervention and practice. Because of the nature of most PDs, these patients meet few, if any, of these criteria. In addition, CBT assumes a degree of flexibility from patients, something not necessarily available in most individuals with PDs. To the contrary, their dysfunctional patterns are rigid, and their repertoire of skills is limited (Millon, 1981; Beck et al., 1990, 2003; Freeman et al., 1990, 2005; Young, 1990).

The first question in considering CBT as a primary modality of intervention relates to "goodness of fit." Inasmuch as the CBT model relies on the awareness and identification of feelings, and the awareness, identification, understanding, and motivation of the patient to change cognitive distortions and irrational thinking, it is questionable whether CBT is an appropriate model for use with patients whose very disorders relate to the absence of these abilities and severe interpersonal deficits. According to the CBT model, the difficulties that these patients experience are the result of their powerful and unyielding schemas, unrealistic beliefs about themselves and others, and their view of the world. All of these ideas culminate in ineffective affective responding, maladaptive behaviors, and interpersonal difficulties. In addition, a CBT approach includes a focus on patients' basic assumptions, their immediate cognitions in problem situations, and their manner of conceptualizing their difficulties, then directing adaptive behavior. Ideally, therapeutic interventions aim to correct existing skills deficits and facilitate new skills acquisition before patients practice the coping behaviors, both within and outside the therapeutic setting.

GROUP THERAPY FOR PDS

The three most commonly practiced group therapy models involve (1) individual therapy within a group context focusing on intrapsychic issues; (2) group dynamics approaches focused on interpersonal issues; and (3) group approaches targeting broad, common symptom problems. In the first model, the therapist works with each participant in the group using a "hot seat" model. He or she addresses each patient, dividing the group time and effort, until all participants are reached. The therapist at times invites group members to respond to, and be involved with, the person currently on the "hot seat." It is, however, the therapist who does the majority of the therapy work. In the group dynamics model, interpersonal issues of group membership, the relationship of members to others in the group, and how one comes across to others are ideally the targets for discussion and clarification. In this model, the group becomes an entity, and one's membership in the group and relatedness to group members (or lack thereof) is the basic issue to be addressed.

The third approach places individuals into the group who, ideally, have similar problems (e.g., depression or anxiety disorders). In some cases, the "shared" problem might be that all of the group members were in the same treatment unit. The "shared problem" groups were generally held in hospitals or community mental health centers and combined both the intrapersonal and interpersonal foci, with the group work specific to some area of mutual concern (e.g., reducing anxiety). In inpatient hospital-based units, for example, patients are automatically entered into a psychoeducational group, even if formal group therapy is not prescribed.

Groups have become, in many settings, a standard part of the treatment protocol. This has emerged for a number of reasons. Group therapy is an economical way to deliver treatment. These groups may be of various types but have the goal of being short-term and problem-oriented. Several of the more important reasons for utilizing groups are now discussed.

Therapeutic Engagement

Individuals may believe that the therapeutic ideal is passivity, and that therapy will be "received." These types of individuals may develop the belief that something will be done "for" or "to" them in therapy, an idea that may even be reinforced by the therapist. Group therapy offers an opportunity to challenge this assumption. The group leaders and the group members endorse the premise that self-control of thoughts, feelings, and behavior is not only possible, but it is also an essential goal of therapy. The group encourages patients to be active participants in their treatment, and the group setting promotes collaboration through a number of procedures, including agenda setting, role playing, and self-help exercises.

Diagnostic Functions

The group experience adds a different dimension to the evaluation process. By directly observing the participant's behavioral interactions with peers on a social level, clinicians are given a glimpse into the participant's repertoire of interpersonal responses. Participants who can appear quite intact in a one-to-one interview may have more trouble maintaining their stability when faced with the added stimuli of a group setting. Conversely, personal strengths, such as empathy skills, that may not be readily apparent in individual therapy may be drawn out in the group.

Universality

Sharing perceptions and reactions in the group allows participants to see that they are not alone in their suffering and that other people have problems of a similar nature. "Normalizing" behavior, what Yalom (1985) observed as a sense of universality, is one of the most helpful features of group therapy. A common theme that surfaces in individual therapy is illustrated by the statement: "You [the therapist] don't understand what I am going through." In a group setting, however, it is far more difficult to dismiss the observations of others who share the similar problems.

Relatedness and Support

The group can help to foster relatedness in the chronically isolated participant and can offer support for an individual who may be going through a personal loss or trauma, or the individual who needs "shoring up" either in decision making or in carrying through on a decision. For individuals who have appropriate social skills but are separated from family and friends, the group can, in many ways, fill the social void. The group can also operate as a support for the participant who faces having to work toward modifying external life stressors.

Psychoeducational Format

The group format is especially well suited for presenting information on specific topics. Special psychoeducational programs can be designed for groups of participants that share psychoeducational issues. Many group programs develop written materials, often combined in a folder or notebook that is presented upon admission to the unit to help participants learn skills in an orderly sequence. The basic principles of CBT approaches are then taught and reinforced in a variety of experiments and group exercises. The basic psychoeducational nature of cognitive therapy is very apparent in the group, inasmuch as the basic principles of the cognitive approach are taught and reinforced in a variety of experiments and group exercises. An excellent workbook in this regard is *Mind over Mood* (Greenberger & Padesky, 1995).

Laboratory for Experimentation

A group can serve as a laboratory in which participants can test out automatic thoughts and experiment with behaviors in a relatively safe environment. It is important to point out that although the group can provide opportunities for a broad range of cognitive and behavioral experiments, it also has the potential to be an area for repeating dysfunctional behaviors or expressing primitive aggressive or narcissistic themes. A structured, problem-oriented approach, under the astute direction of a well-trained leader, tends to avoid these problems.

Modeling and Social Skills Practice

Participants often model the behaviors of other group members or the therapists. In the process, the individual can learn effective coping strategies (e.g., assertiveness, empathic responses, goal setting, and problem solving). Basic social skills can be taught, discussed, and role-played in the group. It is important to practice all of these skills, and the group can provide the opportunity for practice. Those who have severe social skills deficits require the most assistance in building a higher level of social competence.

Motivation for Individual Therapy

Groups can serve as motivators for individual therapy. As group members speak of the help they get in their individual therapy or how they were able to use their therapy for personal gain, all members can profit. Similarly, by offering an opportunity for participants to discuss and process the group experience, the group therapist can offer feedback to the individual therapist, who may be able to work with isolated participants more effectively using the group data. In fact, the participant can use material garnered from the group therapy experience as the grist for the individual therapy mill, rather than reporting old memories and experiences.

Awareness

Awareness, another important facet of group therapy, involves helping group members to be more attentive to data that originate internally (thoughts, percepts) or externally (environmental stimuli). This involves several factors: (1) acknowledging the existence of these data, (2) being primed to act on these data, (3) identifying the source(s) of the data, (4) attempting to view the data as objectively as possible, (5) being aware of how one's earlier learning filters those data, and (6) becoming more aware of past painful experiences, and one's internal representations of those experiences.

Rehearsing New Behaviors

Prior to trying a new behavior in one's environment, an individual can role play and practice in the group before taking the leap to try it out "in real life." The group can offer a vehicle for reality testing and increasing participant responsibility.

Resource Management

Finally, groups offer cost-effectiveness in times of staff, money, and resource shortages. By focusing on present-day life issues and maintaining a firm structure, the therapy addresses the here-and-now issues and saves the participant time, effort, and financial resources. Several participants can be seen in the time usually reserved for two individual sessions.

CBT GROUP TREATMENT OF PATIENTS WITH PDs

Before each disorder is considered separately, a review of the basic components of group CBT is necessary, with specific emphasis on relevant considerations when applying this mode of intervention to patients with PD.
CBT involves the identification and restructuring of irrational or distorted
cognitions and beliefs related to the self, others, and the world, that result in
emotional distress and maladaptive behaviors. Conducting CBT in the group
format maintains the same ultimate goal for each client but provides the
opportunity for clients to experience support, an opportunity for modeling, a
sense of commonality, and an environment in which to practice interpersonal (e.g., appropriate self-disclosure, conflict management) and other skills
learned in the session. For patients with PDs, this social component inherent
in the group modality may be critical for effective treatment. As with CBT
conducted in an individual format, group CBT must encourage the patient to
be active with regard to the direction and process of therapy. Group CBT
relies heavily on the active participation of patients in defining goals, participating in guided discovery of thought patterns and irrational beliefs, practicing skills in group exercises, developing homework to continue practicing new
skills outside of session, and discussing areas of discomfort or difficulty with
the therapist.

Applying these components to a group of patients with PDs may be successful and appreciatively received, but it may also create a situation that is
significantly affected by patients' lack of interpersonal skills, ineffective communication skills, absence of perspective-taking abilities, low frustration tolerance, low motivation, and anxiety, all related to the nature and severity of the
disorder.

Given the previously noted interpersonal problems, it is important that
patients with PDs agree to this intervention prior to being assigned to a group.
The patient who is forced, coerced, or required to meet the demands of some
outside agent or agency will likely do very poorly in the group, regardless of
the diagnosis. Unless the patient is able and willing to work cohesively despite
opposing perspectives of group members' disagreements, group therapy is not
likely to be recommended. The patients must be helped to recognize and
respect the importance of each group member's participation. The group therapy format offers the individual a larger "sounding board" audience to process problematic situations and experiences. Group members can assist one
another in problem-solving discussions, for example, by suggesting multiple
and various alternative solutions and approaches to problems. Patients with
PDs may have a more difficult time accepting suggestions or feedback from
peers (or even the group facilitators) because of the interpersonal difficulties
inherent in Axis II disorders. Some patients may avoid group therapy or reject
it because of distorted cognitions related to interpersonal interactions. This
latter issue is important given the nature of characterological disorders and

the complex modality of group intervention, because it potentially may alter the group process and the likelihood of effective treatment.

CBT TREATMENT ISSUES

In a group for patients with PDs, feedback may be less constructive, and more emotionally charged and self-serving than with other populations. Some patients with PDs may feel insecure and uncertain, or lack skills when giving constructive criticism to others. Dealing with the therapist, inasmuch as he or she is seen in the position of authority, may be especially problematic regarding the fear of rejection or retaliation. On the other hand, other patients with PDs may have difficulty accepting feedback from peers, if part of their pathology relates to narcissistic thinking and an inability to take another's perspective. These patients may also be unable provide constructive feedback to others, potentially limiting the development of a working alliance with the other group members. Patients often assume that they are perceived in a certain way (usually negatively) without ever attempting to verify this in a reliable manner. The group environment allows patients to restructure these strongly held beliefs. The positive aspects of the therapeutic interchange are not limited to the group members who receive feedback; patients often identify their own previously unrecognized abilities when offering support to others.

The conceptualization of PDs through the cognitive-behavioral model allows for an extensive understanding of the affective and interpersonal difficulties of these patients, as well as the historical development of the cognitive style and firmly held schemas that perpetuate pathology. The origins of irrational and distorted belief systems, which are certainly important, are not dismissed in CBT, as is often suggested in the literature that considers psychodynamic conceptualization of PDs more appropriate (Freeman, et al., 1990, 2005; Hoffman, 2002). Accurate conceptualization also allows clinicians to prescribe the appropriate therapeutic intervention for a given patient group, including whether or not group CBT would be beneficial.

Although each patient presents with an individual profile of needs, competencies, maladaptive behaviors, affective difficulties, and cognitive distortions requiring modification, there have been enough documented patterns of functioning and deficits across patients presented in the literature to prompt the development of criteria for distinct PDs. In addition, except for some population-specific examples, most psychotherapy environments rarely have enough patients with the same PD diagnosis for a single-diagnosis therapy group. Another barrier to effective group CBT for patients with PDs relates to the ego-syntonic nature of PDs: Patients with PDs do not see their behavior as problematic. Therefore, and in combination with the nature of their disorder (namely, suspicion and mistrust), these patients rarely present for therapy and do not typically function so poorly that hospitalization is required (Freeman et al., 1990, 2005).

GENERAL STRUCTURE OF CBT SESSIONS

Setting an effective and workable agenda is important to CBT group sessions, inasmuch as the agenda helps to provide both structure and direction for the group work. The issues raised by a group of patients can usually be grouped into categories that are rank-ordered according to their importance and relevance to the group. The therapist directs the group toward development of an agenda that is likely to be manageable for the given session and productive in meeting the overall goals for the group. The agenda-setting process accomplishes much more than just the selection of topics for the session: Patients gain experience in identifying problems, verbalizing their concerns to others, and negotiating within a group. Although an attempt is made to discuss, at least briefly, all chosen agenda items, a majority of the session is devoted to working with a few topics that are of more general interest, highly significant to group members, and illustrative of cognitive therapy principles. It is more important to select a limited number of items that can serve as teaching vehicles for the entire group than to attempt to cover all issues in an evenhanded but superficial manner.

Information on specific topics or skills may be presented, such as problem solving, self-expression and communication, emotional coping, empathic responding, and relationship maintenance—typically areas of deficit for patients with PDs. It is important to point out that although the group can provide opportunities for a broad range of cognitive and behavioral experiments, and social learning, it also has the potential to be an area for repeating dysfunctional behaviors or expressing primitive aggressive or narcissistic themes—an important consideration when working with patients with PD.

The group must maintain a "here-and-now" focus. Although the dysfunctional patterns manifested by patients likely may have their roots in the past, Freeman et al. (2005) suggest that present functioning be the target of treatment interventions. The CBT group adopts the same "here-and-now" focus emphasized in individual CBT, with historical issues coming to light more through the influence of active and pervasive schemas. Some schemas in PDs are very obvious and will be recognized quickly by the therapist and group members. Other schemas are not so clearly delineated and must be inferred from the patient's habitual cognitive style or behavior within the group. Most patients with PDs have such firmly held maladaptive beliefs that reconstructive work is required via referencing historical realities but focusing on the schematic "learning" developed from those early experiences (Beck et al., 1990, 2003; Freeman et al., 1990, 2005). This may strain the ability of the cognitive-behavioral group therapist to remain focused on the present.

DISORDER-SPECIFIC ISSUES

The following cognitive-behavioral conceptualization of each PD is offered to afford clinicians a starting point for intervention and for deciding whether group CBT would be beneficial for a particular patient. For each disorder, specific group treatment suggestions are offered.

Paranoid Personality Disorder

Paranoid personality disorder (PPD) is characterized by a set of unrealistic, extreme beliefs regarding the motivations and actions of others (Beck et al., 1990, 2003; Freeman et al., 1990, 2005). The problems these patients encounter related to their beliefs about others and their interpretations about the actions of others are characteristic of their overall functioning. The hallmark feature of this PPD population is an enduring, pervasive, and unwarranted suspiciousness and mistrust of others (APA, 2000; Freeman et al., 1990, 2005) in situations in which guardedness or mistrust is unjustified and maladaptive. Patients with PPD have great difficulty in challenging their suspicious thinking in the face of contradictory evidence. They typically overlook and reject evidence that may conflict with their mistrust and suspiciousness of others. Their vigilance leads to the continual identification of "evidence" for their assumptions about others, perpetuating a paranoid approach to life. In addition, and as a consideration in therapeutic intervention, patients with PPD are also likely to become suspicious of others who attempt to challenge their long-standing beliefs.

PPD is the result of a once-adaptive need to protect the self through hypervigilance and suspicion related to the ill-intent of others. It is conceptualized cognitive-behaviorally as the result of beliefs about the self as inadequate, insufficient, and imperfect, and subsequent feelings of shame and humiliation (Colby, Faught, & Parkinson, 1979). The paranoid cognitive style is motivated and perpetuated by distress-reducing effects (i.e., the reduction of shameful feelings) (Colby et al., 1979; Freeman et al., 1990). This is why directly challenging specific suspicious assumptions is likely to be difficult, ineffective, and unlikely to address the underlying factors perpetuating the disorder, and produces anger and aggression (or passive–aggressive behavior) because of such "unjustified" intrusions into the patient's personal domain.

These reactions are problematic in a therapy situation, and especially so in a group modality, in which the multiple, potential "attackers" include participants in the hoped-for working alliance: the therapist(s) and other group members.

Therefore, the motivation to change, which is necessary in CBT-oriented therapy, may be lacking in this population, because change is accomplished by challenging the beliefs that, to this point, have proved "successful" for patients with PPD in reducing negative emotions. The challenging process within therapy may produce discomfort and uncertainty—a risk that is often too great for many patients with PPD, given their difficulty with emotional management.

Although, given the cognitive nature of this disorder, the presenting problems of patients with PPD appear to be well suited for intervention with the CBT framework, the primary difficulty lies in patients' interpersonal difficulties. It is unlikely that a psychotherapy practice would treat enough patients with PPD to form a disorder-specific group for this population—if, in fact, this were a good idea in the first place. Including these patients in a multiple-diagnoses PD group would likely be ineffective, given their distrust and suspiciousness of others, and the difficult interpersonal styles of others with PDs (i.e., the seductiveness of patients with histrionic PD and the aggressive, self-centered style of patients with antisocial PD). The expectations of persons with PPD that others are devious, disloyal, deceptive, and even hostile often result in these patients acting toward others as if their assumptions were accurate. As a result, these patients are seen by others as disloyal, deceptive, stubborn, defensive, unwilling to compromise, and even hostile (Freeman et al., 1990, 2005). This compounds their already strained interpersonal relationships and would likely sabotage the therapeutic relationship within group therapy.

Although possible, establishing a trusting, working relationship with patients with PPD is challenging. In fact, these patients are "reluctant to confide in or become too close to others because they fear that the information they share will be used against them" (APA, 2000, p. 634). Persons with PPD are also resistant to rules and structure, which are necessary in group CBT, because they interpret such regulations as restrictions on their freedom and feel vulnerable and trapped. Group CBT is therefore more appropriate after significant individual treatment. When motivation to change is established, and the patient has had an opportunity to experiment with trusting the therapist, group therapy might be useful. Overall, patients with PPD are poor candidates for group work.

Schizoid Personality Disorder

Schizoid personality disorder (SPD) is perhaps one of the most confusing of the PDs, and its definition has been evolving for decades. Historically, persons with SPD presented as shy, reserved, quiet, and "schizophrenic-like" (Freeman et al., 1990, 2005), but the literature also described subtypes who were more formal, "stiff," and socially adept; isolated, eccentric, and socially apathetic or ignorant; and others who were more hypersensitive, fragile, and delicate (Kretschmer, 1936). The fourth edition, text revision of the *Diagnostic and Statistical Manual of Mental Disorders* (DSM-IV-TR; APA, 2000), like its predecessors, views SPD as a distinct disorder, with a personality style that is identified by the patient who is chronically reclusive and isolated, whose basic characteristics include emotional constriction, detachment, and a lack of desire to form interpersonal relationships.

Individuals with SPD typically stand out in generally sociable environments (work settings, neighborhoods, schools) as odd or eccentric, because they are primarily solitary and keep to themselves (Freeman et al., 1990, 2005). Viewed through a cognitive-behavioral conceptualization, the isolative nature and emotional constriction of these patients is the result of a lack of positive beliefs about closeness, along with positive beliefs about being alone (Beck et al., 1990, 2003). These patients see little benefit in social interaction and therefore do not interact socially. They typically deny fears related to having close relationships, but it is possible that their beliefs originate in or persist because of negative social experiences. Goals of intervention are aimed at increasing positive beliefs and disproving negative beliefs about social interaction, and reducing positive assertions related to isolation. A group therapy modality would therefore seem ideal in accomplishing these goals.

However, potential obstacles to inclusion of patients with SPD in group therapy relate to the low likelihood of these patients to seek any therapy. It seems unlikely that in one clinical setting there would be enough of patients with SPD for a diagnosis-specific group. Patients with SPD would therefore be placed in a multiple-diagnosis group. Although a group therapy environment would provide the therapist with observable data related to these patients' social behavior, the group may be aversive to patients who are typically socially unresponsive or avoidant of group involvement given their lack of desire for interpersonal relationships. In addition, other group members may be resistant to collaboration with these patients, who restrict social interaction and emotional closeness, and cannot be equal partners in therapeutic relationship (Freeman et al., 1990, 2005). Whereas this modality may appear to be a positive option for restructuring the cognitions and adjusting maladaptive social behaviors in this population, it is likely an unrealistic option given the nature of the pathology. In addition, patients with SPD would likely have little motivation to change given the ego-syntonic nature of their disorder. Their lack of motivation to engage in any therapeutic process—especially one involving social interaction—would negatively impact the potential for active participation in a group.

Group therapy should only be considered after the patient with SPD learns to develop a successful interpersonal relationship with the therapist, acquires some basic social understanding and skills, and accepts his or her current functioning (the symptoms that usually do result in these patients participating in therapy, i.e., depression or anxiety) as likely related to SPD.

Schizotypal Personality Disorder

Perhaps one of the most difficult persons to engage in the therapeutic process is the individual diagnosed with a schizotypal personality disorder (STPD). Individuals with this disorder present with multiple problematic characteristics that limit the potential for therapeutic success. Their descriptive characteristics relate closely to those evident in schizophrenia, and the differential diagnosis is based on subjective judgment of the severity of symptoms (Beck et al., 2003; Freeman et al., 1990, 2005) or the presence of persistent psychotic symptoms (APA, 2000). It is difficult to present a thorough conceptualization of the cognitive aspects of STPD, because of the combination of exceptional difficulties these patients have in relating coherently to others, and because "the bizarre thought processes characterizing this disorder greatly complicate the process of identifying specific automatic thoughts and underlying assumptions" essential to a course of CBT (Freeman et al., 1990, p. 179). The ability of these patients to relate to others in socially appropriate ways or to communicate effectively is mitigated by their odd beliefs and magical thinking, severe social discomfort in close relationships, unusual cognitive and perceptual distortions, ideas of reference, eccentric behaviors, impoverished speech, inappropriate affect, and suspiciousness (APA, 2000; Freeman et al., 1990, 2005).

Intervention strategies tend to be more behavioral in nature, focusing on the acquisition of social, communication, and problem-solving skills rather than on monitoring or restructuring thought processes (Freeman et al., 1990, 2005). This does not rule out group CBT as an appropriate option, where the focus may be a social skills group that comprises patients with similar difficulties. The group can work on social skills training and provide a social environment to practice the acquired skills. However, a mixed-diagnosis group would be ill-advised given the characteristics of this disorder. In addition, if the group focuses on cognitive distortions and irrational beliefs, it may be unlikely that it would be effective with this population. If participating in a group with multiple PD diagnoses, these patients may be misunderstood, rejected, or even ridiculed by the other patients, increasing their paranoia and social anxiety.

Antisocial Personality Disorder

Antisocial personality disorder (ASPD) is characterized by an enduring pattern of irresponsible, impulsive, and aggressive actions, as well as irritability, a low frustration tolerance, and anger (APA, 1994; Freeman et al., 1990). Patients with ASPD are quick to deny personal problems (it is unlikely that they seek treatment of their own volition) and to blame their difficulties on mistreatment by others. ASPD patients have a pervasive pattern of behavior that includes disregard for and violation of the rights of others, failure to conform to social norms, and manipulation and deceit (Beck et al., 1990; Freeman et al., 1990). These patients are likely not motivated to change their behaviors, because to do so would result in no longer being able to look out for themselves in the hostile world, where others are "out to get what they can for themselves" (Freeman et al., 1990, p. 227). They are most often motivated only by their own self-interest, and effective therapy would likely result from therapists helping them to understand that change is in their best interests (i.e., they would be more apt to obtain their goals if they acquired the skills necessary to become more socially adept, learned to anticipate long-term consequences, etc.).

In addition to a lack of motivation for treatment as an obstacle for inclusion in group CBT, patients with ASPD, similar to patients with PPD, mistrust others, avoid revealing their vulnerabilities, assume that they will be mistreated by others, and avoid closeness. These assumptions and beliefs about others limit their ability to form the trusting relationship necessary for the therapeutic alliance of group therapy; therefore, they are unlikely candidates for this modality of intervention. These patients typically assume the "tough guy" role and refuse to acknowledge their own fears or demonstrate (if felt) caring toward others. Combined, these interpersonal difficulties may invoke discomfort or fear, as well as dislike and anger, in other patients in the group, because patients with ASPD do not offer the emotional or social support inherent in the group process.

Furthermore, individuals with ASPD have difficulty working toward long-term goals (e.g., acknowledging or exhibiting vulnerabilities in a therapeutic situation) due to their impulsivity in response to perceived threat and inability to think of consequences of their actions before behaving erratically. As a result, patients with ASPD are typically unsuccessful at planning ahead and following rules or procedures; these failures support their already negative views regarding norms and rules in general, therefore limiting their responsiveness to the structure of CBT group therapy. Despite these potential obstacles, group CBT may be an effective modality for intervention if the group consists solely of a population with ASPD, because it offers an opportunity for like-minded patients to provide feedback about the impact of each other's behavior and an opportunity for role playing to develop more effective communication and problem-solving skills. In addition, patient with ASPD is likely to be especially "perceptive in confronting other group members' attempts at evasion or manipulation" and "credible in pointing out the ways in which antisocial behavior is counterproductive" (Freeman et al., 1990, p. 234). This modality may even prove superior to individual therapy if, in fact, it is appropriate in the first place.

Borderline Personality Disorder

Although it is possible to write an entire chapter solely on the presentation, clinical conceptualization, and available literature on patients with borderline personality disorder (BPD), we focus here on some of the major themes in CBT treatment for BPD. The essential feature of BPD "is a long-term, pervasive pattern of instability of interpersonal relationships, self-image, and affects, and a marked impulsivity" across functioning (APA, 1994, p. 650). No single feature is invariably present in all cases; however, the most prominent features are what warrant diagnosis of a distinct disorder, and include intensity of reactions and variability and lability of mood (Beck et al., 1990; Freeman et al., 1990; Linehan, 1993). Patients with BPD are not necessarily constantly in crisis, but they typically initiate therapy when they are; as a result, they usually offer a complex and chaotic clinical presentation. Conceptually, these patients' difficulty stems from poorly integrated, extreme, or abusive childhood relationships with caregivers, resulting in equally extreme, unrealistic expectations and assumptions about all interpersonal relationships. These irrational and/or distorted expectations, beliefs, and assumptions result in irrational behavioral and emotional responses. Millon (1981) offered an explanation of the BPD presentation based on social learning theory, suggesting that the patient with BPD lacks a clear and consistent identity and personal goals, and, as a result, lacks impulse control, coordinated efforts, and efficacy from not having achieved goals consistently. Because of this lack of self-efficacy, their insecure identities result in dependence on others and vulnerability to extreme distress should they be separated (voluntarily or otherwise) from these support sources (Freeman et al., 1990).

This issue of separation is characteristic of patients with BPD, in that their fear of, and subsequent emotional and behavioral attempts to avoid abandonment (whether perceived or real) is a significant motivating factor (Linehan, 1993). Because the majority of maladaptive behaviors, emotional dysregulation, and interpersonal difficulties relate to cognitive processes and belief systems, patients with BPD individuals would, ideally, respond positively to CBT. The group modality, however, may pose some challenges and requires some considerations for inclusion related to patient readiness for change, patient emotional lability, interpersonal difficulties, patient safety, and impulse control.

Perhaps the biggest problem for group CBT with patients with BPD is establishing a collaborative working alliance between group members (Freeman et al., 1990). Due to their interpersonal difficulties with trust and fear of abandonment, these patients may have trouble engaging in the intimate exchange typical of group CBT. Paradoxically, they may also disclose personal information too quickly as a means to "test" the other members and the therapist for trustworthiness or rejection. Their interpersonal style, resistance to engagement, and impulsive disclosure likely leave patients with BPD feeling a variety of emotional responses related to suspicion of the other group members or vulnerability, such as anxiety, guilt, shamefulness, anger, and even rejection, if the desired or anticipated response is not received. Another potential problem for the inclusion of patients with BPD in group CBT relates to boundaries and patients' ability and willingness (or lack of both) to accept reasonable limits and structure—components that are important to group CBT in directing treatment and protecting the safety of all group members.

Histrionic Personality Disorder

Patients with histrionic personality disorder (HPD) are lively, dramatic, emotionally excitable, and crave stimulation and constant attention (APA, 1994; Beck et al., 1990; Freeman et al., 1990). These patients are prone to exaggeration and often present excessive emotional and behavioral responses to minor situations (i.e., angry outbursts and tantrums). Their interpersonal difficulties relate to their constant need for attention from others, who typically perceive patients with HPD as shallow, demanding, selfish, immature, and overly dependent. In addition, these patients may appear warm and caring initially, but as their need for attention surfaces, their interactions look more self-focused, superficial, and ingenuine. As with the other PDs, individuals with HPD often do not seek treatment for the PD, but instead for symptoms of depression and intense dissatisfaction or anxiety (Beck et al., 1990; Freeman et al., 1990).

The presentation of the patient with HPD stems from underlying beliefs related to inadequacy and the need to rely on others for care and safety, as well as the need "to be loved by everyone for everything one does" (Freeman et al., 1990, p. 208). They tend to overreact to any perceived rejection, even from people unimportant to them, because it signifies that their existence is vulnerable. Therefore, these patients actively seek to procure their needs through dramatic, attention-seeking means. They are unable to communicate their needs directly for fear of rejection, so they often use manipulation and even threats to elicit what they want from others. Patients with HPD lack an identified sense of self, and place sole emphasis on external approval and the importance of external events. They are unable to define their thoughts and feelings clearly in a detailed fashion, resulting in a global cognitive style and equally global emotional experience—often seen as exaggerated, intense, and labile.

The interpersonal styles of patients with HPD pose a potential obstacle to their inclusion in group therapy, because they would most likely be unable to attend to the needs of others and would attempt to dominate the group, and react with intense, exaggerated emotions if their efforts were unsuccessful. In addition, because their focus is consistently external, they are unaware of their identity, needs, preferences, emotions, or cognitions. Patients with HPD would likely actively avoid attempts to gain self-knowledge, which would produce emotional discomfort they would not know how to manage. As a result, these patients are typically lost when depth of interpersonal relationships is required, such as in the case of the collaborative, working relationship of group therapy. Of greatest concern in considering the patient with HPD for group CBT is the potential for the structured, focused, and systematic nature of the CBT model to be so diametrically opposed to the patient's global, diffuse, and exaggerated approach to life that it results in an ineffective match for treatment (Beck et al., 1990; Freeman et al., 1990). This is not to say that it is impossible to conduct CBT with patients with HPD, but this conflict of styles must be resolved gradually, which requires motivation to change on the part of the patients. In terms of readiness and motivation to change, as in the other PDs, these patients often do not recognize a need to change, and they respond so poorly to emotional discomfort (a natural product of cognitive and behavioral change) that they are not genuinely motivated to engage in the therapeutic process. A benefit of group CBT for patients with HPD, should motivation be adequate, is the availability of a therapeutic, interpersonal environment for feedback about communication style and for role-playing new skills. These patients may also be able to work to define their identity independent of others, through testing competencies and interpersonal skills. The CBT group would also provide enough structure and boundaries to facilitate the growth of these important social skills. But these potential benefits, again, rely completely on the degree of motivation of the patients and the ability to modify their style enough to engage in this process.

Narcissistic Personality Disorder

Similar to patients with ASPD, patients with narcissistic personality disorder (NPD) are inherently self-focused and lack empathy for others; however, these patients also experience grandiose views of themselves and are hypersensitive to the evaluation of others (APA, 1994; Beck et al., 1990; Freeman et al., 1990). They relate to the world in a dramatic, erratic, and emotional way. Individuals with NPD typically present for therapy because of symptoms of depression and anxiety, not their narcissism. These individuals constantly pursue recognition and acknowledgment from others and their environment, which leaves them feeling depressed and unfulfilled because of the expenditure of such efforts. They receive little joy from achievements, because they believe they are entitled to their successes, rather than regarding their success as a sign of their abilities. Interpersonally, they are overreactive toward others, competitive, and jealous of others' accomplishments.

Conceptually, the central dysfunctional belief of patients with NPD is that they are, or must be, "special" people. As a result, any suggestion to the contrary by others is perceived as a personal insult and an obstacle in attaining special treatment, and typically results in anger, frustration, and even acting-out behaviors. These patients also exhibit distorted thinking of the selective abstraction and all-or-nothing styles (Beck et al., 1990; Freeman et al., 1990): They constantly seek, attend only to, and greatly exaggerate "evidence" in their environment to support their superiority. They either ignore evidence of normalcy or respond to being "average" with anxiety, anger, and verbal overcompensation (e.g., exaggerating their accomplishments or "showing off"). This selective view of data results in extreme responses, indicating poor problem-solving and reality-testing abilities.

Patients with NPD are likely not appropriate candidates for group CBT inclusion, because they lack empathy for others, avoid and fear revealing flaws or shortcomings, desire (and expect) special treatment, resist common rules, and engage in power struggles with perceived authority figures (i.e., the therapist). They may believe that people with "problems" are beneath them in status, and may therefore resist even attending a therapy group. They do not participate as active members in a group forum out of a sense of commitment to the other members or the process, because they do not experience a desire to please others or do what is "right." On the other hand, if individual therapy has progressed to the point that the patient's narcissism is moderated and he or she has proven capable of engaging actively in the therapeutic process, the patient with NPD may benefit from the group modality because of the opportunities for genuine skills building and earning the recognition of others by helping them with their problems—a self-serving motivator, but nonetheless one that may facilitate the development of empathic responding and prove a benefit of group therapy.

Avoidant Personality Disorder

Avoidant personality disorder (AVPD) is similar to PPD and SPD in that patients withdraw socially; however, the motive is different. These individuals withdraw due to pervasive timidity, social discomfort, and fear of being negatively evaluated by others (APA, 1994; Freeman et al., 1990). Any criticism or disapproval from others is especially painful, and patients with APD worry so much about being embarrassed in front of others that they avoid social interaction almost entirely. These patients differ from patients with SPD, in that they desire interpersonal relationships, but the risk of rejection or humiliation is too great. This inability to develop relationships further distresses patients with APD and perpetuates the strongly negative self-view and feelings of hopelessness.

Conceptually, individuals with APD believe they are unacceptable to others and will therefore be humiliated, hurt, rejected, and devastated if they attempt to initiate close relationships (Beck et al., 1990; Freeman et al., 1990). They therefore make the active and self-protective decision to withdraw socially and avoid intense pain based on this irrational assumption. Because they are so certain they will be humiliated and hurt, they display hypervigilance with regard to the actions of others, misinterpret innocuous behavior, and ignore entirely any positive responses from others. Their maladaptive cognitions are therefore very resistant to restructuring, because their selective attention is so strong. Also, their self-protection instincts extend to avoiding confrontation of their own painful thoughts and feelings, as a result of the belief that they cannot adequately cope with distress.

The major obstacle to conducting group CBT with patients with APD relates to inability to form the therapeutic working relationship because of patients' cognitive distortions and anxiety related to their negative self-view and expectation of rejection. Patients with APD are unwilling to engage in interpersonal interactions unless they are certain of being liked. It is possible that a group environment with multiple members would be too overwhelming. In addition, because these patients have often resorted to avoidance of interpersonal interactions, they typically lack the basic social skills that are important to simple interaction and communication with others. These patients undoubtedly interpret many of the benign group interactions negatively and as rejection, which makes early termination a risk. Group CBT would be beneficial, although stressful, for these patients after a period of individual therapy has addressed these basic relationship concerns, improved social skills, and begun to restructure distorted cognitions, so that new attitudes and skills may be practiced in a safe, benign environment. It would be important, then, to consider the nature of the group and its members to ensure an accepting and supportive environment.

Dependent Personality Disorder

Dependent personality disorder (DPD) is characterized by a pervasive pattern of dependence and submissiveness, indecisiveness, significant discomfort when alone, and extensive effort to avoid being alone (APA, 1994; Beck et al., 1990; Freeman et al., 1990). Patients with DPD are preoccupied with abandonment, hypersensitive to disapproval, and exhibit exaggerated attempts to gain others' approval. These patients have a negative view of the self; specifically they believe that they are inadequate, helpless, and unable to cope with the lonely, cold, dangerous world. This all-or-none thinking regarding autonomy, the primary cognitive distortion in DPD, results in these patients giving up responsibility for their care and dismissing their own needs, so that someone else will take care of them—someone more competent and capable, in the patient's view. This then limits the opportunities for patients ever to experience themselves as adequate and capable in stressful situations. They have little opportunity to acquire or master skills needed for independence or even to become aware of the skills they do possess. They may sabotage therapeutic intervention by actively avoiding skills acquisition, because they fear that competence leads to abandonment (Freeman et al., 1990).

The maladaptive interpersonal relationship patterns are a significant part of the problem for patients with DPD, and the biggest potential roadblock for this population being included in group CBT. These individuals are overly concerned with pleasing others, which makes the genuineness of their therapeutic bond questionable and minimizes their ability to focus on their own problems. In addition, patients with DPD are overly dependent on the relationships within the therapy context, potentially overwhelming other group members, who are struggling with their own interpersonal and emotional problems and may perceive them as desperate and needy. Because these patients believe they need to depend on others for safety and experience great distress related to developing competencies of their own, their lack of the necessary motivation to change undermines the potential gain from group CBT. These patients may, however, be successful in a group therapy modality once they have acquired some basic skills, as a means not only to reduce the dependence on the therapist and temper the relationship, but also to encourage greater reliance on peers rather than on one person (Beck et al., 1990; Freeman et al., 1990). In addition, other members of group may be able to serve as models for developing and practicing new skills and independence.

Obsessive–Compulsive Personality Disorder

Patients with obsessive–compulsive personality disorder (OCPD) typically enter treatment because of symptoms related to depression, anxiety, or interpersonal problems. Their interpersonal difficulties result from their rigid, ruminative, indecisive style of thinking, and perfectionistic expectations for themselves and others (APA, 1994; Beck et al., 1990; Freeman et al., 1990), which are not problematic for the patients. They are often seen by others as opinionated and dogmatic, and frequently "miss the point" in social situations because they attend intensely and pointedly to one particular detail at a time, often missing the "big picture." These patients experience anxiety related to not following routines strictly, not being deliberate enough, and worrying about trivial "what ifs." They also have difficulty managing the distress they feel when blocked from controlling themselves or their environment—a central "need" in order to avoid making mistakes.

The maladaptive functioning of patients with OCPD is the result of the central distorted assumption that they "must avoid mistakes at all cost," and that every situation has a "right" and "wrong" action. They believe that loss of control or incorrect action is a mistake, and that mistakes absolutely deserve criticism (Freeman et al., 1990). In addition, these patients, if they anticipate not being perfect in their actions, may choose inaction over the risk of making a mistake; they frequently only make choices or act when success is guaranteed. This may pose considerable vocational and interpersonal difficulties. These patients' motivation for change may relate more to their desire to address symptoms of anxiety, interpersonal problems, or to improve performance than to their irrational, distorted views of "right" and "wrong" or success and failure.

With regard to appropriateness for group CBT, their biggest problem (besides lack of motivation for change that negatively impacts therapy in general) likely relates to their lack of tolerance for "beliefs, values, or ways of doing things that differ from (their) own" (Freeman et al., 1990, p. 254). Patients with OCPD possess the unrealistic expectation that others follow the same irrational rules they set for themselves, and a resistance to allowing others to do things because of the conviction that they will not do it correctly. In addition, in a group therapy situation, what is "right" is not necessarily clear, and there may be multiple possible solutions for a group member's problem. In this situation, patients with OCPD would experience a great deal of discomfort and likely withdraw from the situation. Their intense desire to avoid mistakes would also be an impediment to successful group CBT, because of their resistance to trying new approaches to problems. These patients, if able to consider uncertain solutions, may have great difficulty completing tasks because of unrealistically high standards for success (all-or-nothing thinking) and perseveration on the details of the solution's implementation.

EXISTING GROUP CBT APPROACHES WITH PDs

Given the potential obstacles to traditional CBT inherent in including a group modality in the treatment of patients with PD, as well as the presenting characteristics typical in their presentation, CBT has been an infrequent practice in these populations. Although a great deal of the literature (though not abundant) documenting the efficacy of CBT for patients with PD involves group therapy (Leichsenring & Leibing, 2003), these studies are usually limited by sample size or the presence of multiple PD diagnoses in a single group. Any group comprised solely of patients with PD will invariably be composed of individuals with diverse diagnoses, assorted degrees of pathology, and different levels of motivation. In addition, most of the CBT-oriented groups represented in the literature follow basic model principles, not unique, manual-driven programs of intervention for particular disorders.

Diagnostic, terminology, and classification issues have resulted in difficulties within the PD literature, as well as over- and underinclusion within diagnostic categories and a lack of predictive validity regarding the therapeutic approach best suited for different disorders (Higgit & Fonagy, 1992). The most commonly referenced and empirically validated approach is Linehan's dialectical behavior therapy (DBT; Linehan, 1993). A review of this model, the only extensively developed one in practice, may offer some insight into this discussion of the usefulness or benefits of including group therapy as a modality in providing CBT to individuals with PD.

Linehan's Dialectical Behavior Therapy

Despite the documented occurrence of PDs in the treatment-seeking population, few theoretically driven models specifically treat this population of patients, and there is a lack of treatment options and research related to treatment across the PDs (Endler & Kocovski, 2002). The leading CBT model, Linehan's DBT, was originally developed specifically for the treatment of suicidal and parasuicidal women diagnosed with BPD (Endler & Kocovski, 2002; Linehan, 1993; Swales, Heard, & Williams, 2000). Linehan outlined five subsystems or categories of dysregulation into which the diagnostic criteria for BPD can be organized, and by which typical presenting symptomatology may be conceptualized: affective, behavioral, interpersonal, self, and cognitive (Linehan, 1993; Swales et al., 2000). Her biosocial theory that prompted this model's conception proposes that a combination of biological vulnerability to emotional dysregulation and an invalidating environment results in BPD. Essentially, this model emphasizes the importance of both acceptance (of the patient's current life situation as it is, of the patient as he or she is, and of the working relationship as it is) and change (as is necessary for the continuation of treatment) (Linehan, 1993; Swales et al., 2000). It stresses the importance of the patient coming to understand that reality is a continuous process of change, including the relationships within it (which, again, are most difficult for patients with BPD to manage).

The DBT model, as a CBT model, emphasizes the importance of maintaining structure—especially with the BPD population, because these patients often present with crisis after crisis, and without a structured approach to skill development, it is easy for the therapist to lose focus. Linehan's model is adaptable to a variety of settings given that she outlined five primary treatment tasks, regardless of setting: enhance the patient's capabilities, motivate the patient to use these abilities, generalize these skills across relevant contexts, help the patient restructure his or her environment to facilitate progress, and address the motivation and abilities of the therapist (Linehan, 1993; Swales et al., 2000). In addition, Linehan outlined five stages through which treatment should progress, depending on degree of pathology: pretreatment, during which the goal is commitment from the patient to engage actively in therapy; Stage I, which focuses on stability, connection, and safety (for severe pathology, in which suicidal actions may be of concern); Stage II, during which exposure and emotional processing of the past are the focus (i.e., reducing posttraumatic stress); Stage III, which focuses on increasing self-esteem and achieving goals; and Stage IV, which focuses on the capacity to maintain a job (resolving existential life issues) (Linehan, 1993; Swales et al., 2000). To progress through these stages and facilitate change most effectively, Linehan emphasized problem-solving strategies as central to the model. In addition, the main acceptance strategy is validation (Linehan, 1993).

DBT has been shown to be effective in reducing parasuicidal behaviors and hospitalizations, as well as a higher retention rate than standard, nonmanualized treatment (Endler & Kocovski, 2002; Linehan, Armstrong, Suarez, Allmon, & Heard, 1991; Linehan, Heard, & Armstrong, 1993; Linehan, Tutek, Heard, & Armstrong, 1994; Swales et al., 2000). The efficacy of DBT as a group therapy approach with BPD has more recently prompted the expansion of potential populations to include substance abuse, eating disorders, and anger (Endler & Kocovski, 2002). However, literature documenting the efficacy of this model (so that it may become the hallmark of BPD treatment) is still needed. Despite the efficacy of DBT demonstrated in the literature, Hoffman (2002) asserts that when assigned to group therapy, patients with BPD often drop out, and that this form of treatment should not be imposed on this subgroup of the PD population.

ADDITIONAL CONSIDERATIONS

Despite the many obstacles to including patients with PDs in group CBT, some potential benefits are worthy of consideration if the individual patient and the degree of pathology do not rule out the patient's effective participation in the group.

CBT GROUPS FOR SPECIFIC DISORDERS

Direct Interpersonal Observation

Because each disorder we have discussed is characterized by interpersonal difficulties, a benefit of group CBT is that it provides an opportunity for direct observation of the patient's verbal and behavioral interactions with others, and offers the therapist a window into the patient's repertoire of interpersonal responses. The therapist does not have to depend on patients' reports of how others react to them, or how they react to others, inasmuch as the scenario unfolds before the therapist's eyes. It allows for direct interventions in the here-and-now format advocated in CBT. For example, if a patient with DPD indiscriminately and repeatedly agrees with a particularly assertive group member, regardless of topic of discussion, the therapist and peers who may notice can point this out to the patient while it is happening, allowing the patient to gain more than just a hypothetical awareness of his or her interpersonal tendencies. Immediate intervention and alternative responses may also be discussed and practiced through reframing and role playing.

Skills Building and Modeling

In addition to a more advantageous vantage point for the therapist, group CBT would allow more motivated patients with PD a social area to acquire and practice skills related to social awareness, self-expression and communication, assertiveness, empathic responding, problem-solving abilities, and negotiation and interpersonal compromise. The availability of peer feedback would allow for a more realistic understanding of the perceptions others have of the patient, helping to provide evidence for adequacy instead of the initial assumptions of inadequacy. Patients would be able to develop a greater sense of independence and self-efficacy through trial and error, and managing the distress related to that process.

Rotating-Theme Groups

The rotating-theme group was developed specifically for use in hospital settings (Bowers, 1989; Freeman, Schrodt, Gilson, & Ludgate, 1993; Freeman & Morgillo-Freeman, 2005). In this type of group cognitive therapy (GCT), an external structure for the therapy agenda is used in an attempt to circumvent some of the problems encountered due to rapid participant turnover, limited patient motivation, and the broad range of patient pathology inherent in a mixed PD group. Several steps are involved in developing a rotating-theme group. For the sake of illustration, let us assume that the therapy group typically meets once or twice weekly. The theme cycle might change every 12 sessions, so that patients may attend as few or as many sessions as they can (or choose to attend). By focusing each of the 12 sessions on a particular theme (e.g., the stigma of having a PD, dealing with children, coping with parents, problems with school or work, or other common areas of difficulty), the therapist can structure a comprehensive GCT experience. Initially, topics for the sessions can be developed by the group therapists based on their experiences with the range of participants typically encountered in this type of mixed group. The topic list should be matched to the population mix. For example, themes for GCT in a population that presents for therapy with depression might include building self-esteem, choosing pleasurable activities, or coping with loss. On the other hand, themes for GCT in a group whose participants have mostly eating disorders might include body image, meal planning, or thoughts about eating. The topic list evolves as the group therapists have the opportunity to experiment with various group themes.

A shift in the composition of the participant group would suggest that the session themes need to be altered. Most programs experience surges of admissions of certain types of participants. Sometimes the group may be made up of individuals with affective disorders; at another time, personality disorders, chemical dependence, or other conditions may predominate.

The topics for each session are provided to all participants, who are asked to prepare, in advance of each group meeting, two questions, problems, or thoughts relative to the selected theme of that group, and to bring these to the next group session. Index cards are supplied for writing down ideas. Although not every theme is fully relevant to every participant, the topic areas should be of broad interest to capture the attention of most group members. Some participants, however, may have to wait for a future session before dealing with their primary problem. Writing down questions or ideas allows participants who have difficulty being spontaneous in the group, or who have problems in identifying problems, to have a mechanism for expressing themselves.

As the agenda is set, the group therapist or cotherapist reads the cards, and a group "scribe" writes the items on a board. The therapist can then put two or more items of similar meaning together. Alternatively, group members are then asked to read what they have written on their index cards. Usually, 10 members do not generate 20 distinct issues; a good deal of overlap almost always occurs. A hierarchy of agenda items is established, and the group begins to work.

Participants who have been in other therapy groups may have difficulty making the transition to a theme-focused format, because they have become accustomed to a less structured approach. In more traditional forms of group therapy, the outspoken individual may be able to force his or her issues to the forefront and dominate the group.

The therapist prepares psychoeducational materials that are relevant to each theme and may outline the general content and procedure for the session in advance. However, it is also important to involve the group members in setting the agenda and providing input on the direction for therapy. The rotating-theme group is more structured than the open-ended group, but spontaneity and vigorous group interaction are still encouraged.

All of the guidelines and procedures for the open-ended groups described earlier also apply to the rotating-theme group. The only major difference is that a general topic is used to speed the agenda-setting process and to provide a thematic structure for group sessions. For example, see the sample schedule for the first week of a rotating theme group below:

Session 1	Reactions to having a personality disorder
Session 2	Hopelessness versus optimism
Session 3	Accepting who we are
Session 4	Getting motivated again
Session 5	Overcoming fears and anxieties
Session 6	Setting and reaching goals
Session 7	Coping with family and friends
Session 8	Problems of work or school
Session 9	Hopelessness versus optimism
Session 10	Coping with frustration
Session 11	Controlling anger
Session 12	Accepting who we are

A patient joining the group at Session 5 would be in the group for Sessions 5–12 and can then cycle through Sessions 1–4 for the full experience. Because each session is self-contained, the patient will take something away from the session and the therapy experience. Finally, a patient in the group for several months may cycle through the program several times.

CONCLUSIONS

GCT can help participants to engage more fully in the overall treatment process, assist the therapist(s) in obtaining a multifaceted picture of the participant's disorder *in vivo*, and provide peer feedback to group members. This form of cognitive therapy also promotes a sense of universality that helps to ease the participant's isolation and burden of shame and guilt. However, the main contribution of GCT is a resolution of symptoms through the identification and modification of cognitive-behavioral pathology. This chapter has described basic procedures for GCT with patients having PDs. The issues of selecting and preparing participants for group therapy, structuring the length and frequency of sessions, and maintaining a "here-and-now" focus become all the more important with this population. Pacing group sessions is one of the most complex and difficult parts of GCT because of rapid participant turnover and wide variations in levels of symptomatic distress. Nevertheless, cognitive interventions such as identifying automatic thoughts, listing advantages and disadvantages of maintaining particular behaviors, or examining alternatives, can be used with benefit in most group sessions. Standard behavioral procedures such as graded-task assignments and rehearsal are also utilized widely in GCT. Three major categories of GCT are detailed: core groups (open-ended, rotating-theme, and programmed), program–community meetings, and special purpose groups. Factors such the homogeneity of the participant group and availability of other methods of delivering cognitive therapy should be considered in designing the group therapy components of GCT.

The higher the level of structure, the greater the likelihood of group success. Toward this end, the rotating-theme model of group therapy can be of value. This model takes into account the needs of most of the patients (not all, at all sessions). It focuses on the psychoeducational aspects of function without challenging many strongly held and ego-syntonic beliefs.

We conclude that group therapy can be a valuable part of the overall treatment program for patients with PDs. The nature of participants' disorders can mitigate the potential success of the group, so care must be exercised in choosing participants and in focusing the group.

CHAPTER 15

Schizophrenia

David L. Roberts
Amy E. Pinkham
David L. Penn

DESCRIPTION OF SCHIZOPHRENIA

Schizophrenia is a severe and disabling illness that affects approximately 1% of individuals in the population. It is a multidimensional illness characterized by a range of positive symptoms (hallucinations and delusions), negative symptoms (including avolition, affective flattening, and alogia), and cognitive impairments (Andreasen, 1995). Depression and, to a lesser extent, anxiety may also be experienced secondary to the core symptoms of the disease (Siris, 2000; Tollefson & Sanger, 1999). Behavioral correlates of schizophrenia include social withdrawal, bizarre and disorganized behavior, and decline in vocational and social functioning (Mueser & Bellack, 1998). The presentation of schizophrenia is heterogeneous, with affected individuals exhibiting varying combinations of these signs and symptoms, and widely varying levels of impairment. Schizophrenia onset typically occurs between the late teens and late 20s (Gottesman, 1991). Although it was originally viewed as a chronic and degenerative condition, research shows that there is wide variability in the course and outcome of schizophrenia (Carpenter & Strauss, 1991).

Since the 1960s, antipsychotic medication has been first-line treatment for schizophrenia (Smith & Docherty, 1998). Despite its widespread use, medication has several shortcomings. First, although it can reduce positive symptoms and decrease length of hospitalization, it has less of an impact on negative symptoms and other functional consequences of the disorder. For

350

example, there is little evidence that pharmacological treatments can improve social functioning, which is one of the strongest correlates of current functioning and predictors of long-term outcome in schizophrenia (Amminger et al., 1999; Baum & Walker, 1995; Halford & Hayes, 1995; Macdonald, Jackson, Hayes, Baglioni, & Madden, 1998). Second, 25–50% of individuals with schizophrenia continue to experience residual positive symptoms even after stabilizing on an optimal medication regimen (Kane & Marder, 1993; Pantelis & Barnes, 1996; Wiersma, Nienhuis, & Slooff, 1998). And third, between 45 and 60% of patients do not adhere to their medication regimen (Fenton, Blyler, & Heinssen, 1997), often because of troubling side effects (Hoge et al., 1990). Thus, there is a strong need for adjunctive psychosocial interventions, such as CBT for schizophrenia, particularly for treatment-resistant symptoms.

CBT FOR SCHIZOPHRENIA

There is strong rationale for specifically applying CBT to treat the residual symptoms of schizophrenia. First, CBT uses a relatively straightforward problem-solving approach that is consistent with the concrete orientation of many individuals with schizophrenia. Second, cognitive and behavioral treatments are effective with other psychiatric disorders (DeRubeis & Crits-Christoph, 1998), and have already shown some effectiveness at treating the positive symptoms of schizophrenia (Bustillo, Lauriello, Horan, & Keith, 2001; Dickerson, 2004; Gould, Mueser, Bolton, Mays, & Goff, 2001; Jones, Cormac, Mota, & Campbell, 2000; Pilling et al., 2002; Rector & Beck, 2001). Third, CBT can be tailored to the individual needs of clients, which is important because of the heterogeneous presentation of schizophrenia. Fourth, many individuals with schizophrenia already use their own coping strategies to manage symptoms (Falloon & Talbott, 1981; Tarrier, 1987; Tarrier, Harwood, Yusupoff, Beckett, & Baker, 1990), which can be strengthened with CBT approaches (Tarrier et al., 1993). In the paragraphs that follow, we discuss CBT for schizophrenia in more depth.

For the past 50 years, strictly behavioral interventions for schizophrenia have been widespread, particularly in inpatient settings. These treatments typically follow operant conditioning theory, using controlled reinforcement schedules to modify specific behaviors (Curran, Monti, & Corriveau, 1982; Haddock et al., 1998; Mueser, 1993; Paul & Lentz, 1977). Within the past decade, however, interest in cognitive therapy of schizophrenia has grown, in part because the shift to community treatment has highlighted the difficulty of providing behavioral reinforcement in the context of outpatient care. Cognitive therapy of schizophrenia dates back to the early work of Beck (1952), but controlled trials of this intervention have only accrued over the past 10 years. As with cognitive treatments, cognitive theory in schizophrenia is not as well developed as in other disorders, such as depression and anxiety (Morrison, 2001). Nonetheless, cognitive models of schizophrenia are in line with the broader cognitive framework, emphasizing beliefs and attributions as mediators of experience. The following section reviews current cognitive models of schizophrenia.

Consistent with the traditional emphasis in schizophrenia research on positive symptoms, as opposed to negative symptoms and other deficits, cognitive models of schizophrenia have typically focused on hallucinations and delusions. Auditory hallucinations have received special attention because of their high prevalence relative to other symptoms of schizophrenia (Slade & Bentall, 1988). Several researchers have suggested that auditory hallucinations may be misattributions of internal thoughts caused by a speech-processing deficit (David, 1994; Hoffman, 1986), an idea that has received some empirical support (see Haddock et al., 1998). Others hypothesize that speech processing is normal in schizophrenia and that auditory hallucinations are caused entirely by cognitive biases (Bentall, 1990). Etiology aside, cognitive researchers have made important contributions to our understanding of how hallucinations contribute to and maintain dysfunction. For example, hallucinations have been found to be quite prevalent in the general population (nearly 5%; Tien, 1991; van Os, Hanssen, & Vollebergh, 2001; see review in Morrison, 1998), suggesting that some part of the distress and disability associated with schizophrenia may be due to maladaptive reactions to hallucinations.

Several cognitive models of delusions have also been proposed, most of which place a special emphasis on persecutory delusions, because these appear to be more common than other types of delusions (Bentall, Corcoran, Howard, Blackwood, & Kinderman, 2001; Garety, Everitt, & Hemsley, 1988; Garety & Freeman, 1999; Stompe et al., 1999). Bentall, Kinderman, and Kaney (1994) posited that the content of persecutory delusions results from a motivated effort to defend oneself from negative self-evaluation. Other cognitive theories of delusions differ from Bentall's model in that they de-emphasize the motivated/functional role of delusions and the significance of content, while stressing the role of cognitive process. For example, Maher (1988) posited that delusions arise when normal reasoning is used in an attempt to explain anomalous perceptual experiences (e.g., hallucinations). Garety, Hemsley, and Wessely (1991), on the other hand, hypothesized that delusions result from beliefs formed using biased logic.

Drawing on developments in the cognitive theory of other disorders (e.g., anxiety; Wells, 1995), researchers more recently have suggested a prominent role for metacognitive processes in the maintenance of both delusions and hallucinations. "Metacognition" refers to an individual's beliefs about his or her own thoughts and thought processes. Of specific interest in the context of schizophrenia are individuals' beliefs regarding the controllability, power, and beneficence or malevolence of their hallucinations and delusions. For example, Morrison, Haddock, and Tarrier (1995) have hypothesized that individuals' beliefs in their ability to control their thoughts can lead to hallucinations being attributed to external sources in order to reduce cognitive dissonance. This and other theories suggest that one's beliefs about voices and delusions can affect one's emotional reactions to these anomalous experiences, mediating the associated distress and disability.

As cognitive theory and research on schizophrenia have developed, several efforts have been made to synthesize the empirical research and resolve points of theoretical dispute. Bentall and colleagues (2001) have expanded their previous theory of persecutory delusions, incorporating a wider array of research findings and metacognitive theory. Called the "attribution–self-representation cycle," this model posits that individuals with paranoia employ biased causal attributions of events to support an unrealistic self-image, on which they draw to make further biased attributions. This theory is contextualized within a range of experimental findings that links paranoid delusions to low self-esteem (Lyon, Kaney, & Bentall, 1994), jumping to conclusions (Garety et al., 1991; Huq, Garety, & Helmsley, 1988), externalizing (Kaney & Bentall, 1989) and personalizing attributional biases (Kinderman & Bentall, 1997), and attentional bias toward threatening information (Bentall & Kaney, 1989; Fear, Sharp, & Healy, 1996). Morrison (2001), on the other hand, has suggested an integrated model of positive symptoms in schizophrenia that shares similarities with cognitive models of other disorders, such as anxiety, panic, and hypochondriasis. In this model, hallucinations are treated as intrusions into awareness that are experienced by a significant minority of normal individuals. These intrusions may be caused by a wide range of factors, including sleep deprivation, biological abnormalities, and interactions between personal and environmental factors. Delusions occur when intrusions are interpreted in culturally unacceptable ways. Distress and disability result, in turn, when intrusions and delusions are interpreted in the context of dysfunctional metacognitions that at once perpetuate delusional reactions and heighten distress. Both the Bentall and the Morrison theories have integrated an impressive amount of empirical research. Although these two theories posit differing explanations and have different foci, they also overlap significantly, which suggests that cognitive theories of schizophrenia may be converging.

INDIVIDUAL CBT FOR SCHIZOPHRENIA

As with cognitive theories of schizophrenia, the bulk of CBT for schizophrenia has focused on delusions and hallucinations. Several treatment-specific considerations have contributed to this focus. First, CBT is designed to treat disordered thought, and as such lends itself more to treatment of delusions and hallucinations than to negative symptoms. Second, early case reports and case series using CBT for these symptoms were generally successful (e.g., Beck, 1952; reviewed in Haddock et al., 1998). Third, many individuals with schizophrenia already use CBT-style techniques to manage positive symptoms (Falloon & Talbott, 1981). In the following section, we provide a brief overview of the literature that is limited to randomized, controlled trials. Comprehensive reviews of the literature are available elsewhere (Bouchard, Vallieres,

Roy, & Maziade, 1996; Dickerson, 2000; Garety, Fowler, & Kuipers, 2000; Gould et al., 2001; Pilling et al., 2002; Rector & Beck, 2001).

Five trials have compared CBT to nonspecific interventions for individuals with medication-resistant positive symptoms. Kuipers and colleagues (1997) compared CBT plus treatment as usual (TAU) to TAU alone in a 9-month outpatient trial (n = 60). CBT was superior in reducing overall symptomatology and producing clinical improvement, but trends favoring CBT in the reduction of delusions and hallucinations were not significant. At 9-month follow-up (n = 47), the CBT group remained less symptomatic overall, and their gains over the control group in delusion-related distress and frequency of hallucinations had reached significance (Kuipers et al., 1998). Tarrier and colleagues (1998) compared CBT plus TAU to supportive counseling (SC) plus TAU, and to TAU alone in a 10-week outpatient trial (n = 87). The CBT group showed significantly greater improvement between baseline and 3 months posttreatment on measures of severity and number of positive symptoms. At 12- and 24-month follow-ups, the significant advantage of CBT over SC disappeared, while its advantage over TAU remained (Tarrier et al., 1999, 2000). Sensky and colleagues (2000) compared CBT plus TAU to a nonspecific befriending intervention plus TAU in a trial of up to 9 months (n = 90). The interventions both showed significant improvements in positive symptoms at the end of treatment; however, at 9-month follow-up, only the CBT condition retained these benefits. Pinto, La Pia, Mennella, Giorgio, and DeSimone (1999) found CBT plus social skills training to be superior to SC in outpatients in terms of overall symptomatology at termination of treatment and at 12-month follow-up (n = 37). Finally, Rector, Seeman, and Segal (2003) compared CBT plus "enriched" TAU to enriched TAU alone in a 6-month trial (n = 42). CBT showed nonsignificant trends toward improved symptoms at termination of treatment and at 6-month follow-up.

Other studies have examined the effectiveness of CBT in recovery from acute psychosis, relapse prevention, as a brief intervention, and in early psychosis. Drury, Birchwood, Cochrane, and MacMillan (1996a, 1996b) found CBT to be superior to recreational activities plus informal support in speed and extent of symptom recovery after acute relapse (n = 40). A prospective randomized controlled study by Gumley et al. (2003) compared CBT to TAU in preventing relapse over 12 months. The CBT group had significantly fewer relapses and significantly fewer psychotic and overall symptoms. As a brief intervention, Turkington, Kingdon, and Turner (2002) compared 6 weeks of CBT provided by psychiatric nurses to TAU among 422 outpatients. Brief CBT was found to be significantly better in reducing overall symptomatology and depression, and improving insight, but not in reducing psychotic symptomatology. Finally, Haddock, Tarrier, et al. (1999) compared brief CBT to SC and psychoeducation among 21 recent-onset inpatients. Over a maximum treatment period of 5 weeks, the groups exhibited no differences in terms of length of hospital stay, relapse within 2 years, or psychotic symptomatology. In a similar 5-week trial with greater power (n = 315; Lewis et al., 2002a,

2002b), the same research group found CBT to be associated with speedier improvements than SC in terms of auditory hallucinations. This advantage held at 18-month follow-up, but CBT was not significantly superior on other outcome or follow-up measures. Both groups were superior to TAU.

In summary, research supports the use of adjunctive CBT in schizophrenia. A recent meta-analysis of studies comparing CBT to control conditions calculated a mean effect size difference of 0.65 for reduction of positive symptoms, and of 0.93 for showing continued gains in symptomatology at follow-up (Gould et al., 2001). Thus, CBT appears to be more effective than other interventions in treating residual positive symptoms. There is also evidence that CBT reduces negative symptoms better than other psychological interventions, especially at follow-up analysis (Drury et al., 1996b; Pinto et al., 1999; Rector et al., 2003; Sensky et al., 2000; Tarrier et al., 1999, 2001), as well as overall symptomatology and depression (Sensky et al., 2000). In terms of technique, it remains unclear whether specific interventions within the CBT armamentarium are more effective than others, or whether the broader approach shared by all CBT interventions is the key to effectiveness. That said, an innovative recent analysis of available studies suggests that more behaviorally oriented CBT interventions (emphasizing behavioral experiments and the setting of behavioral goals) may be more effective than cognitively focused interventions (i.e., emphasizing schema formation in earlier life, recording of automatic thoughts, etc.; Tarrier & Wykes, 2004).

GROUP CBT FOR SCHIZOPHRENIA

The success of individual CBT has prompted researchers to examine more efficient means of administering CBT for residual psychotic symptoms. One such way is to present the intervention in a group format. Gledhill, Lobban, and Sellwood (1998) pointed out that sharing similar experiences with members of the group may help individuals feel less isolated by their symptoms, and that the presence of other members may allow for positive peer pressure to comply with homework assignments. The group setting may also allow participants to model positive coping strategies and to learn from and reinforce each other (Johns, Sellwood, McGovern, & Haddock, 2002). Thus, beyond general social support, group approaches to schizophrenia treatment appear to have many benefits that are not easily afforded by individual treatments.

Studies that have examined the efficacy of group CBT interventions for schizophrenia have reported positive findings for a variety of symptoms (See Table 15.1 for details of group CBT studies). For instance, in a study that used group CBT to address general symptomatology, mood, self-esteem, and knowledge, half of the group members felt better able to cope with their symptoms, all individuals reported less depression, and the majority of group members had higher self-esteem and greater knowledge about schizophrenia at the end of treatment (Gledhill et al., 1998).

TABLE 15.1. Studies of Group CBT for Schizophrenia

Study	Participants	Design	Results
Daniels (1998)	40 outpatients (27 male) with schizophrenia (15) or schizoaffective disorder (12); mean age = 33.7 years	16-session CBT plus group process intervention versus wait-list control	CBT group showed significant increase in global, psychosocial, and occupational functioning, and trend toward decreased negative symptoms; wait list had no significant changes.
Gledhill, Lobban, & Sellwood (1998)	4 consecutively referred outpatients (2 male) with schizophrenia, stabilized on medication; median age = 41 years	Uncontrolled pre- to poststudy of 8-week CBT	Half of Ps reported improved symptom coping; all reported less depression; a majority reported better knowledge of schizophrenia and self-esteem.
Lecomte et al. (1999)	95 inpatients and outpatients (72 male) with schizophrenia (85) or schizoaffective disorder (10); mean age = 40.6 years	Randomized, controlled 12-week trial of self-esteem/ empowerment groups plus TAU (n = 51) versus TAU (n = 44); includes follow-up assessment	Experimental group showed significant short-term reduction in positive symptoms and significant improvement in active coping skills relative to control group.
Wykes, Parr, & Landau (1999)	21 patients with schizophrenia and distressing, medication resistant AH; mean age = 40 years; all Ps on medication	Controlled study of 6 sessions of CBT versus wait-list condition; includes follow-up assessment	Relative to wait-list condition, significant reduction in experience of AH, maintained at follow-up, and increase in perception of control over AH.
Andres, Pfammatter, Garst, Teschner, & Brenner (2000)	32 consecutive patients (21 male) with schizophrenia (22) or schizoaffective disorder (10); mean age = 31.5 years	Controlled comparison of coping-oriented therapy (n = 17) to supportive therapy (n = 15) over 24 sessions; includes follow-up assessments	Both groups showed medium effect sizes in improving cognizance, general psychopathology, and negative symptoms; effects were larger in the coping-oriented group.
Chadwick, Sambrooke, Rasch, & Davies (2000)	22 patients with schizophrenia or schizoaffective disorder and distressing, medication-resistant AH; all Ps on medication	Uncontrolled pre- to poststudy of 8-session group CBT for AH	Significantly reduced beliefs in omnipotence of AH and in beliefs that AH were uncontrollable.
Halperin, Nathan, Drummond, & Castle (2000)	20 outpatients (13 males; mean age = 39.6 years)	8 weekly sessions of CBT, and 6-week follow-up	Significant improvement in social anxiety and avoidance, mood, and quality of life; gains maintained at follow-up; 7 Ps reported increased symptom control and decreased AH-related distress and distraction.

(continued)

356

TABLE 15.1. *(continued)*

Study	Participants	Design	Results
Perlman & Hubbard (2000)	9 outpatients (3 male) with schizophrenia; age range, 35–50 years; all on medication	Uncontrolled pre- to poststudy of 23-session, CBT-based self-control skills group	
Johns, Sellwood, McGovern, & Haddock (2002)	4 patients with schizophrenia, reporting distressing negative SX and no prominent positive SX	Uncontrolled pre- to poststudy of 16-session CBT	Significant reduction in avolition/apathy, and trend toward reduced negative SX; half of Ps reported reduced negative-symptom-related distress.
Kingsep, Nathan, & Castle (2003)	33 outpatients	24-session CBT versus wait-list control group	Significant reductions in social anxiety, general psychopathology, and quality of life relative to wait-list.
Bechdolf et al. (2004)	88 consecutive acute-admission inpatients (48 female) with ICD schizophrenia or related disorder; mean age = 32 years	Ps randomized to 8 weeks of CBT (16 sessions; $n = 40$) or psychoeducation (8 sessions; $n = 48$); 6-month follow-up assessment	Both groups had significantly improved PANSS scores; CBT was nonsignificantly better in overall relapse (13 vs. 20%) and compliance, significantly better in relapse during follow-up (0 vs. 12.5%).
Pinkham, Gloege, Flanagan, & Penn (2004)	11 inpatients (8 male) with chronic schizophrenia (5) or schizoaffective disorder (6) experiencing distressing, medication-resistant AH; mean age = 39.6 years; all Ps on medication	Uncontrolled, pre- to postcomparison of 7-week ($n = 5$) and 20-week ($n = 6$) AH-focused CBT	No outcome differences between groups; combining groups, subjects reported significant decrease in distressing beliefs about AH; trend toward reduced frequency of AH in 20-week group.
Newton et al. (2005)	22 outpatients (17 female) with medication-resistant AH that began before age 18 and lasted less than 3 years; no diagnostic requirement; mean age = 17 years	Wait-list control (6 weeks), followed by 6-week treatment and 12-week posttreatment. "Total treatment phase" = Week 6 to Week 24	PSYRATS-AH showed no change over wait-list period or treatment period, but significant reduction over total treatment phase. Perceived control over AH and reduced distress were significantly correlated.

Note. Studies are listed in chronological order.
AH, auditory hallucinations; P, participant; ICD, *International Clarification of Diseases*; TAU, treatment as usual; SX, symptoms.

In addition, several studies have also found that group CBT can be particularly helpful in learning to cope with persistent auditory hallucinations. In a controlled trial that utilized a wait-list control group, Wykes, Parr, and Landau (1999) found that following group CBT, participants reported a reduction in the experience of auditory hallucinations and an increased perception of control over the voices. Likewise, seven of nine individuals who participated in a CBT-based self-control skills group reported that their voices were less distressing and less distracting at the end of treatment (Perlman & Hubbard, 2000). Chadwick, Sambrooke, Rasch, and Davies (2000) found that individuals who participated in their group CBT for auditory hallucinations achieved a significantly reduced conviction in beliefs that the voices were omnipotent and that they had no control over the voices. Two more recent studies used the Wykes et al. (1999) protocol to target auditory hallucinations in diverse patient groups. One study with an inpatient sample noted significant decreases in distressing beliefs about voices, as well as a reduction in the frequency of auditory hallucinations (Pinkham, Gloege, Flanagan, & Penn, 2004). A second study used a wait-list control design among individuals younger than 21 who had been experiencing voices for less than 3 years (Newton et al., 2005). This study found a significant reduction in Psychotic Symptoms Rating Scales (PSYRATS; Haddock, McCarron, Tarrier, & Faragher, 1999) auditory hallucination scores over the total study phase, and noted a significant relationship between perceived control over hallucinations and reduced distress. Thus, evidence supports the positive impact of group CBT on auditory hallucinations among first-episode youth and chronically ill inpatients, as well as higher-functioning outpatients.

Fewer studies have examined group CBT for negative symptoms. Johns et al. (2002) found that following a group CBT intervention that primarily sought to increase motivation, participants showed a reduction in avolition and a trend toward reduced overall negative symptoms. Two of the four members of their group also reported a reduction in the distress associated with their negative symptoms. Despite the extremely small sample size of this study ($n = 4$) and the caution that should accompany it, these findings gain additional support from two studies that have combined CBT with other group psychotherapy approaches to treat negative symptoms. Daniels (1998) found that individuals who participated in a combined CBT and interactive behavioral training group showed a trend toward decreased negative symptoms, whereas individuals who were in a wait-list group did not. Similarly, Andres, Pfammatter, Garst, Teschner, and Brenner (2000) found reductions in negative symptoms in individuals who participated in a coping-oriented group therapy; the effect size of this improvement was larger for the coping-oriented group (1.46) than for a supportive treatment group (0.80).

CBT-oriented group interventions have also been tailored to address comorbid social anxiety (Halperin, Nathan, Drummond, & Castle, 2000; Kingsep, Nathan, & Castle, 2003), low self-esteem (Lecomte et al., 1999), and first-episode schizophrenia (Lecomte, Leclerc, Wykes, & Lecomte, 2003). In their study with 20 outpatients, Halperin and colleagues (2000) observed significant reductions in social anxiety and avoidance, mood, and quality of life in the CBT group relative to a wait-list control group. In a similarly designed study with 33 outpatients, the same research group (Kingsep et al., 2003) observed significant reductions in social anxiety, general psychopathology, and quality of life in the CBT condition relative to the wait-list control group. In a study with 95 patients, Lecomte and colleagues (1999) incorporated cognitive techniques into a group self-esteem and empowerment module. Participants receiving this module plus regular treatment exhibited significantly reduced positive symptoms and increased coping ability compared to participants receiving regular treatment alone. No differences were observed in self-esteem. Finally, Lecomte and colleagues (2003) have developed a first-episode intervention that targets coping with symptoms, as well as collateral difficulties, such as stress, anxiety, and substance abuse. Qualitative results from a small trial are promising, but they require replication.

In a relatively large randomized, controlled study, Bechdolf and colleagues (2004) used CBT techniques developed by Tarrier and colleagues (1990, 1993) to target relapse, symptomatology, and medication compliance among individuals who had experienced recent symptom relapses. Compared to a time-matched psychoeducation group (8 weeks), individuals in the group CBT condition showed a trend toward fewer relapses and better medication compliance at posttreatment, and had significantly fewer relapses between posttreatment and 6-month follow-up. Both groups showed significant improvement in symptomatology, as measured by the Positive and Negative Syndrome Scale (PANSS; Kay, Fizbein, & Opler, 1987).

All in all, group CBT for schizophrenia appears to be a promising intervention for both positive and negative symptoms; however, these studies are not without limitations. Only one controlled trial (Wykes et al., 1999) has targeted these symptoms, and only one study (Pinkham et al., 2004) has utilized group CBT with an inpatient sample. Additionally, many of the studies mentioned have utilized small, homogenous samples that make it difficult to generalize to the average individual with schizophrenia. Despite these limitations, however, the heuristic value of these studies should not be ignored, and group CBT for schizophrenia should be considered a viable and promising treatment.

ASSESSING SUITABILITY FOR GROUP CBT AND TREATMENT GAINS

Assessing Suitability for Participation

Schizophrenia is a heterogeneous condition, and manifestations of the illness vary widely. To maximize the effectiveness and appropriateness of the intervention, group CBT practitioners should target specific domains for treatment and recruit patients with demonstrable need in the targeted area. Targets of treatment may include (but are not limited to) severity or frequency of hallucinations; conviction associated with delusional beliefs; distress and/or disability directly associated with hallucinations or delusions, negative symptoms (e.g., motivation), coping abilities, problem solving, relapse prevention, social functioning, social skills, insight, self-esteem, and disease-related anxiety or depression. Additionally, because presentation, deficits, and treatment needs differ across the course of the illness, it is best to compose groups of individuals within the same phase of the illness (i.e., prodromal, first episode, acute, chronic and stable, or residual). Reducing "noise" in these ways should maximize the members' level of shared experience and their perception of "being in the right place," which in turn should increase opportunities for social learning and level of engagement. Additionally, it should decrease heterogeneity of in-session presentation—a key consideration in this population.

Because schizophrenia also differentially affects basic cognitive abilities (including attention, concentration, and executive functioning), efforts should be made to compose groups of individuals of similar intellectual ability. Whereas some individuals may have only slight cognitive deficits, others may be profoundly cognitively impaired. And because educational attainment tends to be lower in schizophrenia than in most patient groups (Hafner et al., 1995; Isohanni et al., 2001), variability in this domain can also widen the gulf between group members. Thus, we recommend screening individuals with an abbreviated IQ measure (e.g., the Wide Range Achievement Test—Reading [WRAT-R] or two subtests of the Wechsler Abbreviated Scale of Intelligence [WASI]) to minimize heterogeneity in cognitive ability in the group. Depending on the patient population, separate groups may be run for individuals with normal and subnormal IQ.

Motivation for treatment is another key domain in schizophrenia treatment. Unlike many individuals with mental illnesses, people with schizophrenia frequently suffer from poor insight into their condition. They may not recognize that they have an illness or that they are in need of treatment. Indeed, individuals may have negative associations with mental health workers and be hostile to treatment. Because many group treatments for schizophrenia are conducted in inpatient settings in which some group members participate involuntarily, it would be unrealistic to suggest recruiting only motivated individuals. That said, we do suggest counterbalancing unmotivated individuals with motivated individuals within a group when possible. It is possible that motivated, optimistic members can positively influence less motivated members and serve as role models for individuals who may be less engaged in treatment. We are aware of one measure of motivation for treatment, the Daiuto Treatment Questionnaire, that is appropriate for use among inpatients with limited cognitive ability and varying levels of insight and psychotic symptomatology (Jennifer Snyder, personal communication, November 2004).*

*Inquiries about the Daiuto Treatment Questionnaire should be directed to Jennifer Snyder at jennifer.snyder@ncmail.net.

Another issue that relates to both cognitive ability and motivation for treatment is cognitive flexibility. Because of the nature of CBT, we have found that individuals with very limited cognitive flexibility are poor candidates for the cognitive components of this intervention. Many cognitive exercises, such as generating alternative explanations for events, tend to be too difficult for these individuals and are of limited utility. Finally, we suggest excluding from group participation members who are chronically highly disorganized in behavior and/or speech, or who are aggressive. It is to be expected that some members will become disorganized during periods of symptom exacerbation; however, patients who are chronically disorganized stand to benefit less from CBT, and can hinder the progress of others by derailing and intruding in conversation.

To illustrate these group recruitment principles, we review our criteria for inclusion in a recent CBT group. This group was designed to target frequency, severity, and symptom-related distress associated with medication-resistant auditory hallucinations among chronic but stable outpatients with schizophrenia or schizoaffective disorder. Community providers familiar with the treatment goals referred candidates. Candidates were then interviewed to confirm diagnosis and to ensure that they experienced at least moderate auditory hallucinations (as measured by the PANSS. Participants also needed to report that their hallucinations were problematic in their lives, and that they would like to address them in treatment. We also screened these individuals with an abbreviated IQ measure (the WRAT-R), and included only those with an estimated IQ above 70.

Assessing Treatment Outcome

As discussed earlier, developments in the cognitive theory of psychosis have led to an increase in specific targets for intervention and a corresponding proliferation of outcome instruments. Because it is beyond the scope of this chapter to review all potentially useful outcome measures, we provide an overview of key considerations, outcome domains, and instruments that we have found useful in assessing the effectiveness of group CBT for schizophrenia.

As in all treatment interventions, outcome assessment should measure change in the specific domains targeted by the intervention. The most frequently targeted domains in CBT for schizophrenia are delusions and hallucinations. Over the past 20 years, conceptualization of these symptoms has become increasingly complex as researchers have moved away from viewing them as present versus absent, toward a more dimensional approach, and have established the importance of multiple dimensions within each of these symptom types (Garety, Dunn, Fowler, & Kuipers, 1998). Thus, delusions can now be assessed in terms of a patient's conviction in the delusion, preoccupation with it, distress experienced as a result of it, and action taken in response to the delusion. The multidimensional view of hallucinations allows for measurement of frequency, degree of interference in daily functioning, distress caused by hallucinations, and omnipotence and omniscience attributed to hallucinated voices.

In our experience, the PSYRATS is a useful instrument for assessing the multiple dimensions of hallucinations and delusions (and as an instrument to complement information obtained on the PANSS). The PSYRATS is administered as a structured interview and includes separate versions for delusions and hallucinations. Each version takes 20–30 minutes to administer. The Beliefs about Voices Questionnaire—Revised (BAVQ-R; Chadwick, Lees, & Birchwood, 2000) is a self-report measure that assesses the individual's beliefs, emotions, and behavior related to auditory hallucinations. The participant is asked to state to what degree he or she agrees with statements such as "My voice is punishing me for something I have done" and "My voice makes me feel down." This measure is particularly useful for assessing delusion-related distress and beliefs rather than frequency. Thus, by using this measure, one can examine improvements in coping with voices rather than a simple decrease in symptomatology.

Social functioning, an outcome domain that has received increasing attention, remains difficult to assess validly. The Social Functioning Scale (SFS; Birchwood, Smith, Cochrane, Wetton, & Copestake, 1990), is a semi-structured interview that lasts between 15 and 45 minutes and does not require specialized training, measures activities of daily living, self-care, vocational readiness, and social integration. This instrument is more useful for outpatients than for inpatients because of its emphasis on community-based indicators of functioning (e.g., shopping and seeking employment, and varied recreational activities). A disadvantage of the SFS as an outcome measure is that it may not reflect certain ecologically significant changes in an individual's social functioning. For example, an individual who, over the course of treatment, gains one new friend may experience a substantial increase in the quality of his or her social life despite the relatively small quantitative change reflected in the SFS.

Finally, outcome assessments should include a general measure of schizophrenia symptomatology. The most commonly used measures are the PANSS (Kay et al., 1987) and the Brief Psychiatric Rating Scale (BPRS; Ventura, Green, Shaner, & Liberman, 1993). Both the PANSS and the BPRS are semistructured interviews that can be administered in 30–60 minutes by an interviewer who has been trained to reliability. In settings in which use of the PANSS or BPRS is not feasible, the Brief Symptom Inventory (a 53-item self-report measure; Derogatis, 1993) can provide a broad index of symptoms and symptom-related distress.

When planning an assessment battery, researchers should keep in mind that long assessments can be overly demanding, frustrating, and aversive to individuals with schizophrenia. For this reason, and because many measures for this population require substantial time to administer, we typically conduct baseline and endpoint assessments, but seldom assess clients more than once during the course of treatment. For researchers and clinicians interested in process variables, this caution should be balanced against the necessity of collecting data with greater frequency.

Finally, it should be noted that because of the nature of schizophrenia, including variable insight, paranoia, and positive psychotic symptoms, self-report measures may be of questionable validity in this population. Thus, if possible, it is useful to solicit information from family members and other care workers who are familiar with the client. This can provide a measure of convergent validity to support client reports and increase the ecological validity of findings, particularly when measuring level of functioning. In addition to clinical measures and family or staff reports, broad indices of functioning in schizophrenia that are often informative include number of relapses (i.e., significant worsening of symptoms), number of hospitalizations, and number of days spent in the hospital.

SAMPLE CBT PROTOCOL FOR AUDITORY HALLUCINATIONS GROUP

In this section (and in Table 15.2) we present a sample protocol used in a CBT intervention for auditory hallucinations. Regardless of the specific focus of the group CBT intervention, we recommend adhering to several broad guidelines. These guidelines are similar to those used in CBT groups for nonpsychotic clinical samples. In general, the first session should be devoted to introductions, providing an overview of the group content and goals, and setting ground rules. A structured treatment manual should guide subsequent sessions. Within each session, the following structure should be followed: (1) greetings; (2) setting the agenda; (3) reviewing homework; (4) working through content for that session; (5) summarizing content; (6) soliciting participant feedback; and (7) assigning homework for the next session.

One of the authors (Penn) of this chapter revised and expanded the CBT manual developed by Wykes et al. (1999) to better meet the clinical needs of an inpatient population.* This revised manual extended the format of the intervention from 7 to 12 sessions. Only minor alterations were made to the content of the original manual; the main changes included spending more time on difficult topics and assigning additional homework.

The overall goal of the intervention is to apply cognitive-behavioral techniques to auditory hallucinations. The group comprised two therapists, one of whom took primary responsibility for facilitating discussion, while the other assisted with role plays and in administrative duties (e.g., writing down coping strategies generated by the group on a flip chart). The group was intentionally

---

*A revised manual is available upon request.

TABLE 15.2. Sample Outline of Treatment Protocol for Group CBT of Voices in Schizophrenia

Session	Strategies covered

Session 1	Establishing a therapeutic alliance
	• Introduction of group members (including therapists):
	  1. Name and where from.
	  2. Why each person wants to participate in the group.
	• Review of group frequency and format:
	  1. Discussion of the purpose of the group: to help people better cope with their voices and to enhance the quality of their lives.
	  2. The group meets weekly, for 1-hour sessions, for a total of 12 meetings.
	  3. Overview of the topics/phases of treatment.
	  4. Address group questions.
	• Determine group ground rules.

Session 2	Education about voices and sharing voice experiences • Show first half of film, *Hearing Voices* (Session 2). Stop film periodically and ask group members for their reactions to what they are seeing in the film. • Ask group members to comment on similarities of their experiences with those depicted in the film. Do any of the experiences reported in the film seem familiar?

Session 3	Education about voices and sharing voice experiences
	• Show second half of film.
	• Introduce normalizing rationale (Session 3).
	  1. Note the wide experiences of the voice hearers in the videotape.
	  2. Introduce normalizing "continuum of experience": A fair percentage of the general population reports hearing voices; hearing voices or sounds can occur when falling asleep, when waking up, during sensory deprivation, etc.
	• Review basic psychoeducation discussed in film.
	  1. Models of hearing voices (e.g., medical and psychological models).
	  2. Role of medication.
	  3. Treatment for hearing voices.

Sessions 4–5	Content of voices
	• Solicit group members' experiences with voices.
	• Use the following probes to help elicit the voice themes:
	  1. Are the voices friendly or not friendly?
	  2. What do they typically say to you?
	  3. How do the voices make you feel?
	  4. Do you view the voices as strong or weak?
	  5. What you happen if you ignored or disobeyed them?
	• Elicit reactions from the group concerning the common voice themes.
	• Ask clients to record the content of their voices on the Voice Content Form.

Sessions 6–7	Behavioral analysis of voices
	• Teach the ABC model.
	  1. Use flip chart to illustrate the model.
	  2. Provide a general example of how one's belief (B) system, in response to an event (A) can lead to negative consequences (C).

(continued)

TABLE 15.2. *(continued)*

Session	Strategies covered

Sessions 6–7 *(cont.)*	• Ask group members to provide daily (but not psychotic) examples of the ABC model.
	• Shift the model to discussion of voices.
	  1. Ask for a volunteer and ask him or her for an example of where he or she was, what he or she was doing, and what time, he or she heard the voice.
	  2. See if you can clarify what was happening *before* the client heard the voice. This can include behaviors, thoughts, and/or feelings.
	  3. Identify the consequences of the member hearing voices (i.e., behavioral, cognitive, and emotional). The consequences will be an area to be addressed when discussing coping strategies.
	• Assign homework to group members in which they have to monitor, on a daily basis, the ABC's of when their voices occurred.

Sessions 8–9	Increasing and decreasing strategies
	• Review the key antecedents for each group member and discuss:
	  1. What situations/events make the voices worse?
	  2. What makes them better?
	• Assign "Better/Worse" form for homework to help people monitor factors that affect their voices' intensity.

Sessions 10–12	Coping strategies
	• Ask each group member for some alternative coping strategies he or she could use. Write these on a flip chart.
	  1. What are the strategies that consistently work?
	  2. In which situations do they work?
	  3. Summarize findings on the flip chart.
	  4. Ask the group members to rate each of the strategies and see if there is any consistency.
	• After a list is compiled, ask each member what strategy he or she is currently using and work with him or her to come up with a new strategy.
	• Have the group members break into pairs and role-play coping with voices.
	• Assign practice of coping strategies for homework (and have group members complete Coping Strategies Worksheet).
	• Get feedback on coping strategies.
	  1. Review with each group member coping strategies that were attempted and whether they were successful.
	  2. Identify alternative strategies if implemented ones were not successful. Ask for group feedback and help in this process.
	  3. Continue with in-session role plays.

kept small (i.e., five to seven clients), so that relatively "individualized" attention could be given to all group members.

The first five sessions focused on building rapport among the group members, providing basic education about auditory hallucinations, and exploring the content of members' voices. First, all participants, including the therapists, were asked to introduce and tell a bit about themselves. Second, the group viewed *Hearing Voices*. The BBC-produced film presents both individuals with a psychiatric disorder and those without, who hear voices. The film was frequently paused by the therapist, so that the group could discuss how the experiences of people in the film matched those of group members. Third, following the film, group members were encouraged to discuss their own experiences with hearing voices. Particular attention was given to the content of the voices, and members were asked to comment on common themes within the content of the voices. Some content themes that emerged were negative and degrading statements, and commentary on activities. Other themes related to the experience of hearing voices that were distracting, stigmatizing, and frightening. Finally, the group leader facilitated a discussion of how voices occur, the stress-vulnerability model, and how the voices may be understood as lying on a continuum (e.g., from hearing sounds when one is falling asleep to hearing a loud voice when no one is in the room).

Sessions 6 and 7 were devoted to discussion of the ABC model of voices: understanding the *antecedents* of voices, individual *beliefs* or reactions to the voices, and the *consequences* of the voices. This behavioral analysis helped group members to understand that their voices were not random but occurred in a specific context. To identify the ABC's of voices, each group member was asked to monitor his or her voices for at least 1 or 2 weeks. For example, one client reported that her voices seemed to occur when she was lying in bed at night, worrying that the voices would emerge (antecedents). Then, after negative, berating voices became manifest, she would think that she was being punished for actions over the course of the previous day (beliefs). This resulted in fear, anxiety, and insomnia (consequences).

The remaining sessions were spent on developing and practicing coping strategies. This involves both a better understanding of what makes voices worse, and what makes them better. For example, in a session, therapists assessed whether each group member could do something that would make the voices worse. If a client reported that the voices were worse when he or she was alone, that client was asked to see whether he or she could make the voices worse by isolating him- or herself. The second aim was to develop strategies that would reduce the intensity or frequency of voices. To do this group members were first asked to describe the current strategies they used and to evaluate their effectiveness. If members did not have a sense of what reduced the intensity of the voices, they were encouraged to monitor, for 1 week, times when they felt good, and when the voices were not bothering them. If a strategy that clients were using was evaluated to be ineffective or maladaptive (e.g., yelling at voices), alternative strategies were identified, typically with the help of the group. For example, a client whose voices bothered her at night had difficulty identifying helpful coping strategies. Each group member was asked to identify a strategy that client might use.

In keeping with a problem-solving approach, brainstorming was encouraged, and coping strategies were not evaluated until a full list had been compiled. Thus, for this client, potential coping strategies included (1) sleeping in a different bed, (2) going to bed at a different time, (3) ignoring the voices, (4) arguing with them, and (5) using relaxation techniques.

Once coping strategies were identified, the next task was to put them into action. Thus, each client was asked to practice, for homework, his or her new coping strategy and to report on its effectiveness. All efforts at following through with homework were reinforced with praise. If a client had difficulty completing the assignment (or even attempting it), then possible obstacles were identified, and the homework was reassigned.

As reported in a recent article (Pinkham et al., 2004), this uncontrolled group CBT intervention was associated with a reduction in distressing voices, as measured by the PSYRATS for hallucinations, and in beliefs in the strength and power of voices, as measured by the BAVQ-R (Chadwick, Lees, et al., 2000). These findings suggest that group CBT for inpatients with persistent auditory hallucinations is feasible and has promise as an adjunctive psychosocial treatment.

GROUP PROCESS IN CBT FOR SCHIZOPHRENIA

Because of the nature of the illness, schizophrenia presents a unique set of obstacles and opportunities that affect group process. Obstacles to consider include (1) cognitive disability and negative symptoms; (2) limited insight, paranoia, and defensiveness (often associated with experiences of stigma and self-stigma); and (3) in-session exacerbations of hallucinations and delusions. A crucial opportunity presented by group CBT is its creation of a social space for individuals who often struggle with isolation and loneliness.

Cognitive deficits in attention, concentration, and abstract thinking are likely to be present in most, if not all, group members. Even after working to maximize homogeneity in cognitive abilities, significant heterogeneity should be expected. Overlapping with cognitive deficits are negative symptoms, including avolition, alogia, anhedonia, and affective flattening, as well as medication side effects (e.g., drowsiness). These deficits have several implications. First, they contribute to group members' difficulty in grasping the concepts of CBT. Thus, repetition, concrete explanation, and active rehearsal of psychoeducational components of the intervention should be used. Materials should be presented in multiple formats, including verbal didactics, visual presentation with a flip chart, dry-erase board or blackboard, and handouts provided to members.

A second obstacle is that cognitive deficits and negative symptoms can result in individuals' withdrawal from active participation, which affects mastery of the material, alliance formation, and general social integration. Secondary effects may also include demoralization, poor attendance, and poor homework adherence. Therefore, efforts should be made to maximize engagement in the group at various levels. At the most basic level, we recommend providing light snacks during each group to maximize attendance. At the level of basic communication, when engaging lower-functioning clients, use of simple, closed-ended prompts (yes–no questions) lessens clients' chances of becoming overwhelmed or frustrated and increases the likelihood that they will respond. At the level of conceptual didactics, one can maximize engagement by focusing on group members' own lives and experiences. Thus, after describing abstract concepts, such as the antecedents–beliefs–consequences (ABC) model, events from group members' lives are solicited to use as examples that further illustrate the concept. And last, group leaders should remain mindful of the amount of input given by each member during each session, and endeavor to balance participation as much as possible. As in any group, some members are inclined to talk a great deal, whereas others are quiet. It is the job of the group leader both to create a space for the reticent members to express themselves and the expectancy in each member that he or she will speak at each meeting.

Despite their best efforts, group leaders should expect variable levels of motivation both among different members and within individual members from week to week. Therapists should remain watchful for indicators of disengagement and attempt to reengage clients via eye contact or soliciting response to a question. One should keep in mind, however, that cognitive deficits and negative symptoms will likely lead to some individuals *appearing* uninterested in the group despite actually being very interested and committed. Thus, whereas a group member may contribute very little to conversation and appear to be uninterested in the group, upon questioning, the group leader may find that the group members looked forward to the group all week and cherishes the social contact it provides.

Another common obstacle in schizophrenia treatment, poor insight, may be associated with defensiveness if clients resent being told that they have an illness that they do not recognize having. A defensive stance may be further exacerbated if the individual suffers from paranoia. Group CBT offers a powerful opportunity to improve insight; however, group leaders should balance this goal against the risk of damaging the therapeutic alliance. First, group leaders should be sensitive to the very real role that stigma can play in creating defensive denial in persons with schizophrenia. Given the level of alienation that schizophrenia can induce, it follows that some individuals may protect their self-esteem by denying the existence of the illness (Bentall et al., 1994).

The group process in CBT offers an opportunity for compassionate normalization to decrease the need for this form of self-protection. Group leaders should encourage individuals with greater insight to share their experiences and model ways of acknowledging the illness that are consistent with good self-esteem and healthy disease management.

A key principle in working with individuals with poor insight is "meeting the client where he is." In the context of group CBT, this includes noting and mirroring the language that each individual uses to describe his or her illness-related experiences. For example, many people choose not to apply the word "schizophrenia" to their experiences, opting instead to refer to "my episode" or "my illness." The delicate balance between fostering insight and cultivating client comfort is highlighted during sessions focusing on psychoeducation. In our experience, individuals with poor insight typically can tolerate the dissonance brought about by psychoeducation. However, group leaders should avoid using a heavy-handed approach when presenting facts on schizophrenia. For example, although Socratic questioning is useful in this context, one should not use it to trap a client into admitting that he or she has schizophrenia. A better, gentler approach would be to inquire whether the individual has had any of the experiences associated with the illness, and to reflect his or her response nonjudgmentally. This shows that the group leader is prepared to accept the group member's report of his or her own experience at face value, setting the stage for collaborative amelioration of the symptoms.

A third potential obstacle in group treatment is disruptive in-session exacerbations of positive symptoms. Although group participants typically are on a stable medication regimen, periods of symptom worsening are common. For some, positive symptoms tend to be worse at certain times of day, whereas for others, severity of symptoms corresponds to stress levels. Such exacerbations can lead individuals to speak loudly, out of turn, incoherently, or offensively. They can also lead to bizarre, offensive, or otherwise disruptive behaviors. We recommend that CBT groups collaboratively establish a set of "group guidelines" or rules during the first or second session, and that these be posted on the wall of the meeting room throughout the treatment course. While the group is devising this list, the group leader may raise the issue of how to handle it when somebody experiences symptom exacerbation during group. Unless the group consists of first-episode or otherwise treatment-naive individuals, most members will have experience with their own or others' symptom exacerbation, and will recognize the usefulness of addressing this issue. Guidelines may include others pointing out the disruption to the person and reminding him or her of an agreement not to disrupt the class; the person excusing him or herself from the meeting; the person taking a short break outside; or the group leader asking the individual if he or she is able to control the disruptive behavior, then collaboratively deciding whether the member should remain in the room. Whatever protocol the group decides on, the group leader's goal should be to minimize the disruption caused to the group, while retaining a respectful posture toward the individual experiencing the exacerbation.

Before concluding this section on group process, it is important to emphasize a key advantage of this modality of schizophrenia treatment, namely, that group treatments for schizophrenia appear to confer benefits just by providing social contact. A recent review comparing supportive therapy and CBT for schizophrenia found that the two interventions yield roughly equivalent outcomes (Penn et al., 2004). Additionally, studies of patient requests in therapy indicate that social functioning is one of the most important domains for individuals with schizophrenia (Coursey, Keller, & Farrell, 1995; Slade, Phelan, Thornicroft, & Parkman 1996), many of whom consider social functioning to be a key area of unmet needs (Middelboe et al., 2001). Thus, one should keep in mind that even if it appears that individuals may not fully understand the concepts and techniques taught in treatment, mere attendance and basic participation in a group can still afford substantial benefits to many individuals with schizophrenia.

CONCLUSIONS

The bulk of research into group CBT for schizophrenia has involved small, uncontrolled trials. Results from these trials have been promising, suggesting that group CBT may help individuals cope with symptoms and secondary distress associated with the disease. The literature on individual CBT is more robust and indicates that durable improvements in various symptom and functioning domains can be achieved as a result of CBT. Taken together, these bodies of research suggest that large-scale, controlled studies of group CBT should be conducted.

Beyond these data on CBT, there is a strong rationale for continuing research into the group modality of psychotherapy for schizophrenia. First, interpersonal deficits are a hallmark of this illness, and the group setting provides an important, if nonspecific, venue for the development of social skills. Second, the group setting provides an opportunity for individuals to develop relationships with others, to increase their social networks, and to experience meaningful human interaction. Self-report data suggest that interventions that include substantial social opportunities are likely to be appreciated by many individuals with schizophrenia, which may limit attrition and maximize engagement. Third, group therapy is more cost-effective than individual therapy, which, again, takes on special meaning among individuals with schizophrenia, because they are more likely to receive publicly funded treatment.

In addition to improved methodological rigor, we suggest that future research on group CBT for schizophrenia address several key domains. First, to determine whether the group modality does indeed help to address the stated social needs of individuals with schizophrenia, group cohesion or alliance measures should be included in future assessment batteries. Similarly, social functioning measures should be included to assess the nonspecific impact on this illness-related domain. Future research should also compare rates of attrition from group CBT versus individual psychotherapy. Finally, we recommend that future investigations continue to focus on circumscribed illness domains (e.g., hallucinations or social functioning), and use a manualized approach that follows the generic CBT model.

PART III

Comorbidity and Future Directions

CHAPTER 16

Comorbidity and CBT Groups

Comorbidity, defined here as the co-occurrence of two or more Axis I DSM psychiatric conditions, is of critical importance for CBT because of its impact on the process of treatment and outcomes. Comorbidity is common in most mental health settings; findings in various clinics and settings suggest astonishingly high rates of co-occurrence among Axis I disorders in psychiatric populations (e.g., Bieling, Summerfeldt, Israeli, & Antony, 2004). In a recent comprehensive study of comorbidity rates in 670 outpatients seen in an anxiety disorders specialty clinic, only 5% of individuals diagnosed with a primary depressive illness *had not been* diagnosed with an anxiety disorder at some point in their lifetime (Brown, Campbell, Lehman, Grisham, & Mancill, 2001). Also, 73% of patients with generalized anxiety disorder (GAD) had a lifetime additional diagnosis of mood disorder, and this figure was 71% for obsessive–compulsive disorder (OCD; Brown, Campbell, et al., 2001).

Comorbidity is important, because it affects a host of variables related to treatment, including techniques used and process factors in groups. Treatment outcomes may also be affected. In individual CBT, comorbidity has been shown to impact treatment response negatively. Studies in this area typically compare patients with and without comorbidity in the context of treatment studies examining the efficacy of CBT for a primary condition; this allows for a direct comparison of treatment response and/or symptomatic changes in those with and without comorbidity. Overall, patients with comorbid conditions respond less robustly to CBT, though the degree of impact differs between studies (Brown, Antony, & Barlow, 1995; Erwin, Heimberg, Juster, & Mindlin, 2002; Newman, Moffitt, Caspi, & Silva, 1998). Comorbidity of social phobia and mood disorders appears to be associated with ongoing impairment after group CBT for social phobia (Erwin et al., 2002). In a treatment study of panic disorder, participants with comorbidity were more likely to seek further treatment when the study treatment ended. Moreover, although the treatment did reduce level of comorbidity acutely, over 24 months of follow-up, comorbidity rates returned to pretreatment levels, suggesting a lack of long-term improvement in comorbid patients (Brown et al., 1995). Comorbidity of depression and OCD appears to result in fewer treatment gains in CBT involving exposure and response prevention; those with comorbid depression had higher posttreatment OCD symptom scores (Abramowitz & Foa, 2000; Abramowitz, Franklin, Street, Kozak, & Foa, 2000). In a broad review of treatment outcome studies, personality disorder comorbidity has been shown to have a detrimental impact on the outcome of CBT for panic disorder compared to patients without personality comorbidity (Mennin & Heimberg, 2000). Equally striking in these studies of comorbidity and CBT is that despite the presence of multiple conditions, CBT nonetheless makes a significant clinical impact that improves symptoms and functioning (Barlow et al., 2004). This finding, along with studies of the latent structure underlying common Axis I conditions, has prompted some writers to describe a broad "negative affect syndrome" (Barlow et al., 2004), which is thought to benefit from the common treatment strategies present in most CBT protocols.

Clearly, the presence of multiple disorders is related to not only different kinds of symptoms and symptom severity but also to other kinds of psychopathology indicators. For example, patients with social phobia with comorbid GAD have been found to have more severe levels of social anxiety, greater depressed mood, and more functional impairment than those without GAD (Mennin, Heimberg, & MacAndrew, 2000). Moreover, the impact of comorbidity is not simply additive. In a study of the cognitive profiles of patients with panic alone, depression alone, and comorbid panic and depression, patients with single disorders endorsed thoughts and beliefs consistent with their disorder. The comorbid patients endorsed additional, distinct cognitions related to evaluative fears that the pure disorder groups did not (Woody, Taylor, McLean, & Koch, 1998). Comorbidity is also associated with a high level of maladaptive perfectionism, which may not only indicate vulnerability to further distress and symptoms but may also be a focus of treatment (Bieling et al., 2004).

These studies of comorbidity suggest that multiple conditions may not only result in fewer treatment gains but will also be associated with other individual differences that impact on treatment process. We suggest further that studies to date likely underestimate the implications of multiple disorders; most treatment efficacy studies exclude patients with significant levels of comorbidity, especially combinations of Axis I and Axis II conditions, and situations in which there are two coprincipal Axis I diagnoses. In real-world clinical practice, clinicians are faced with patients who, having much more confounding diagnostic profiles, would almost certainly be excluded from efficacy trials. Thus, difficult decisions need to be made about what type of CBT strategies should be used and whether single-disorder protocols are even appropriate in such cases. Comorbidity issues therefore raise a number of interesting questions and dilemmas: When patients have multiple Axis I problems, how are these best understood, and what problems are treated first? Should patients with comorbidity be treated in a group context? What is the impact of these comorbidities on the techniques that will be used in the group? How is group process altered when patients have multiple disorders? In this chapter, we address each of these questions in turn, recognizing that data in this area are still in early development.

RECOGNIZING AND TREATING COMORBIDITY

Key to managing comorbidity correctly is proper recognition, diagnosis, and prioritizing of disorders. In everyday practice, a clinical interview focusing on patients' key complaints (i.e., what brought them to the clinic for treatment) is likely to be driven by efficiency concerns, as well as the desire to begin treatment expeditiously. In these interviews, the main point may be to establish whether the individual has the disorder of interest (inclusion) that is treated in the clinic or in the group. But such a delimited clinical interview can also be a serious obstacle to recognizing comorbidity, since it may not include a thorough and broad range of questions about all categories of disorders (which may or may not be exclusions). A complete structured or semistructured interview is likely to yield considerably more information and is thus much more likely to identify comorbidity.

The last 20 years have seen tremendous advances in diagnostic interviews, moving from dissatisfaction with open-ended clinical interviews to the development of specific diagnostic criteria and questions, to a complete and comprehensive standardized interview that has both clinical and research validity (Nezu et al., 2000). In clinical settings, the gold standard for comprehensive diagnostic interviews is the Structured Clinical Interview for DSM-IV (SCID-IV; First, Spitzer, Gibbon, & Williams, 1997). The SCID is a semistructured interview designed to be consistent with DSM-IV disorders, with questions and decision rules designed to arrive at a formal diagnosis and therefore fully operationalize Axis I disorders. The limitation of the SCID in clinical practice is that it requires both specific training and a considerable amount of time to administer, usually 60–90 minutes, but as much as 2 hours in individuals with multiple disorders. Alternatives to a complete SCID do involve some compromises but can be more efficient.

For example, the Mini-International Neuropsychiatric Interview (MINI; Sheehan et al., 1998) is also a clinician-administered, structured interview that provides diagnoses for both DSM-IV and the 10th edition of the *International Classification of Diseases* (ICD-10; World Health Organization, 1993). Most anxiety and mood disorders are covered in this interview, along with several other Axis I categories. The advantage of the MINI is that it is very brief, taking 10–15 minutes to complete, and was designed with epidemiological studies and multicenter trials in mind (Summerfeldt & Antony, 2002). A second alternative that is more efficient than the SCID is the Primary Care Evaluation of Mental Disorders (PRIME-MD; Spitzer et al., 1994), which was designed to assess five types of disorders (mood, anxiety, somatoform, alcohol, and eating) commonly found in primary care. It uses a two-stage process, a patient questionnaire containing yes–no screening questions, and a clinician follow-up interview that inquires about 18 diagnostic categories. The entire process takes less than 20 minutes (Spitzer et al., 1994). Either of these more simple instruments may be quite useful in identifying, or at least in screening for, possible diagnoses to be followed up in a more comprehensive clinical interview.

Beyond these interviewing strategies, there are also a wealth of self-report scales that screen for, or even assess in detail, a variety of Axis I and II conditions. A full discussion of these instruments, and the construction of a complete testing battery, is beyond the scope of this chapter. Nonetheless, for those practitioners engaged in screening for and conducting CBT groups, a thorough diagnostic procedure and at least screening for comorbidity is likely to be of considerable value. Accurate assessment helps the clinician to avoid a number of difficult clinical situations in which comorbidity is only discovered after a treatment has already started, or worse yet, has failed to produce any meaningful result because the complexity of the patient was simply not appreciated.

Establishing the existence of multiple diagnoses is only the first phase for optimizing treatment with CBT. The next challenge is to use the carefully gleaned clinical information to determine a treatment plan that best recognizes the multiple disorders and maximizes potential change in all of them. A first step is to clarify which diagnosis is *primary*, that is, the diagnosis that accounts for the greatest level of impairment and distress. In some cases, this is abundantly clear. The patient, in the way he or she conveys information about symptoms and functioning, may make plain which disorder causes the most difficulties. Other times, the patient (and therapist) may have some difficulty specifying which of multiple disorders is most troubling and how to prioritize it.

The CBT treatment-planning literature can be very useful to sift through various domains and assist in decision making. For example, Woody, Detweiler-Bedell, Teachman, and O'Hearn (2003) have described a number of domains that are important to consider when making decisions about what to treat; most relevant for a CBT group approach are the following:

1. The extent to which the client acknowledges the existence of a need to change a specific problem.
2. The impact of the problem on significant others (and, we would add, the extent to which the issues causes problems within the person's psychosocial system, including occupation).
3. The probability of success in tackling a specific problem and the generalizability of this success.
4. Level of motivation to change a specific problem.

These points may be useful to discuss with a case example:

> John, a 43-year-old man with a history of various anxiety- and mood-related problems, is recently divorced but able to work and pursue a limited set of social relationships with his family. A SCID has identified the presence of panic disorder with agoraphobia, a generalized social phobia, and major depression. John says his biggest problem is that he needs to find a new relationship, because he feels intensely lonely, but he feels lost. He struggles to leave his house at all and is intensely anxious when meeting new people. Any of the disorders mentioned could easily be primary, but at the diagnostic feedback session, John disbelieves the depression diagnosis. To John, his low mood is what anyone who has just had a major stressor and such a high level of anxiety would experience. Thus, he neither acknowledges nor does he seem likely to be motivated to tackle the depression in its own right (issues 1 and 4). Consider also what CBT treatment for depression might involve, particularly in a group that might start with behavioral activation. Since John leaves his house only to go to work and strictly limits other social activities, behavioral activation is likely to meet with stiff resistance (issue 3). Similarly, in exposure to social situations in a social phobia group, John would first have to overcome his reluctance to go out, since he fears having a panic attack (issue 3). On the other hand, working on the agoraphobia and panic would help him to be able to go out of his house more, and this could readily generalize to social events (issues 2 and 3). Finally, if John believes his depression is caused by anxiety problems, treating the anxiety first seems the most acceptable option. Once this phase of treatment is completed, the depression could be reassessed and, if it is not resolved, John might then be motivated to tackle this remaining problem.

Thus, in this particular instance, it may not even be strictly necessary to declare that the panic disorder with agoraphobia is the primary diagnosis. Rather, treating this disorder first seems the most logical and functional point of departure. Also, resolving "easier" (but still significant) problems can often set the stage for tackling more difficult issues later (Woody et al., 2003). Prioritizing disorders, whether based on primacy or a more sophisticated functional analysis, sets the stage for choosing which type of treatment to offer and consideration of an individualized treatment plan.

TREATMENT PLANNING FOR COMORBID PATIENTS

To date, little has been written about treatment planning that is specific to a group modality. This is likely because treatment planning is maximally flexible in individual therapy and seemingly inflexible when considering group treatments. Theoretically, a therapist working in a one-on-one format can allocate any number of sessions for a specific issue, then change to a second area, then a third, when each preceding issue has been addressed. When considering a CBT group, making these kinds of determinations usually involves placing the individual in one type of single-disorder group or another for the duration of the protocol. Thus, treatment planning in a group setting could involve simple decisions about what type of group should be first, second, and so on. However, these issues may be much more subtle and complex than they at first appear.

For example, there may be settings in which both individual and group CBT are offered. If that is possible, a combination of modalities may be indicated, usually in a preplanned sequence. For example, prior to beginning a group, the comorbid patient might need to be seen individually for motivational interviewing and motivational enhancement to help him or her understand the need to treat a specific problem first. In other situations, the patient might be asked to attend a group first, followed by some individualized intervention to work through a problem that was not addressed in the group, and that is more unique to that patient. This kind of approach can help to strike a compromise in a setting where groups are conducted because of their inherent efficiency, while still recognizing the specific needs of individuals who have multiple presenting problems that can only be addressed by offering at least some individual therapy.

It may also be the case that a patient will be assigned to multiple groups set in a certain sequence. Concurrent groups are typically not recommended, because this might require patients to spread their attention across two sets of group members and techniques, and this could be very confusing from a group process perspective. Nonetheless, a plan to attend two groups in sequence can be formulated, and a reinterview is recommended to assess progress after one group protocol has ended and another is set to begin. This can establish whether priorities have changed, and whether treatment gains from one approach have generalized to other domains.

Whether a comorbid case is assigned to multiple modalities or potentially a sequence of groups, the therapist should also review the protocol for a specific disorder group and consider how the patient might react to each of the interventions being considered. This can require some considerable detail and case formulation but essentially involves evaluating the interaction between the patient's presentation, symptoms, and the techniques used in the group. A therapist ought also to consider how that patient's particular set of problems and presentation would impact on the group, especially when there is a high probability that the group will not be meeting all of the person's needs. Consider again our case example. If the patient with depression and agoraphobia were assigned to a depression treatment, would it seem likely that he could complete behavioral activation without activating avoidance patterns and anxiety? How would the presence of a patient with agoraphobia, who may not be able to comply with behavioral activation, or who has panic attacks when he does, influence the other members of the depression group? Does this have the potential to make the depression group less effective for its members? Likewise, what would be the impact of a patient's depression on an agoraphobia group? These questions must be answered uniquely for each case; the answers depend on a number of specific factors, including the severity and level of impairment from each disorder. Based on that individualized analysis, it may then be useful to begin with the protocol that seems to be the best fit and has the fewest obstacles—both for the patient and for the group in which he or she will be placed.

Sequencing two or more different kinds of protocols is likely the most common solution to address comorbidity, but other possibilities exist. In some cases, it may actually be possible and reasonable to construct *specific* comorbidity groups, for example, in tertiary care clinics that identify many cases with similar comorbidity. Such groups can involve a sequence or, more likely, an integration of two protocols for those who have two co-occuring disorders. Some protocols lend themselves to this process readily, especially combining two kinds of anxiety disorders or an anxiety disorder and depression.

For illustrative purposes, we describe an integrated depression–social phobia protocol and outline the session structure in Table 16.1. The protocol combines aspects of the depression treatment, including behavioral activation and cognitive strategies aimed at automatic thoughts and negative belief systems. At the same time, it integrates the three components of anxiety; elements of exposure, including hierarchy construction and simulations in groups; and cognitive strategies for disputing anxiety cognitions. Because it is integrated, the number of sessions is 19, three more sessions than a standard depression protocol but fewer than a standard depression protocol plus a social anxiety protocol. This is possible due to the fact that some of the techniques and discussion, for example, around automatic thoughts and disputation, as well as deep cognition, can occur simultaneously for both depression and anxiety content.

Similar integrations are possible for two anxiety disorders. This could involve variants on exposure for each (e.g., interoceptive exposure for panic symptoms and social exposure for social phobia symptoms). However, some disorders are difficult to treat with a combination of protocols. For example, an OCD group protocol might not include thought disputation strategies, and it might then be difficult to construct a combined depression and OCD protocol, because thought disputation is such a central and necessary feature of depression treatment. The net result could be inconsistency, confusion, and the potential for patients to use the wrong response strategy, for example, trying to dispute their obsessions.

A second difficulty with integrating protocols for two disorders is that this approach relies on having many patients with a specific combination of problems and therapists trained to deliver various protocols. Moreover, even this approach does not get around the difficulty of two patients with the same diagnoses not reacting similarly to the same treatment. Much depends on the functional relationship between the two disorders and the other factors described earlier, before decisions can be made about sequential or integrated treatment. A more general, non-disorder-specific group approach might be considered as an alternative.

TABLE 16.1. Sample Outline of Treatment Protocol for Group CBT for Comorbid Depression and Social Phobia

Session	Strategies covered

Session 1	• Introduction of therapists and group members.
	• Group "rules."
	  1. Confidentiality.
	  2. Check-in and rating scales.
	  3. Homework.
	  4. Missing appointments.
	• Introducing the CBT approach to depression and social phobia.
	  1. Behavioral interventions: Activation and exposure.
	  2. Cognitive interventions.
	• Describing the biopsychosocial model of depression and social phobia, and introducing the five components.
	  1. Behavior.
	  2. Thoughts.
	  3. Emotions.
	  4. Biology.
	  5. Environment.
	• Overview of social phobia, including:
	  1. The nature of fear and social anxiety (e.g., occasional social anxiety is normal and has a survival function).
	  2. Myths and misconceptions regarding fear and social anxiety.
	  3. The three components of fear (i.e., physical, cognitive, behavioral).
	• Homework: Complete biopsychosocial model and purchase companion manual.

Session 2	• Goal setting.
	  1. Eliciting goals from patients.
	  2. Specifying behavioral changes to meet goals.
	  3. How to track goals and monitor progress.
	• Outline relationship between mood state and behavior.
	• Introduce mood/emotion rating system.
	• Demonstrate relationship between activities and mood (i.e., what activities improve mood, what activities decrease mood).
	• Homework: Complete activity schedule with activities and mood ratings.

Session 3	• Behavioral interventions: Modifying activities to improve mood. • Introduce the concepts of mastery (sense of accomplishment) and pleasure, using examples from past to illustrate these types of activities. • Focus on adding mastery and pleasurable activities to establish balance of reinforcement. • Homework: Complete activity schedule with new activities added in and rate mood.
Session 4	• Examine outcome of behavioral modifications and adjust where needed. • Identify "mood shifts" and "anxiety shifts" to target with cognitive interventions. • Label and rate emotion(s) experienced in difficult situations from examples.

(continued)

TABLE 16.1. *(continued)*

Session	Strategies covered
Session 4 *(cont.)*	• Describe common information-processing biases (e.g., black-and-white, arbitrary inference, selective abstraction, and catastrophic thinking); the patient is taught how to identify his or her anxious and depressive thoughts. • Homework: First two columns of dysfunctional thought record (DTR; situation and emotion) to be completed.
Session 5	• Review examples of thought records: Situation description and emotion identification. • Describe interpretation and "self-talk" as the link between situation and emotions of depression and anxiety, using patient examples. • Automatic and "hot thoughts": Focus on the thought most related to the emotion. • Introduce the three components of the anxiety monitoring form. • Homework: First three columns of the DTR, and anxiety monitoring form.
Session 6	• Review examples from thought records: Situation, mood, and thoughts description. • Introduce cognitive restructuring for anxious and depressive thoughts. • Introduce the evidence technique and finding evidence "for" and "against" the hot thought. • Dispute handles and other thought challenge techniques. • Homework: Evidence gathering and disputation of thoughts.
Session 7	• Review examples from thought records: Situation, mood, thoughts, and evidence for and against automatic thoughts. • Review and practice thought disputation strategies. • Use patients' examples to illustrate questioning to elicit evidence for and against automatic thoughts. • Homework: Complete thought record, including thought disputation.
Session 8	• Rationale and general principles of effective exposure are provided. • Development of exposure hierarchies: Group members and therapists develop a detailed hierarchy of situations used to plan exposure practices conducted for homework and during in-session exposures. • Discussion of in-session exposures. • Homework: Continue practicing cognitive restructuring.

Sessions 9–12	• In-session exposures may include:
	  1. Role-play simulations (e.g., a simulated job interview).
	  2. Public speaking.
	  3. Simulated social settings.
	• Exposures followed by discussion of tracked automatic thoughts and group discussion of disputation as well as feedback.
	• Discussion of social skills as needed.

Session 13	• Introduce action plans/problem solving for ongoing stressors. • Discuss problems that need to be solved and steps to creating solutions. • Homework: Construct a problem-solving plan.

(continued)

TABLE 16.1. (continued)

Session	Strategies covered
Session 14	• Introduce "deep cognition" concepts of conditional assumptions and core beliefs in social anxiety and depression. • Illustrate deep cognition using downward arrow technique. • Describe downward arrow technique as used for conditional assumptions about self, others, and the world. • Homework: Complete a downward arrow.
Session 15	• Explain connection between conditional assumptions and core beliefs. • Illustrate "continuum" model of core beliefs and emphasize prospective techniques to change core beliefs. • Describe evidence gathering, experiments, and problem-solving plans for changing typical patterns of coping and collecting information to support alternative core beliefs. • Emphasis on ongoing exposure to change anxiety beliefs. • Homework: Generate a continuum of core belief and keep track of evidence concerning alternative core belief.
Session 16	• Introduce coping strategies associated with core beliefs. • Use patients' examples to illustrate the potential self-defeating nature of coping strategies. • Propose alternative coping strategies for patients. • Homework: Implement alternative coping strategies and monitor outcome of the alternatives.
Session 17	• Biweekly booster session to integrate and implement skills learned, as directed by patients.
Session 18	• Biweekly booster session to integrate and implement skills learned, as directed by patients.
Session 19	• One-month booster session. • Introduce the concepts of lapse and relapse. • Introduce strategies for dealing with lapse and relapse. • Plan patient-specific strategies for coping in relapse. • Wrap-up.

A GENERAL CBT GROUP APPROACH

The alternative approach to working with patients with multiple disorders and an array of different symptoms is to take the focus of the group away from syndromes, or clusters of symptoms, and focus instead on techniques and skills that lend themselves to multiple domains. This approach draws on the tradition of scholarship concerning CBT that focuses on techniques, including Beck's (1995) technique- and case-based approaches to CBT (Persons, 1989). It is also consistent with a more recent emphasis on the many commonalities of different disorders, as well as latent structure of negative emotionality (Barlow et al., 2004). Barlow and colleagues have also argued that treatment for one disorder often has some effect on another, and that many emotional disorders have similar underlying etiologies. This has led to the notion of a unified treatment model of emotional disorders (Barlow et al., 2004) that emphasizes three "fundamental therapeutic components": (1) changing cognitive appraisals of events, (2) reducing emotional and behavioral avoidance, and (3) facilitating action that counters the negative emotional state. To a large extent, these three components represent the latent structure of CBT; each is evident in combination and admixtures in the protocols described in this volume for specific disorders.

It is therefore possible to develop a group protocol based on these CBT "common factors." Each component may be introduced to a group as a set of techniques that is appropriate for certain kinds of domains. For example, cognitive appraisal techniques may be applied to situations involving not only sadness but also anxiety, anger, and any other strong negative affect. Specific strategies included in this component involve teaching patients the value of monitoring and recording their thoughts, creating a more objective appraisal, and identifying distortions that lead to distress. The second component focuses on exposure to affect-inducing experiences, including not only anxiety-provoking situations but, more broadly, also the notion of acceptance of emotionality rather than misplaced—and ultimately unsuccessful— attempts to suppress such emotions. This component of treatment facilitates approach rather than avoidance or withdrawal from experiences and situations—avoidance that is likely to have important consequences for the patient's ability to function. The final component of treatment involves changing usual behaviors that undermine coping and functioning, and substituting more positive behaviors. Action plans, or problem solving, more generally fall under this category, as would behavioral experiments. Underlying all of these interventions is working around the usual responses that exacerbate problems and strengthening the type of behavior that leads to a reduction or resolution of a problem. In Table 16.2 we outline a protocol that contains these three components, and also includes familiar and traditional CBT techniques that can be applied across various kinds of symptom presentation. The overall flow of this approach is first to teach patients to take a different perspective on their experiences, to move toward rather than away from situations that engender strong affect, and to take action in those domains that create and maintain their difficulties.

The first session provides a general overview, followed by four sessions on cognitive strategies. These sessions do not focus on any single affective domain; rather, they focus on recording situations and thoughts related to any experience of negative emotionality. Traditional techniques, including evidence gathering, labeling distortions, and experiments, are taught. In practice, therapists move readily between situations that have resulted in depression, anxiety, or anger by applying the common techniques to all these types of affect. Thus, there is no "pull" in the group for discussion of a particular domain, as there would be in a traditional anxiety disorder or depression

**TABLE 16.2. Sample Outline of Unified Treatment Protocol
for Multiple Presentations**

Session	Strategies covered
Session 1	• Introduction of therapists and group members. • Group "rules." 1. Confidentiality. 2. Check-in and rating scales. 3. Homework. 4. Missing appointments. • Introduce the CBT approach to problems of living. • Describe the three components of the treatment: 1. Cognitive strategies. 2. Exposure and acceptance. 3. Problem solving. • Discuss individual goals, problem domains. • Homework: Complete worksheet on personal goals and problem/symptom domains to be worked on.
Session 2	• Review goals and domains. • Identify situations with negative affect and "mood or anxiety shifts" to target with cognitive interventions. • Label and rate emotion(s) experienced in difficult situations from examples. • Describe interpretation and "self-talk" as the link between situation and use examples to help group members articulate thoughts. • Homework: First three columns of dysfunctional thought record (DTR; situation, emotion, thoughts) to be completed.
Session 3	• Review examples of thought records: Situation, emotion, and thought identification. • Automatic and "hot thoughts": Focusing on the thought most related to the emotion. • Describe common information-processing biases (e.g., black-and-white, arbitrary inference, selective abstraction, and catastrophic thinking), and teach patient how to identify his or her anxious and depressive thoughts. • Homework: First three columns of the DTR, and identifying distortions.
Session 4	• Review examples from thought records: Situation, mood, thoughts, and distortions. • Introduce the evidence technique, finding evidence "for" and "against" the hot thought. • Dispute "handles" and other thought challenge techniques. • Homework: Evidence gathering and disputation of thoughts on DTR.
Session 5	• Review examples of evidence gathering. • Introduce experiments to verify automatic thoughts. • Construct sample experiments for group members. • Homework: Experiment based on a DTR.
Session 6	• Describe withdrawal, avoidance, and suppression strategies, and their ineffectiveness. • Psychoeducation concerning anxiety and "false-alarm" response.

(continued)

TABLE 16.2. (continued)

Session	Strategies covered
Session 6 (cont.)	• Provide rationale and general principles of exposure. • Discuss domains of avoidance. • Homework: List areas for exposure exercises.
Session 7	• Development of exposure hierarchies: Group members and therapists develop a detailed hierarchy of situations that will be used to plan exposure practices. • In-session exposures followed by discussion of tracked automatic thoughts and group discussion of disputation as well as feedback. • Homework: First steps of hierarchies.
Sessions 8–10	• Discuss exposures from hierarchies. • In-session practices and discussion. • Problem solving around exposure and motivation. • Homework: Movement through hierarchy.
Session 11	• Introduce action plans/problem solving for ongoing stressors. • Identify individual problem areas. • Describe problem solving, action plans, and assertiveness for each area. • Homework: Construct problem-solving goals.

Session 12	• Introduce problem-solving techniques:
	  1. Identification.
	  2. Brainstorming.
	  3. Pros and cons of alternatives.
	  4. Action and follow-up.
	• Discuss group members' examples.
	• Homework: Problem-solving steps.

Session 13	• Introduce action plans and obstacles to positive behaviors. • Use of action plan worksheets with group members' examples. • Homework: Individual action plans.
Session 14	• Introduce rationale for assertiveness. • Discuss assertiveness domains. • Refusing unreasonable requests. • Asking to have needs met. • Describe assertiveness steps and skills. • Discuss group members' examples. • Homework: Assertiveness practice.
Session 15	• Wrap-up and summary. • Review of the three areas addressed in treatment. • Application of skills to novel problems.

group. Also, each patient is able to discuss examples from week to week, some of which may be manifestations of one disorder, such as depression, whereas the next week, the same patient may wish to discuss panic-related thoughts. In this sense, such a group allows for comorbidity and group therapists can in fact go out of their way to work with different kinds of examples that cover the spectrum of problems in the group.

Next, Sessions 6 through 10 shift the discussion to exposure, or approach, rather than withdrawal or avoidance. This begins with psychoeducation about the behavioral model, habituation, and the need for exposure. Group participants are asked to choose an anxiety, or exposure, domain that is unique to them and, as in any group with mostly anxiety disorders, a hierarchy is constructed for each member. The subsequent sessions need to be fluid but have the overall focus of working through group members' hierarchies, some of which may involve in-session exposures, whereas others involve support and discussion of *in vivo* exposures. Flexibility is the key; for some group members, interoceptive exposures might be indicated, whereas exposures for others could involve social situations.

The final five sessions focus on coping and to some extent take a longer range view of resolving issues that make the individual vulnerable to negative emotionality. In these sessions, patients consider their usual ways of responding to life circumstances and are encouraged to broaden their perspective and consider other ways of responding to stressing or upsetting situations. Problem-solving and action plan strategies are intended to resolve real problems that likely were identified in the first two phases of treatment. Assertiveness, or lack of the same, is so often an issue in individuals with Axis I conditions that one session focuses on this area. The overall thrust of these last five sessions is for patients to make particular changes in their lives that will create a healthier and more positive set of circumstances for them.

This "unified" or "generic" approach to treating individuals with multiple and heterogeneous conditions has advantages and disadvantages. One advantage is that it has flexibility by design; it can not only be used to treat patients who each have multiple conditions but it can also be used in a group of people with single but heterogeneous conditions. A second advantage is that this single protocol might be easier to learn and train in than multiple protocols for different disorders (Barlow et al., 2004). However, therapists still need an excellent knowledge of different disorders and techniques. Therapists need to have the skills to dispute negative thoughts in the depression domain and also know how to structure an interoceptive exposure hierarchy for panic. There are also numerous instances in which this group would not be sufficient for patients with comorbidity. For example, this approach may not be suitable for OCD or eating disorders, because exposure–response prevention or nutritional principles could be difficult to integrate into this protocol. Substance abuse is not likely to be adequately addressed here, and personality disorder features could also be challenging.

A unified approach likely works best when there are combinations of various mood and anxiety disorders.

The appearance of a unified protocol may prove to be a watershed moment for CBT, and its application to groups involves a significant departure from the more traditional and empirically validated protocols for single disorders. Certainly, before such an approach can be fully understood and endorsed, significant research evidence on efficacy should be accumulated. Nonetheless, when considering comorbidity, CBT therapists are often forced to operate in areas where there are as yet few studies that would help them make treatment decisions. Clearly, comorbidity in CBT will emerge as a significant area of research in its own right. Until those studies become available, therapists must rely on careful clinical judgment and careful tracking of outcomes for each individual.

COMORBIDITY AND GROUP PROCESS

Comorbidity poses a number of challenges in a group format. In Chapter 6, this volume, we describe the impact that unrecognized comorbidity has on a group. Even in cases in which comorbidity is well understood, it is inevitable that individuals engaged in group treatment for one disorder will describe symptoms of their other disorder. For example, an individual in a social phobia group may have a worsening of a coexisting depressive disorder, such that he or she becomes hopeless and suicidal. Where such a change in symptom severity, or rather symptom primacy, seems lasting, current treatment has to be reconsidered and may involve discontinuing participation in the group and offering whatever treatment is more appropriate. In addition to exacerbation of a mood disorder and suicidal risk, relapse of a substance use disorder, onset of a bipolar episode, or acute psychotic symptoms may also warrant discontinuation of group treatment for a patient with significant comorbidity. When symptoms of different disorders wax and wane, perhaps the most important question the group practitioner should ask him- or herself is "Would I elect to put the patient into this group if he or she came to the assessment now?" If the answer is "no," alternative strategies should be put in place. However, often comorbidity is well understood before the group begins and is simply a fact of that patient's presentation in the group. In that case, it becomes important to consider how that comorbidity can contribute to, or undermine, positive group functioning.

The most obvious way that comorbidity impacts group CBT is when the person with a comorbid condition raises issues related to a disorder for which the group is not intended. For example, in a depression group that is working on evidence gathering for negative thoughts, a patient with major depression and OCD might present an example of an obsessive thought rather than a negative automatic thought. A patient with comorbid depression in a social phobia group might describe a loss of motivation prior to doing a social exposure exercise. In some cases, this mismatch between a technique and a patient may not necessarily present a problem. For example, thought disputation strategies in depression and a number of the anxiety disorders are quite similar, even if the exact content of the thought varies according to different disorders. In some instances, even therapists have difficulty distinguishing a thought related to one disorder versus another. Worry thoughts common in GAD and pessimistic thoughts common in depression can be handled with the same techniques, so that overall group learning is relatively unaffected. Similar processes occur in behavioral strategies. The social exposure hierarchy of a patient with social phobia and panic disorder may appear similar enough to the hierarchy of a patient with pure social phobia, such that group members are not aware of the possible subtle differences.

However, patients' use of examples that "cross" categories represents an interesting challenge to the group and its members. Returning to the example of depression plus OCD versus depression alone, someone with OCD may present an obsessional thought as an example for disputation. In OCD, this technique generally is not endorsed, because it represents reassurance seeking. Moreover, an obsessive thought about contamination will have unusual qualities to which group members with depression may not be able to relate. The best course of action is for group therapists to identify the origin of this thought and, if necessary, provide some psychoeducation to the group member, and to the group, on why this thought cannot be disputed. This needs to be done efficiently, so that the group can return to the work it was intended to do, but also sensitively, so that the group member with OCD is helped and feels that his or her example was welcomed and taken seriously.

At other times, issues related to a comorbid disorder can trigger a useful discussion. In a panic disorder group, a group member who also has depression might raise a question about low mood and how this is interfering with exposure. Other group members, even if they do not have clinical depression, may readily be able to relate to low motivation; thus, this more general issue can be discussed within the group. This can help both the individual with comorbidity and the group as a whole.

Patients with significant comorbidity are also sometimes singled out by other group members because of their unusual presentations. A group of depressed people may not readily identify with the one group member who also has OCD and describes a preoccupation with contamination and cleaning. Similarly, a person in a social phobia group with significant substance use may get little sympathy if others in the group do not use substances. Here, the group therapists must do extra work to emphasize the universality of group members' experiences and heterogeneity in people's symptoms. Group members who have comorbidity could be asked to describe the nature of these other problems, supplemented by psychoeducation from therapists. By openly discussing comorbidity, group members are more likely to be understanding and empathic rather than exclusionary or stigmatizing.

CONCLUSIONS

Comorbidity is still a somewhat underexplored frontier in CBT, though clinicians have long recognized the need to tailor interventions to those with multiple diagnoses. Recognition is the key to developing effective contingencies for the patient with comorbidity, and treatment planning for multiple disorders may be challenging and require considerable creativity in the ordering of treatment, or in determining whether multiple modalities are indicated. Sequencing of treatments likely represents the most common practice, but it is also possible to integrate multiple approaches into a single group protocol that addresses multiple domains. Much work still needs to be done to validate approaches for multiple disorders, thus moving toward the empirically validated algorithms for making treatment decisions in those who present with multiple conditions on Axis I. Very little work has yet addressed broader definitions of comorbidity, for example, when Axis I conditions co-occur with Axis II conditions, organic and medical problems, or developmental disorders. These really represent comorbidity in special populations for which a host of adaptations and modifications clearly need to be made. Undoubtedly, the tailoring of CBT to these kinds of more complex types of comorbidity will be a major area of growth in the coming years, and this area of research will do much for group therapists who must make challenging treatment decisions.

CHAPTER 17

The FAQs of CBT
Group Intervention

Our goals for this book have been threefold. First, we attempted to integrate concepts from the group process literature into the CBT model of group intervention in a comprehensive manner. We made the first attempt that we know of to lay out and carefully define a discrete set of interpersonal, interactional factors that we believe are the hallmarks of a well-functioning CBT group. Second, we provided a number of disorder- or problem-specific examples of group protocols that describe both the specific CBT techniques to be implemented and process issues that arise in such groups. Third, we tried to attend to common examples of challenges and issues that can undermine positive outcomes in group CBT, such as problematic in-group behavior and comorbidity. In the process of working toward these goals or answering the questions we had set for ourselves, many more questions arose. Other issues were raised during the review and editing process, and we are grateful to several anonymous reviewers who brought up many of these issues.

Some of the unanswered questions we encountered are very important, and few concrete answers are available. In closing this volume, this chapter summarizes some of the important remaining questions or issues that need to be resolved in the future. Most of these, sadly, cannot yet be answered adequately with data. In some cases, this is because such studies would be difficult to design or carry out; in other cases, it is because the work simply does not exist yet. In the pages that follow, we pose what we think are the five most important questions, describing what is already known in the area, and also proposing what might be done to answer these questions more comprehensively. We begin with perhaps the single, most important question.

1. Is CBT group as effective as individual CBT, all other things being equal? This question reflects a theme that is basic to this work: There is little point in discussing details of group process and how to conduct a CBT group if this approach is clearly inferior to individual CBT. But to what extent can we answer this question, and to what extent do the data give us a clear and interpretable signal? The example of depression is illustrative in part because depression treatment studies are some of the most common. Yet even here a direct comparison between group and individual CBT is difficult to make. Very comprehensive meta-analyses and box score reviews of CBT versus other kinds of treatments, and group versus individual treatments, do exist (Burlingame et al., 2004; McDermut, Miller, & Brown, 2001; Robinson et al., 1990). However, these reviews generally do not answer the question directly, because the comparison of most interest is not group versus individual CBT. What they do tell us is that CBT is generally effective, and that group therapy, generally, is effective for depression. On the more specific question of group versus individual CBT, our group has conducted a meta-analysis of the only seven studies we could find with this "head-to-head" approach (Grant, Bieling, Antony, & McCabe, 2006). Overall, effect size difference between modalities slightly favored individual CBT in an absolute sense, but more importantly, this difference was not large enough to be considered significant; that is, the confidence interval for the difference included zero (effect size for individual CBT was 1.20 and 0.79 for group CBT; Grant et al., 2006). Importantly, this is what most reviewers have concluded: Individual CBT for depression seems to be slightly better than group intervention, but that difference is either barely significant or is, just as often, a statistical trend.

A similar pattern can be discerned for other disorders. For example, in social anxiety disorder (SAD), three head-to-head comparisons (described in detail in Chapter 9, this volume) also result in mixed findings. Although the three studies we reviewed do suggest slight superiority for individual CBT treatment for SAD, the most well established group treatment (Heimberg's cognitive-behavioral group therapy) was not studied in any of these three trials. Also, we reviewed two studies of "head-to-head" group versus individual CBT for panic disorder in Chapter 7, this volume. Here, too, there was some slight superiority for individual treatment, but this was inconsistent over different outcome measures and follow-up periods.

Our intent in summarizing these findings here is not to detail exhaustively each of these studies and reach definitive conclusions about which treatment is better, but to discern some general patterns. What we conclude is that, across all disorders, there are simply too few head-to-head comparisons of group versus individual CBT to declare a "winner" or a "loser." Both approaches are clearly efficacious, though. It is important to make three additional points about this area of research.

First, the lack of true head-to-head studies is probably not surprising in light of the politics and usual paradigms of clinical trials design. Most studies of two or more treatments are likely to pit two different modalities against one another, for example, a medication versus a form of psychotherapy. The question of whether group and individual CBT are different is likely to be something of a niche interest, relevant only to the CBT community and perhaps group therapy researchers. Funders of clinical trials may not be convinced that this question is of particular import, a position with which we disagree.

Second, it does seem that when individual and group CBT are compared, there is a slight advantage for individual in terms of some outcomes, but it is slight enough that the difference might actually be nonsignificant. This begs the question of the importance, clinically and in a real-world effectiveness context, of the difference observed in clinical trials that compare group and individual CBT. If the differences were larger, or if group CBT was not efficacious but individual was so, then clinicians, clinics, and their stakeholders would likely gravitate to an individual format based on that evidence. But what if individual CBT really is only "slightly" better than group CBT? In settings where time and therapists are in short supply, is this slight difference enough to cause a shift in policy about the use of a group modality? Where individual therapy simply is not possible, for example, in public health settings or countries with universal health care, the difference between group and individual approaches would have to be large and obvious for individual treatment to be favored. Certainly, advocates of group CBT would have no difficulty demonstrating that this approach is efficacious in a clinically meaningful way. Nonetheless, having more definitive, large population studies that are properly powered to detect small differences in effect sizes could answer the "head-to-head" questions in a more decisive way. At very least, they would inform the clinical community about what, if anything, we give up in terms of outcomes by choosing to use a group modality. That outcome difference would then have to be balanced against cost-saving and efficiency arguments.

Finally, we would add that future studies comparing group versus individual CBT need to take into account the group process factors described in this volume. Others have argued the same point, namely, that studies of group CBT have not yet maximized the impact of this approach, because CBT researchers and clinicians have not sufficiently leveraged the power of group process alongside their very potent techniques (Burlingame et al., 2004). Thus, in head-to-head trials, it will be important that all conditions be implemented in the best possible way, employing the most studied and robust group protocol, with carefully trained clinicians and investigators whose experience and allegiance is balanced with equal representation for both group and individual CBT on the research team.

2. How important is CBT technique compared to process in predicting outcomes? Another theme that runs through this volume is the extent to which "variance explained in outcome" is due to group process issues versus specific CBT techniques. Of course, the group CBT literature is not alone in this. A similar debate smolders in individual CBT, where questions remain about "effective ingredients." Some scholars question the extent to which change in symptoms is due to cognitive mediation and actual changes in information processing or style versus therapeutic alliance factors such as empathy, hopefulness, and directed changes in behavior. No doubt these questions are important and can be operationalized in studies. The quality of techniques offered, and the extent to which patients implement these strategies, could be measured alongside parallel measures of group process, and both sets of measure could be allowed to compete for variance in symptom change.

However important this question is conceptually, we believe that this issue is clinically moot. Put simply, we contend that good techniques and good process are highly correlated, and both are important components of good clinical practice. Presenting a technique in a noninteractive way, one that ignores the current experience of group members, or in which the group leader lectures to 10 different individuals, is not likely to be scored by an expert rater as "good use of technique." Similarly, good group process does not exist, unless some CBT technique is being discussed; effective CBT groups do not contain random self-disclosure, emotional confrontation among group members, or straying into deep affective expressions in the absence of a CBT strategy or technique. Just as good techniques are linked to good process, when there are no CBT techniques on the group's agenda, process cannot be "good." Thus, clinically, the technique versus process debate is, to us, something of an artificial debate, in which one is set up to win and the other loses. In practice, the two act in harmony, and this needs to be reflected in the approach to treatment and the training of CBT clinicians.

3. What are the most important CBT process factors? We recognize that we have just begun describing CBT process factors. Distilling our own clinical experience, and carefully sifting the work of Yalom and Burlingame, which we believe to have the most kinship with process in the context of CBT, we derived seven process factors (summarized in Table 2.1 in Chapter 2, this volume). To what extent do these seven factors describe the universe of process issues in CBT? Is the list too large? Are some factors redundant or so highly correlated with one another that no distinction needs to be drawn? Likewise, have we missed some aspects of process in our taxonomy? The answer to both questions is likely "yes." As in any first attempt, we hope that our scheme and definitions are fodder for writers and researchers. We certainly believe that one of the next steps in this work will be to measure the constructs of interest and to use the usual kinds of psychometric analyses to derive a true factor structure of process and establish a better sense of relations among these constructs. Indeed, this step is absolutely necessary, because, unfortunately, a lack of scientific scrutiny is acknowledged as a major problem with group process issues in general (Burlingame et al., 2004). Given the fact that so many aspects of CBT have been carefully studied in the past, we believe that the field will take up this kind of challenge readily.

We also believe that process issues can go beyond this taxonometric kind of approach, and that group dynamics, the patterns of interactions among individuals and leaders over time, are also an important issue to study.* In Chapter 6, this volume, we described aspects of particular individuals in groups that can lead to problems with group process. At the same time, group dynamics occur not only because of one individual and the "ripple" effects initiated by that member but also from the group as a whole. These more complex dynamics represent a particular pathway that a group takes, determined by many forces, including not only each of its members, the overall pattern of interaction, and the impact of leaders but also other, external circumstances and changes over time. For example, Motherwell and Shay (2005) describe a host of potentially destructive group dynamics (and potential solutions) that are rooted in particular leadership approaches, therapist level of disclosure, boundary issues, countertransference reactions, and destructive group trajectories. There is no reason to believe that these same issues do not play some role in CBT as well. And although Motherwell and Shay tend to focus more on traditional, in some cases, very long-term treatment groups, their work is still important reading for CBT group therapists. Certainly future work could address these kinds of "group dynamic" issues from a CBT perspective.

4. What are the important questions for which we lack research evidence in group CBT? In writing this book, we frequently confronted the need to make specific suggestions for "best practice" when conducting CBT groups. And although the global issue of the efficacy and effectiveness of CBT groups is largely settled by existing research, there are considerable gaps in our knowledge. In those cases, we relied on standard clinical wisdom, our own experiences, and the recommendations of other experts. Nonetheless, it is still striking how little we know, and how basic some of the questions are.

First, what is an ideal CBT group size? Although this might vary for specific disorders, there is almost no research base for making this recommendation. Certainly one can cite the number of participants per group from efficacy trials, and in the absence of other information, this would offer the best possibility for replicating effects in the real world. However, it is not clear that these kinds of studies tell us much about the "ceiling" or "floor" in terms of numbers of individuals in groups. Clinically, when a group grows larger than 12 members it is a fact that in a 2-hour group session, some members may not ever have a chance to speak, and that in a group of six members, there will almost inevitably be time and space for every member to have the floor. Whether this truly makes a difference to outcome is not yet known, yet this is a rudimentary question that we need to answer daily in clinical settings.

---

*We wish to thank an anonymous reviewer for this suggestion and feedback.

Another issue for which few explicit data exist concerns the composition of a CBT group. We have generally argued that some amount of heterogeneity is best for most groups, but this is based on clinical experience. Individuals with different backgrounds and experiences, different status and socioeconomic standings, who recognize through group that they all have the same kinds of problems, connect with one another in ways that appear to us to be meaningful and lead to enhanced motivation and more symptom change. Having individuals of both sexes, where possible, can be useful, because relationships with the opposite sex almost invariably arise as a group learns CBT techniques and shares examples and experiences. Having both men and women in a group creates a sex and gender sounding board that would not exist in a group that comprises only men or only women. However, we would also argue that some differences between group members, too much heterogeneity, can be insurmountable. In one recent example, one of us ran a group in which, by a series of events, a woman whose difficulties were sparked by domestic violence was in the same depression group as a man with a history of arrest for assault, although of a different kind. When these issues emerged in group, the results were dire. The group as a whole banded together around the woman who had been assaulted and asked, as a group, for the male member of the group to be removed. While the group therapists tried to maintain the group for several more sessions, eventually it was necessary to divert the man to individual treatment.

Studying these issues would, of course, be difficult, but not impossible. Individual differences on any number of dimensions could be assessed prior to treatment, and variability in these dimensions could be used to predict process or outcome variables. Unfortunately, we are not aware of any studies on this issue in CBT.

Another issue that remains understudied is suitability for CBT group and treatment matching. In Part II of this volume, we described some criteria that can be used for screening group members and helping to determine the fit between the person and the CBT group approach. However, most of this depends on clinical wisdom and experience rather than data. A research agenda in this area would be relatively simple. Putative suitability criteria could be assessed carefully prior to treatment, and these variables could be used to try to predict outcome, attendance, compliance with treatment and homework, and dropout. Of course, some of these same questions remain largely unanswered for individual CBT, and for most psychotherapies, for that matter.

But perhaps the most important question to which we have no answer is, "Does paying attention to group process matter in CBT?" Again, our fundamental argument in this book is that process does occur in such groups, that it has been undervalued in the CBT group literature, and that supporting and enhancing good group process leads to better outcomes. Yet, to our knowledge, there is no substantive research or tradition of inquiry on this issue in the CBT literature. In addition to questions about the impact of process variables on outcome, research in this area could examine other variables, including dropout rates, motivation for change, as well as client and therapist satisfaction with treatment.

*5. How do we best train future CBT group therapists to consider both technique and process?** A primer on training issues in CBT is beyond the scope of this volume. But it is important to note that determining "competence" in conducting individual CBT, and what training it takes to reach this point, is itself a difficult issue. There is broad agreement that to become a skilled, accredited therapist in CBT, one needs a combination of didactic training and direct supervision on some number of cases. And we would argue that the same holds true for group CBT. We also would suggest that knowledge and ability to conduct individual CBT be a prerequisite for conducting groups, because there is simply more inherent complexity in tracking process issues in a group compared to one individual, although the techniques delivered are the same. Ideally, CBT therapists learning to conduct groups would be expending less mental energy on the mechanics of the CBT techniques, because this is already well learned. This would allow them to devote attention to the group modality, including how to present material didactically to a group, how to track process issues, and how to devise interventions that enhance positive process. But this training also needs to occur within the context of exposure to seminal texts on group process issues.

In an ideal setting, a trainee would first be a cotherapist, with his or her supervisor acting as primary therapist. This would allow for not only "live" supervision but also observational learning from a more seasoned therapist. Over time, the trainee would be required to do more and more of the clinical work, based on his or her competence and confidence. Time for planning each session and debriefing after a group has occurred are also very valuable to consolidate learning. Once a trainee is at the point of leading a group without his or her supervisor present, videotaping of group sessions, where possible, would be the ideal mode of supervision.

FINAL THOUGHTS

We believe that this volume offers the beginning of an integration of CBT group protocols and group process factors. But it is only a beginning and cannot be a definitive statement. The issues we have described will, we hope, be subject to further academic inquiry by theorists and researchers alike. In addition, as the field of CBT groups develops, so too will these ideas about process. The emerging "third-wave" of approaches that build on CBT, for exam-

---

*We are grateful to an anonymous reviewer for encouraging us to address this question.

ple, mindfulness-based approaches or acceptance and commitment therapy, include a host of new strategies and techniques that are gaining ground and popularity for a number of disorders. Interestingly, mindfulness approaches tend to be group-based by definition. These interventions, with their roots in Buddhist meditation practices, take a unique approach to the benefits of group practice and interaction that is quite unlike more traditional CBT groups, or even psychotherapy group structures. These third-wave approaches will represent new and different kinds of challenges for CBT therapists and the group processes involved.

References

Abramowitz, J. S. (1996). Variants of exposure and response prevention in the treatment of obsessive–compulsive disorder: A meta-analysis. *Behavior Therapy, 27*, 583–600.

Abramowitz, J. S. (1997). Effectiveness of psychological and pharmacological treatments for obsessivecompulsive disorder: A quantitative review. *Journal of Consulting and Clinical Psychology, 65*, 44–52.

Abramowitz, J. S. (1998). Does cognitive-behavioral therapy cure obsessive–compulsive disorder?: A meta-analytic evaluation of clinical significance. *Behavior Therapy, 29*, 339–355.

Abramowitz, J. S., & Foa, E. B. (2000). Does major depressive disorder influence outcome of exposure and response prevention for OCD? *Behavior Therapy, 31*, 795–800.

Abramowitz, J. S., Franklin, M. E., Street, G. P., Kozak, M. J., & Foa, E. B. (2000). Effects of comorbid depression on response to treatment for obsessive–compulsive disorder. *Behavior Therapy, 31*, 517–528.

Agras, W. S. (1987). *Eating disorders: Management of obesity, bulimia, and anorexia nervosa.* Oxford, UK: Pergamon Press.

Akiskal, H. S., & Pinto, O. (1999). The evolving bipolar spectrum: Prototypes I, II, III, and IV. *Psychiatric Clinics of North America, 22*, 517–534.

Alcoholics Anonymous. (1999). 1998 membership survey: A snapshot of AA membership. In *About AA.* New York: Alcoholics Anonymous World Services, Inc.

Allen, J. P. (Ed.). (2003). *Assessing alcohol problems: A guide for clinicians and researchers* (2nd ed.) (National Institutes of Health Publication No. 03-3745).

Allison, D. B. (Ed.). (1995). *Handbook of assessment methods for eating behaviors and weight-related problems.* Thousand Oaks, CA: Sage.

Alloy, L. B., & Abramson, L. Y. (1999). The Temple–Wisconsin Cognitive Vulnerability to Depression Project: Conceptual background, design, and methods. *Journal of Cognitive Psychotherapy, 13*, 227–262.

Alloy, L. B., Abramson, L. Y., Hogan, M. E., Whitehouse, W. G., Rose, D. T., Robinson, M. S., et al. (2000). The Temple–Wisconsin Cognitive Vulnerability to Depression Project: Lifetime history of Axis I psychopathology in individuals at high and low cognitive risk for depression. *Journal of Abnormal Psychology, 109,* 403–418.

American Psychiatric Association. (1987). *Diagnostic and statistical manual of mental disorders* (3rd ed., rev.). Washington, DC: Author.

American Psychiatric Association. (1994). *Diagnostic and statistical manual of mental disorders* (4th ed.). Washington, DC: Author.

American Psychiatric Association. (2000). *Diagnostic and statistical manual of mental disorders , 4th ed., text rev.). Washington, DC: Author.*

Amminger, G. P., Pape, S., Rock, D., Roberts, S. A., Ott, S. L., Squires-Wheeler, E., et al. (1999). Relationship between childhood behavioral disturbance and later schizophrenia in the New York High-Risk Project. *American Journal of Psychiatry, 156,* 525–530.

Andreasen, N. C. (1995). Symptoms, signs and diagnosis of schizophrenia. *Lancet, 346,* 477–481.

Andres, K., Pfammatter, M., Garst, F., Teschner, C., & Brenner, H. D. (2000). Effects of a coping-oriented group therapy for schizophrenia and schizoaffective patients: A pilot study. *Acta Psychiatrica Scandinavica, 101,* 318–322.

Antony, M. M. (2001a). Measures for panic disorder and agoraphobia. In M. M. Antony, S. M. Orsillo, & L. Roemer (Eds.), *Practitioner's guide to empirically-based measures of anxiety* (pp. 95–126). New York: Kluwer Academic/Plenum Press.

Antony, M. M. (2001b). Measures for obsessive–compulsive disorder. In M. M. Antony, S. M. Orsillo, & L. Roemer (Eds.), *Practitioner's guide to empirically-based measures of anxiety* (pp. 219–244). New York: Kluwer Academic/Plenum Press.

Antony, M. M. (2004). *10 simple solutions to shyness: How to overcome shyness, social anxiety, and fear of public speaking.* Oakland, CA: New Harbinger.

Antony, M. M., Bieling, P. J., Cox, B. J., Enns, M. W., & Swinson, R. P. (1998). Psychometric properties of the 42-item and 21-item versions of the Depression Anxiety Stress Scales in clinical groups and a community sample. *Psychological Assessment, 10,* 176–181.

Antony, M. M., Brown, T. A., Craske, M. G., Barlow, D. H., Mitchell, W. B., & Meadows, E. B. (1995). Accuracy of heart beat perception in panic disorder, social phobia, and nonanxious subjects. *Journal of Anxiety Disorders, 9,* 355–371.

Antony, M. M., Downie, F., & Swinson, R. P. (1998). Diagnostic issues and epidemiology in obsessive compulsive disorder. In R. P. Swinson, M. M. Antony, S. Rachman, & M. A. Richter (Eds.), *Obsessive–compulsive disorder: Theory, research, and treatment* (pp. 3–32). New York: Guilford Press.

Antony, M. M., Ledley, D. R., Liss, A., & Swinson, R. P. (2006). Responses to symptom induction exercises in panic disorder. *Behaviour Research and Therapy, 44,* 85–98.

Antony, M. M., & McCabe, R. E. (2002). Empirical basis of panic control treatment. *Scientific Review of Mental Health Practice, 1,* 189–194.

Antony, M. M., & McCabe, R. E. (2005). *Overcoming animal and insect phobias: How to conquer fear of dogs, snakes, rodents, bees, spiders, and more.* Oakland, CA: New Harbinger.

Antony, M. M., Purdon, C. L., Huta, V., & Swinson, R. P. (1998). Dimensions of perfectionism across the anxiety disorders. *Behaviour Research and Therapy, 36,* 1143–1154.

Antony, M. M., & Roemer, L. (2003). Behavior therapy. In A. S. Gurman & S. B. Messer (Eds.), *Essential psychotherapies: Theory and practice* (2nd ed., pp. 182–223). New York: Guilford Press.

Antony, M. M., Roth, D., Swinson, R. P., Huta, V., & Devins, G. M. (1998). Illness intrusiveness in individuals with panic disorder, obsessive–compulsive disorder, or social phobia. *Journal of Nervous and Mental Disease, 186,* 311–315.

Antony, M. M., Rowa, K., Liss, A., Swallow, S. R., & Swinson, R. P. (2005). Social comparison processes in social phobia. *Behavior Therapy, 36,* 65–75.

Antony, M. M., & Swinson, R. P. (2000a). *Phobic disorders and panic in adults: A guide to assessment and treatment.* Washington, DC: American Psychological Association.

Antony, M. M., & Swinson, R. P. (2000b). *The shyness and social anxiety workbook: Proven, step-by-step techniques for overcoming your fear.* Oakland, CA: New Harbinger.

Antony, M. M., & Swinson, R. P. (2001). Comparative and combined treatments for obsessive–compulsive disorder. In M. T. Sammons & N. B. Schmidt (Eds.), *Combined treatments for mental disorders: A guide to psychological and pharmacological interventions* (pp. 53–80). Washington, DC: American Psychological Association.

Antony, M. M., & Watling, M. (2006). *Overcoming medical phobias: How to conquer fear of blood, needles, doctors, and dentists.* Oakland, CA: New Harbinger.

Apanovitch, D. P. (1998). Religion and rehabilitation: The requisition of God by the State. *Duke Law Journal, 47,* 785–852.

Aranda, F. F., Villar, M. B., Murcia, S. J., Gil, V. T., Ruiloba, J. V., & Vilches, I. G. (1997). Outpatient group psychotherapy for anorexia nervosa. *Anales de Psiquiatria, 13,* 236–242.

Ashbaugh, A. R., Antony, M. M., McCabe, R. E., Schmidt, L. A., & Swinson, R. P. (2005). Self-evaluative biases in social anxiety. *Cognitive Therapy and Research, 29,* 387–398.

Baer, L. (2000). *Getting control: Overcoming your obsessions and compulsions* (rev. ed.). New York: Plume.

Bailer, U., de Zwaan, M., Leisch, F., Strnad, A., Lennkh-Wolfsberg, C., El-Giamal, N., et al. (2004). Guided self-help versus cognitive behavioral group therapy in the treatment of bulimia nervosa. *International Journal of Eating Disorders, 35,* 522–537.

Bakker, A., van Balkom, A. J. L. M., & Spinhoven, P. (2002). SSRIs vs. TCAs in the treatment of panic disorder: A meta-analysis. *Acta Psychiatrica Scandinavica, 106,* 163–167.

Ballenger, J. C. (1993). Panic disorder: Efficacy of current treatments. *Psychopharmacology Bulletin, 29,* 477–486.

Ballenger, J. C. (1997). Panic disorder in the medical setting. *Journal of Clinical Psychiatry, 58*(Suppl. 2), 13–17.

Ballenger, J. C., & Fyer, A. J. (1996). Panic disorder and agoraphobia. In T. A. Widiger, A. J. Frances, H. A. Pincus, R. Ross, M. B. First, & W. W. Davis (Eds.), *DSM-IV sourcebook* (Vol. 2, pp. 411–471). Washington, DC: American Psychiatric Association.

Barlow, D. H. (1988). *Anxiety and its disorders: The nature and treatment of anxiety and panic.* New York: Guilford Press.

Barlow, D. H. (2002). *Anxiety and its disorders: The nature and treatment of anxiety and panic* (2nd ed.). New York: Guilford Press.

Barlow, D. H., Allen, L. B., & Choate, M. L. (2004). Towards a unified treatment for emotional disorders. *Behavior Therapy, 35,* 205–230.

Barlow, D. H., & Cerny, J. A. (1988). *Psychological treatment of panic.* New York: Guilford Press.

Barlow, D. H., & Craske, M. G. (2000). *Mastery of your anxiety and panic: Client workbook for anxiety and panic* (3rd ed.). New York: Oxford University Press.

Barlow, D. H., Gorman, J. M., Shear, M. K., & Woods, S. W. (2000). Cognitive-behavioral therapy, imipramine, or their combination for panic disorder: A randomized controlled study. *Journal of the American Medical Association, 283,* 2529–2536.

Basco, M. R., & Rush, A. J. (1996). *Cognitive-behavioral therapy for bipolar disorder.* New York: Guilford Press.

Bateman, A., & Fonagy, P. (2000). Effectiveness of psychotherapeutic treatment of personality disorder. *British Journal of Psychiatry, 177,* 138–143.

Bauer, M. S., Crits-Christoph, P., Ball, W., Dewees, E., McAllister, T., Alahi, P., et al. (1991). Independent assessment of manic and depressive symptoms by self-rating scale. *Archives of General Psychiatry, 48,* 807–812.

Bauer, M. S., Vojta, C., Kinosian, B., Altschuler, L., & Glick, H. (2000). The Internal State Scale: Replication of its discriminating abilities in a multisite, public sector sample. *Bipolar Disorders, 2,* 340–346.

Baum, K. M., & Walker, E. F. (1995). Childhood behavioral precursors of adult symptom dimensions in schizophrenia. *Schizophrenia Research, 16,* 111–120.

Bechdolf, A., Knost, B., Kuntermann, C., Schiller, S., Klosterkotter, J., Hambrecht, M., et al. (2004). A randomized comparison of group cognitive-behavioural therapy and group psychoeducation in patients with schizophrenia. *Acta Psychiatrica Scandinavica, 110,* 21–28.

Beck, A. P., & Lewis, C. M. (Eds.). (2000). *The process of group psychotherapy: Systems for analyzing change.* Washington, DC: American Psychological Association.

Beck, A. T. (1952). Successful outpatient psychotherapy of a chronic schizophrenic with a delusion based on borrowed guilt. *Psychiatry, 15,* 305–312.

Beck, A. T. (1996). Beyond belief: A theory of modes, personality, and psychopathology. In P. Salkovskis (Ed.), *Frontiers of cognitive therapy* (pp. 1–25). New York: Guilford Press.

Beck, A. T., Brown G. K., Steer, A. N., & Weissman, A. N. (1991). Factor analysis of the Dysfunctional Attitude Scale in a clinical population. *Psychological Assessment, 3,* 478–483.

Beck, A. T., Freeman, A., & Associates. (1990). *Cognitive therapy of personality disorders.* New York: Guilford Press.

Beck, A. T., Freeman, A., Davis, D. D., & Associates. (2003). *Cognitive therapy of personality disorders* (2nd ed.). New York: Guilford Press.

Beck, A. T., Rush, A. J., Shaw, B. F., & Emery, G. (1979). *Cognitive therapy of depression.* New York: Guilford Press.

Beck, A. T., Steer, R. A., & Brown, G. K. (1996). *Beck Depression Inventory: Second edition manual.* San Antonio, TX: Psychological Corporation.

Beck, A. T., & Weishaar, M. E. (2000). Cognitive therapy. In R. J. Corsini & D. Wedding (Eds.), *Current psychotherapies* (6th ed., pp. 241–272). Itasca, IL: Peacock.

Beck, A. T., Wright, F. D., Newman, C. F., & Liese, B. S. (1993). *Cognitive therapy of substance abuse*. New York: Guilford Press.

Beck, A. T., & Young, J. E. (1985). Cognitive therapy of depression. In D. Barlow (Ed.), *Clinical handbook of psychological disorders: A step-by-step treatment manual*. New York: Guilford Press.

Beck, J. G., Stanley, M. A., Baldwin, L. E., Deagle, E. A., III, & Averill, P. M. (1994). Comparison of cognitive therapy and relaxation training for panic disorder. *Journal of Consulting and Clinical Psychology, 62*, 818–826.

Beck, J. S. (1995). *Cognitive therapy: Basics and beyond*. New York: Guilford Press.

Belzer, K. D., D'Zurilla, T. J., & Maydeu-Olivares, A. (2002). Social problem solving and trait anxiety as predictors of worry in a college student population. *Personality and Individual Differences, 33*, 573–585.

Bender, D. S., Dolan, R. T., Skodol, A. E., Sanislow, C. A., Dyck, I. R., McGlashan, T. H., et al. (2001). Treatment utilization by patients with personality disorders. *American Journal of Psychiatry, 158*, 295–302.

Bentall, R. P. (1990). The illusion of reality: A review and integration of psychological research on hallucinations. *Psychological Bulletin, 107*, 82–95.

Bentall, R. P., Corcoran, R., Howard, R., Blackwood, N., & Kinderman, P. (2001). Persecutory delusions: A review and theoretical integration. *Clinical Psychology Review, 21*, 1143–1192.

Bentall, R. P., & Kaney, S. (1989). Content-specific information processing and persecutory delusions: An investigation using the emotional Stroop test. *British Journal of Medical Psychology, 62*, 355–364.

Bentall, R. P., Kinderman, P., & Kaney, S. (1994). Cognitive processes and delusional beliefs. *Behaviour Research and Therapy, 32*, 331–341.

Bernstein, D. A., Borkovec, T. D., & Hazlett-Stevens, H. (2000). *New directions in progressive relaxation training: A guidebook for helping professionals*. Westport, CT: Praeger.

Beutler, L. E., Engle, D., Mohr, E., Dalrup, R. J., & Bergan, J. (1991). Predictors of differential response to cognitive, experiential, and self-directed psychotherapeutic procedures. *Journal of Consulting and Clinical Psychology, 59*, 333–340.

Beutler, L. E., Machado, P. P., Engle, D., & Mohr, D. (1993). Differential patient treatment maintenance among cognitive, experiential, and self-directed psychotherapies. *Journal of Psychotherapy Integration, 3*, 15–31.

Bieling, P. J., & Antony, M. M. (2003). *Ending the depression cycle: A step-by-step guide for preventing relapse*. Oakland, CA: New Harbinger.

Bieling, P. J., & Kuyken, W. (2003). Is cognitive case formulation science or science fiction? *Clinical Psychology: Science and Practice, 10*, 52–69.

Bieling, P. J., & MacQueen, G. M. (2004). Bipolar disorder and personality: Constructs, findings, and challenges. In M. Rosenbluth, S. H. Kennedy, & R. M. Bagby (Eds.), *Depression and personality: Conceptual and clinical challenges* (pp. 187–227). Washington, DC: American Psychiatric Press.

Bieling, P. J., Rowa, K., Antony, M. M., Summerfeldt, L. J., & Swinson, R. P. (2001). Factor structure of the Illness Intrusiveness Rating Scale in patients diagnosed with anxiety disorders. *Journal of Psychopathology and Behavioral Assessment, 23*, 223–230.

Bieling, P. J., Summerfeldt, L. J., Israeli, A. L., & Antony, M. M. (2004). Perfectionism as an explanatory construct in comorbidity of Axis I disorders. *Journal of Psychopathology and Behavioral Assessment, 26*, 193–201.

Birchwood, M., Smith, J., Cochrane, R., Wetton, S., & Copestake, S. (1990). The Social Functioning Scale: The development and validation of a new scale of social adjustment fo ruse in family intervention programmes with schizophrenic patients. *British Journal of Psychiatry, 157*, 853–859.

Black, D. W., & Blum, N. S. (1992). Obsessive–compulsive disorder support groups: The Iowa model. *Comprehensive Psychiatry, 33*, 65–71.

Bloch, S., & Crouch, E. (1985). *Therapeutic factors in group psychotherapy.* New York: Oxford University Press.

Blomhoff, S., Haug, T. T., Hellström, K., Holme, I., Humble, M., Madsbu, H. P., et al. (2001). Randomized controlled general practice trial of sertraline, exposure therapy and combined treatment in generalised social phobia. *British Journal of Psychiatry, 179*, 23–30.

Bögels, S. M., & Mansell, W. (2004). Attention processes in the maintenance and treatment of social phobia: Hypervigilance, avoidance, and self-focused attention. *Clinical Psychology Review, 24*, 827–856.

Bouchard, S., Vallieres, A., Roy, M., & Maziade, M. (1996). Cognitive restructuring in the treatment of psychotic symptoms in schizophrenia: A critical analysis. *Behavior Therapy, 27*, 257–277.

Bourque, P., & Ladouceur, R. (1980). An investigation of various performance-based treatments with acrophobics. *Behaviour Research and Therapy, 18*, 161–170.

Bowers, W. A. (1989). Cognitive therapy with inpatients. In A. Freeman, K. M. Simon, H. A. Arkowitz, & L. E. Beutler (Eds.), *Comprehensive handbook of cognitive therapy* (pp. 583–596). New York: Plenum Press.

Bowers, W. A. (2001). Cognitive model of eating disorders. *Journal of Cognitive Psychotherapy, 15*, 331–340.

Boyd, J. H. (1986). Use of mental health services for the treatment of panic disorder. *American Journal of Psychiatry, 143*, 1569–1574.

Boylan, K. R., Bieling, P. J., Marriott, M., Begin, H., Young, L. T., & MacQueen, G. M. (2004). Impact of co-morbid anxiety disorders on outcome in a cohort of patients with bipolar disorder. *Journal of Clinical Psychiatry, 65*, 1106–1113.

Brieger, P., Ehrt, U., & Marneros, A. (2003). Frequency of comorbid personality disorders in bipolar and unipolar affective disorders. *Comprehensive Psychiatry, 44*, 28–34.

Brown, J. M., & Miller, W. R. (1993). Impact of motivational interviewing on participation in residential alcoholism treatment. *Psychology of Addictive Behaviors, 7*, 211–218.

Brown, T. A., Antony, M. M., & Barlow, D. H. (1995). Diagnostic comorbidity in panic disorder: Effect on treatment outcome and course of comorbid diagnoses following treatment. *Journal of Consulting and Clinical Psychology, 63*, 408–418.

Brown, T. A., & Barlow, D. H. (1995). Long-term outcome in cognitive behavioral treatment of panic disorder: Clinical predictors and alternative strategies for assessment. *Journal of Consulting and Clinical Psychology, 6*, 754–765.

Brown, T. A., Campbell, L. A., Lehman, C. L., Grisham, J. R., & Mancill, R. B. (2001). Current and lifetime comorbidity of the DSM-IV anxiety and mood disorders in a large clinical sample. *Journal of Abnormal Psychology, 110*, 585–599.

Brown, T. A., Di Nardo, P., & Barlow, D. H. (1994). *Anxiety Disorders Interview*

Schedule for DSM-IV (Lifetime version). San Antonio, TX: Psychological Corporation.

Brown, T. A., O'Leary, T. A., & Barlow, D. H. (2001). Generalized anxiety disorder. In D. H. Barlow (Ed.), *Clinical handbook of psychological disorders* (3rd ed., pp. 154–208). New York: Guilford Press.

Burlingame, G. M., Fuhriman, A., & Johnson, J. E. (2002). Cohesion in group psychotherapy. In J. C. Norcross (Ed.), *Psychotherapy relationships that work: Therapist contributions and responsiveness to patients* (pp. 71–87). New York: Oxford University Press.

Burlingame, G. M., MacKenzie, K. R., & Strauss, B. (2004). Small-group treatment: Evidence for effectiveness and mechanisms of change. In M. J. Lambert, A. E. Bergin, & S. L. Garfield (Eds.), *Bergin and Garfield's handbook of psychotherapy and behavior change* (5th ed., pp. 647–696). New York: Wiley.

Bustillo, J. R., Lauriello, J., Horan, W. P., & Keith, S. J. (2001). The psychosocial treatment of schizophrenia: An update. *American Journal of Psychiatry, 158,* 163–175.

Bystritsky, A., Ackerman, D. L., Rosen, R. M., Vapnik, T., Gorbis, E., Maidment, K. M., et al. (2004). Augmentation of serotonin reuptake inhibitors in refractory obsessive–compulsive disorder using adjunctive olanzepine: A placebo-controlled trial. *Journal of Clinical Psychiatry, 65,* 565–568.

Calvocoressi, L., Lewis, B., Harris, M., Trufan, S. J., Goodman, W. K., McDougle, C. J., et al. (1995). Family accommodation in obsessive–compulsive disorder. *American Journal of Psychiatry, 152,* 441–443.

Carey, K. B., Purnine, D. M., Maisto, S. A., & Carey, M. P. (1999) Assessing readiness to change substance abuse: A critical review of instruments. *Clinical Psychology: Science and Practice, 6,* 245–266.

Carpenter, W., & Strauss, J. (1991). The prediction of outcome in schizophrenia: Eleven year follow-up of the Washington IPSS cohort. *Journal of Nervous and Mental Disease, 179,* 515–525.

Carroll, K. M. (1998). *A cognitive-behavioral approach: Treating cocaine addiction* (National Institute on Drug Abuse Treatment Manual 1, NIH Publication 98-4308). Rockville, MD: National Institute on Drug Abuse.

Carter, F. A., McIntosh, V. V. W., Joyce, P. R., Sullivan, P. F., & Bulik, C. M. (2003). Role of exposure with response prevention in cognitive-behavioral therapy for bulimia nervosa: Three year follow up results. *International Journal of Eating Disorders, 33,* 127–135.

Cassano, G. B., Pini, S., Saettoni, M. B., & Dell'Osso, L. (1999). Multiple anxiety disorder co-morbidity in patients with mood spectrum disorders with psychotic features. *American Journal of Psychiatry, 156,* 474–476.

Castonguay, L. G., Pincus, A. L., Agras, W. S., & Hines C. E. (1998). The role of emotion in group cognitive-behavioral therapy for binge eating disorder: When things have to feel worse before they get better. *Psychotherapy Research, 8,* 225–238.

Cerny, J. A., Barlow, D. H., Craske, M. G., & Himadi, W. G. (1987). Couples treatment of agoraphobia: A two-year follow-up. *Behavior Therapy, 18,* 401–415.

Chadwick, P., Lees, S., & Birchwood, M. (2000). The Revised Beliefs about Voices Questionnaire (BAVQ-R). *British Journal of Psychiatry, 177,* 229–232.

Chadwick, P., Sambrooke, S., Rasch, S., & Davies, E. (2000). Challenging the omnipotence of voices: Group cognitive behavior therapy for voices. *Behaviour Research and Therapy, 38,* 993–1003.

Chambless, D. L., Caputo, G. C., Bright, P., & Gallagher, R. (1984). Assessment of fear of fear in agoraphobics: The Body Sensations Questionnaire and the Agoraphobic Cognitions Questionnaire. *Journal of Consulting and Clinical Psychology, 52,* 1090–1097.

Chambless, D. L., Caputo, G. C., Jasin, S. E., Gracely, E. J., & Williams, C. (1985). The Mobility Inventory for Agoraphobia. *Behaviour Research and Therapy, 23,* 35–44.

Chambless, D. L., Tran, G. Q., & Glass, C. R. (1997). Predictors of response to cognitive-behavioral group therapy of for social phobia. *Journal of Anxiety Disorders, 11,* 221–240.

Channon, S., de Silva, P., Hemsley, D., & Perkins, R. E. (1989). A controlled trial of cognitive-behavioural and behavioural treatment of anorexia nervosa. *Behaviour Research and Therapy, 27,* 529–535.

Charpentier, P., Marttunen, M., Fadjukov, S., & Huttunen, A. (2003). CBT for adolescent eating disorder patients: Literature review and a report of an open trial of group CBT for adolescent outpatients with eating disorder. In J. Lönnqvist, M. Heikkinen, M. Marttunen, & T. Partonen (Eds.), *Psychiatria Fennica, 2003* (Vol. 34, pp. 80–98). Helsinki: Psychiatria Fennica Oy.

Chen, E., Touyz, S. W., Beumont, P. J. V., Fairburn, C. G., Griffiths, R., Butow, P., et al. (2003). Comparison of group and individual cognitive-behavioral therapy for patients with bulimia nervosa. *International Journal of Eating Disorders, 33,* 241–254.

Chorpita, B. F., & Taylor, A. A. (2001). Behavioral assessment of anxiety disorders. In M. M. Antony, S. M. Orsillo, & L. Roemer (Eds.), *Practitioner's guide to empirically-based measures of anxiety* (pp. 19–24). New York: Kluwer Academic/Plenum Press.

Chudzik, S. M., McCabe, R. E., Antony, M. M., & Swinson, R. P. (2001, November). *The effect of a comorbid mood disorder on treatment outcome for panic disorder.* Paper presented at the meeting of the Association for the Advancement of Behavior Therapy, Philadelphia, PA.

Clark, D. A. (2004). *Cognitive-behavioral therapy for OCD.* New York: Guilford Press.

Clark, D. A., Antony, M. M., Beck, A. T., Swinson, R. P., & Steer, R. A. (2005). Screening for obsessive and compulsive symptoms: Validation of the Clark–Beck Obsessive–Compulsive Inventory. *Psychological Assessment, 17,* 132–143.

Clark, D. A., & Beck, A. T. (2002). *Manual for the Clark–Beck Obsessive–Compulsive Inventory.* San Antonio, TX: Psychological Corporation.

Clark, D. A., Beck, A. T., & Alford, B. A. (1999). *Scientific foundations of cognitive theory and therapy of depression.* New York: Wiley.

Clark, D. M. (1986). A cognitive approach to panic. *Behaviour Research and Therapy, 24,* 461–470.

Clark, D. M., Salkovskis, P. M., Hackmann, A., Middleton, H., Anastasiades, P., & Gelder, M. (1994). A comparison of cognitive therapy, applied relaxation and imipramine in the treatment of panic disorder. *British Journal of Psychiatry, 164,* 759–769.

Clark, D. M., Salkovskis, P. M., Hackmann, A., Wells, A., Ludgate, J., & Gelder, M. (1999). Brief cognitive therapy for panic disorder: A randomized controlled trial. *Journal of Consulting and Clinical Psychology, 67,* 583–589.

Clark, D. M., & Wells, A. (1995). A cognitive model of social phobia. In R. G.

Heimberg, M. R. Liebowitz, D. A. Hope, & F. R. Schneier (Eds.), *Social phobia: Diagnosis, assessment, and treatment* (pp. 69–93). New York: Guilford Press.

Cloitre, M., Cancienne, J., Heimberg, R. G., Holt, C. S., & Liebowitz, M. (1995). Memory bias does not generalize across anxiety disorders. *Behaviour Research and Therapy, 33,* 305–307.

Clomipramine Collaborative Study Group. (1991). Clomipramine in the treatment of patients with obsessive–compulsive disorder. *Archives of General Psychiatry, 48,* 730–738.

Clum, G. A., Broyles, S., Borden, J., & Watkins, P. L. (1990). Validity and reliability of the Panic Attack Symptoms and Cognitions Questionnaires. *Journal of Psychopathology and Behavioral Assessment, 12,* 233–245.

Cochran, S. D. (1984). Preventing medical noncompliance in the outpatient treatment of bipolar affective disorders. *Journal of Consulting and Clinical Psychology, 52,* 873–878.

Colby, K. M., Faught, W. S., & Parkinson, R. C. (1979). Cognitive therapy of paranoid conditions: Heuristic suggestions based on a computer simulation model. *Cognitive Therapy and Research, 3,* 5–60.

Connor, K. M., Davidson, J. R. T., Churchill, L. E., Sherwood, A., Foa, E., & Wesler, R. H. (2000). Psychometric properties of the Social Phobia Inventory (SPIN). *British Journal of Psychiatry, 176,* 379–386.

Cooke, R. G., Robb, J. C., Young, L. T., & Joffe, R. T. (1996). Well-being and functioning in patients with bipolar disorder assessed using the MOS 20-item Short Form (SF-20). *Journal of Affective Disorders, 39,* 93–97.

Cooper, M. (1993, May). A group for families of obsessive–compulsive persons. *Families in Society: The Journal of Contemporary Human Services,* pp. 301–307.

Cooper, Z., & Fairburn, C. (1987). The eating disorder examination: A semistructured interview for the assessment of the specific psychopathology of eating disorders. *International Journal of Eating Disorders, 6,* 1–8.

Cordioli, A. V., Heldt, E., Bochi, D. B., Margis, R., de Sousa, M. B., Tonello, J. F., et al. (2003). Cognitive-behavioral group therapy in obsessive–compulsive disorder: A randomized clinical trial. *Psychotherapy and Psychosomatics, 72,* 211–216.

Cordioli, A. V., Heldt, E., Bochi, D. B., Margis, R., de Sousa, M. B., Tonello, J. F., et al. (2002). Cognitive-behavioral group therapy in obsessive–compulsive disorder: A clinical trial. *Revista Brasileira de Psiquiatria, 24,* 113–120.

Corey G. (2000). *Theory and practice of group counseling* (5th ed.). Belmont, CA: Wadsworth/Thomson Learning.

Corey, G., Corey, M. S., Callanan, P., & Russell, J. M. (2004). *Group techniques* (3rd ed.). Pacific Grove, CA: Brooks/Cole.

Cottraux, J., Note, I., Yao, S. N., Lafont, S., Note, B., Mollard, E., et al. (2001). A randomized controlled trial of cognitive therapy versus intensive behavior therapy in obsessive–compulsive disorder. *Psychotherapy and Psychosomatics, 70,* 288–297.

Coursey, R. D., Keller, A. B., & Farrell, E. W. (1995). Individual psychotherapy and persons with serious mental illness: The clients' perspective. *Schizophrenia Bulletin, 21,* 283–301.

Cox, B. J., Fergus, K. D., & Swinson, R. P. (1994). Patient satisfaction with behavioral treatments for panic disorder with agoraphobia. *Journal of Anxiety Disorders, 8,* 193–206.

Craske, M. G. (1999). *Anxiety disorders: Psychological approaches to theory and treatment.* Boulder, CO: Westview Press.

Craske, M. G., & Barlow, D. H. (2001). Panic disorder and agoraphobia. In D. H. Barlow (Ed.), *Clinical handbook of psychological disorders* (3rd ed., pp. 1–59). New York: Guilford Press.

Craske, M. G., Brown, T. A., & Barlow, D. H. (1991). Behavioral treatment of panic: A two year follow-up. *Behavior Therapy, 22,* 289–304.

Craske, M. G., DeCola, J., Sachs, A,D., & Pontillo, D. C. (2003). Panic control treatment for agoraphobia. *Journal of Anxiety Disorders, 17,* 321–333.

Craske, M. G., Street, L., & Barlow, D. H. (1989). Instructions to focus upon or distract from internal cues during exposure treatment of agoraphobic avoidance. *Behaviour Research and Therapy, 27,* 663–672.

Crow, S. J., Agras, S., Halmi, K., Mitchell, J. E., & Kraemer, H. C. (2002). Full syndromal versus subthreshold anorexia nervosa, bulimia nervosa, and binge eating disorder: A multicentre study. *International Journal of Eating Disorders, 32,* 309–318.

Curran, J., Monti, P., & Corriveau, D. (1982). Treatment of schizophrenia. In A. S. Bellack, M. Hersen, & A. E. Kazdin (Eds.), *International Handbook of Behavior Modification and Therapy* (pp. xx–xx). New York: Plenum Press.

Daniels, L. (1998). A group cognitive-behavioral and process-oriented approach to treating the social impairment and negative symptoms associated with chronic mental illness. *Journal of Psychotherapy Practice and Research, 7,* 167–176.

David, A. (1994). The neuropsychological origin of auditory hallucinations. In A. David & J. Cutting (Eds.), *The neuropsychology of schizophrenia* (pp. 269–313). Hove, UK: Erlbaum.

Davidson, J. R. T. (2003). Pharmacotherapy of social phobia. *Acta Psychiatrica Scandinavica, 108*(Suppl. 417), 65–71.

Davidson, J. R. T., Foa, E. B., Huppert, J. D., Keefe, F. J., Franklin, M. E., Compton, J. S., et al. (2004). Fluoxetine, comprehensive cognitive behavioral therapy, and placebo in generalized social phobia. *Archives of General Psychiatry, 61,* 1005–1013.

Davidson, J. R. T., & Meltzer-Brody, S. E. (1999). The underrecognition and undertreatment of depression: What is the breadth and depth of the problem? *Journal of Clinical Psychiatry, 60*(Suppl. 7), 4–9.

Davidson, J. R. T., Potts, N. L. S., Richichi, E. A., Ford, S. M., Krishnan, R. R., Smith, R. D., et al. (1991). The Brief Social Phobia Scale. *Journal of Clinical Psychiatry, 52*(Suppl. 11), 48–51.

Davila, J., Hammen, C., Burge, D., Paley, B., & Daley, S. E. (1995). Poor interpersonal problem solving as a mechanism of stress generation in depression among adolescent women. *Journal of Abnormal Psychology, 104,* 592–600.

Dawson, D. A. (1996). Correlates of past-year status among treated and untreated persons with former alcohol dependence: United States, 1992. *Alcoholism: Clinical and Experimental Research, 20,* 771–779.

de Silva, P., & Rachman, S. (1984). Does escape behaviour strengthen agoraphobic avoidance?: A preliminary study. *Behaviour Research and Therapy, 22,* 87–91.

Denys, D., Tenney, N., van Megen, H. J. G. M., de Geus, F., & Westenberg, H. G. M. (2004). Axis I and II comorbidity in a large sample of patients with obsessive–compulsive disorder. *Journal of Affective Disorders, 80,* 155–162.

Derogatis, L. R. (1993). *Brief Symptom Inventory: Administration scoring and procedures manual* (3rd ed.). Minneapolis, MN: National Computer Systems.

DeRubeis, R. J. & Crits-Christoph, P. (1998). Empirically supported individual and group psychological treatments for adult mental disorders. *Journal of Consulting and Clinical Psychology, 66*, 37–52.

DeRubeis, R. J., Gelfand, L. A., Tang, T. Z., & Simons, A. D. (1999). Medications versus cognitive behavior therapy for severely depressed outpatients: Mega-analysis of four randomized comparisons. *American Journal of Psychiatry, 156*, 1007–1013.

Devins, G. M. (1994). Illness intrusiveness and the psychosocial impact of lifestyle disruptions in chronic life-threatening disease. *Advances in Renal Replacement Therapy, 1*, 251–263.

Diaferia, G., Sciuto, G., Perna, G., Bernardeschi, L., Battaglia, M., Rusmini, S., & Bellodi, L. (1993). DSM-III-R personality disorders and panic disorder. *Journal of Anxiety Disorders, 7*, 153–161.

Dickerson, F. B. (2000). Cognitive-behavioral psychotherapy for schizophrenia: A review of recent empirical studies. *Schizophrenia Research, 43*, 71–90.

Dickerson, F. B. (2004). Update on cognitive behavioral psychotherapy for schizophrenia: Review of recent studies. *Journal of Cognitive Psychotherapy, 18*, 189–205.

DiClemente, C. C., & Hughes, S. O. (1990). Stages of change profiles in alcoholism treatment. *Journal of Substance Abuse, 2*, 217–235.

DiClemente, C. C., & Prochaska, J. O. (1998). Toward a comprehensive, transtheoretical model of change: Stages of change and addictive behaviors. In W. R. Miller & N. Heather (Eds.), *Treating addictive behaviors* (2nd ed., pp. 3–24). New York: Plenum Press.

Di Nardo, P., Brown, T. A., & Barlow, D. H. (1994). *Anxiety Disorders Interview Schedule for DSM-IV*. San Antonio, TX: Psychological Corporation.

Donovan, D., & Marlatt, G. A. (Eds.). (2005). *Assessment of addictive behaviors* (2nd ed). New York: Guilford Press.

Dougherty, D. D., Baer, L., Cosgrove, G. R., Cassem, E. H., Price, B. H., Nierenberg, A. A., et al. (2002). Prospective long-term follow-up of 44 patients who received cingulotomy for treatment-refractory obsessive–compulsive disorder. *American Journal of Psychiatry, 159*, 269–275.

Drury, V., Birchwood, M., Cochrane, R., & MacMillan, F. (1996a). Cognitive therapy and recovery from acute psychosis: A controlled trial. *British Journal of Psychiatry, 169*, 593–601.

Drury, V., Birchwood, M., Cochrane, R., & MacMillan, F. (1996b). Cognitive therapy and recovery from acute psychosis: A controlled trial. II. *British Journal of Psychiatry, 169*, 602–607.

D'Zurilla, T. J,. & Goldfried, M. R. (1971). Problem-solving and behavior modification. *Journal of Abnormal Psychology, 78*, 107–126.

D'Zurilla, T. J., & Nezu, A. M. (1998). *Problem-solving therapy* (2nd ed.). New York: Springer.

Eaton, W. W., Kessler, R. C., Wittchen, H. U., & Magee, W. J. (1994). Panic and panic disorder in the United States. *American Journal of Psychiatry, 151*, 413–420.

Eddy, K. T., Dutra, L., Bradley, R., & Westen, D. (2004). A multidimensional meta-analysis of psychotherapy and pharmacotherapy for obsessive–compulsive disorder. *Clinical Psychology Review, 24*, 1011–1030.

Ehlers, A., & Breuer, P. (1992). Increased cardiac awareness in panic disorder. *Journal of Abnormal Psychology, 101*, 371–382.

Ehlers, A., & Breuer, P. (1996). How good are patients with panic disorder at perceiving their heartbeats? *Biological Psychology, 42*, 165–182.

Einstein, D. A., & Menzies, R. G. (2004). The presence of magical thinking in obsessive compulsive disorder. *Behaviour Research and Therapy, 42*, 539–549.

Eldredge, K. S., Agras, W. S., Arnow, B., Telch, C. F., Bell, S., Castonguay, L., et al. (1997). The effects of extending cognitive-behavioral therapy for binge eating disorder among initial treatment nonresponders. *International Journal of Eating Disorders, 21*, 347–352.

Ellis, A. & MacClaren, C. (2005). *Rational emotive behavior therapy: A therapist's guide* (2nd ed.). Atascadero, CA: Impact.

Emmelkamp, P. M. G., & Wessels, H. (1975). Flooding in imagination vs. flooding *in vivo*: A comparison with agoraphobics. *Behaviour Research and Therapy, 13*, 7–15.

Endicott, J., Nee, J., Harrison, W., & Blumenthal, R. (1993). Quality of Life Enjoyment and Satisfaction Questionnaire: A new scale. *Psychopharmacology Bulletin, 29*, 321–326.

Endler, N. S., & Kocovski, N. L. (2002). Personality disorders at the crossroads. *Journal of Personality Disorders, 16*, 487–502.

Enright, A. B., Butterfield, P., & Berkowitz, B. (1985). Self-help and support groups in the management of eating disorders. In D. M. Garner & P. E. Garfinkel (Eds.), *Handbook of psychotherapy for anorexia nervosa and bulimia* (pp. 491–512). New York: Guilford Press.

Erwin, B. A., Heimberg, R. G., Juster, H., & Mindlin, M. (2002). Comorbid anxiety and mood disorders among persons with social anxiety disorder. *Behaviour Research and Therapy, 40*, 19–35.

Evans, L., Holt, C., & Oei, T. P. (1991). Long term follow-up of agoraphobics treated by brief intensive group cognitive behavioural therapy. *Australian and New Zealand Journal of Psychiatry, 25*, 343–349.

Everaerd, W. T. A. M., Rijken, H. M., & Emmelkamp, P. M. G. (1973). A comparison of "flooding" and "successive approximation" in the treatment of agoraphobia. *Behaviour Research and Therapy, 11*, 105–117.

Fairburn, C. G. (1981). A cognitive behavioural approach to the management of bulimia. *Psychological Medicine, 11*, 707–711.

Fairburn, C. G. (1985). Cognitive-behavioral treatment for bulimia. In D. M. Garner & P. E. Garfinkel (Eds.), *Handbook of psychotherapy for anorexia nervosa and bulimia* (pp. 160–192). New York: Guilford Press.

Fairburn, C. G., & Beglin, S. J. (1994). Assessment of eating disorders: Interview or self-report questionnaire? *International Journal of Eating Disorders, 16*, 363–370.

Fairburn, C. G., & Cooper, P. J. (1993). The Eating Disorder Examination. In C. G. Fairburn & G. T. Wilson (Eds.), *Binge eating: Nature, assessment, and treatment* (pp. 317–360). New York: Guilford Press.

Fairburn, C. G., Cooper, Z., & Shafran, R. (2003). Cognitive behaviour therapy for eating disorders: A "transdiagnostic theory" and treatment. *Behaviour Research and Therapy, 41*, 509–528.

Fairburn, C. G., Marcus, M. D., & Wilson, G. T. (1993). Cognitive-behavioral therapy for binge eating and bulimia nervosa: A comprehensive treatment manual. In

C. G. Fairburn & G. T. Wilson (Eds.), *Binge eating: Nature, assessment, and treatment* (pp. 361–405). New York: Guilford Press.

Fairburn, C. G., Shafran, R., & Cooper, Z. (1999). A cognitive behavioural theory of anorexia nervosa. *Behaviour Research and Therapy, 37,* 1–13.

Falloon, I. H. R., & Talbott, R. E. (1981). Persistent auditory hallucinations: Coping mechanisms and implications for management. *Psychological Medicine, 11,* 329–339.

Fals-Stewart, W., Marks, A. P., & Schafer, J. (1993). A comparison of behavioral group therapy and individual behavior therapy in treating obsessive–compulsive disorder. *Journal of Nervous and Mental Disease, 181,* 189–193.

Fear, C. F., Sharp, H., & Healy, D. (1996). Cognitive processes in delusional disorder. *British Journal of Psychiatry, 168,* 61–67.

Federoff, I. C., & Taylor, S. (2001). Psychological and pharmacological treatments of social phobia: A meta-analysis. *Journal of Clinical Pharmacology, 21,* 311–324.

Fenton, W. S., Blyler, C. R., & Heinssen, R. K. (1997). Determinants of medication compliance in schizophrenia: Empirical and clinical findings. *Schizophrenia Bulletin, 23,* 637–651.

Ferrans, C. E., & Powers, M. J. (1985). Quality of Life Index: Development and psychometric properties. *ANS Advances in Nursing Science, 8,* 15–24.

Feske, U., & Chambless, D. L. (1995). Cognitive behavioral versus exposure only treatment for social phobia: A meta-analysis. *Behavior Therapy, 26,* 695–720.

Fiegenbaum, W. (1988). Long-term efficacy of ungraded versus graded massed exposure in agoraphobics. In I. Hand & H. -U. Wittchen (Eds.), *Panic and phobias: 2. Treatments and variables affecting course and outcome* (pp. 83–88). New York: Springer-Verlag.

First, M. B., Spitzer, R. L., Gibbon, M., & Williams, J. B. W. (1996). *Structured Clinical Interview for DSM-IV Axis I Disorders—Patient Edition (SCID-I/P, Version 2. 0).* New York: Biometrics Research Department, New York State Psychiatric Institute.

First, M. B., Spitzer, R. L., Gibbon, M., & Williams, J. B. W. (1997). *Structured Clinical Interview for DSM-IV Axis I Disorders (SCID-I)—Clinician Version.* Washington, DC: American Psychiatric Press.

Foa, E. B., Blau, J. S., Prout, M., & Latimer, P. (1977). Is horror a necessary component of flooding (implosion)? *Behaviour Research and Therapy, 15,* 397–402.

Foa, E. B., & Franklin, M. E. (2001). Obsessive–compulsive disorder. In D. H. Barlow (Ed.), *Clinical handbook of psychological disorders* (3rd ed., pp. 209–263). New York: Guilford Press.

Foa, E. B., Gilboa-Schechtman, E., Amir, N., & Freshman, M. (2000). Memory bias in generalized social phobia: Remembering negative emotional expressions. *Journal of Anxiety Disorders, 14,* 501–519.

Foa, E. B., Jameson, J. S., Turner, R. M., & Payne, L. L. (1980). Massed versus spaced exposure sessions in the treatment of agoraphobia. *Behaviour Research and Therapy, 18,* 333–338.

Foa, E. B., & Kozak, M. J. (1996). Psychological treatment for obsessive–compulsive disorder. In M. R. Mavissakalian & R. F. Prien (Eds.), *Long-term treatment of anxiety disorders* (pp. 285–309). Washington, DC: American Psychiatric Press.

Foa, E. B., Kozak, M. J., Salkovskis, P. M., Coles, M. E., & Amir, N. (1998). The validation of a new obsessive–compulsive disorder scale: The Obsessive–Compulsive Inventory. *Psychological Assessment, 10,* 206–214.

Foa, E. B., & Rothbaum, B. O. (1998). *Treating the trauma of rape: Cognitive-behavioral therapy for PTSD*. New York: Guilford Press.

Foa, E. B., & Wilson, R. (2001). *Stop obsessing! How to overcome your obsessions and compulsions* (rev. ed.). New York: Bantam Books.

Franklin, M. E., & Foa, E. B. (2002). Cognitive behavioral treatments for obsessive compulsive disorder. In P. E. Nathan & J. M. Gorman (Eds.), *A guide to treatments that work* (2nd ed., pp. 367–386). New York: Oxford University Press.

Franko, D. L. (1997). Ready or not?: Stages of change as predictors of brief group therapy outcome in bulimia nervosa. *Group, 21*, 39–45.

Freeman, A., & Morgillo-Freeman, S. (2005). Cognitive behavior therapy in group treatment settings. In S. Morgillo Freeman & A. Freeman (Eds.), *Cognitive behavior therapy in nursing practice* (pp. 295–324). New York: Springer.

Freeman, A., Pretzer, J., Fleming, B., & Simon, K. M. (1990). *Clinical applications of cognitive therapy*. New York: Plenum Press.

Freeman, A., Pretzer, J., Fleming, B., & Simon, K. M. (2005). *Clinical applications of cognitive therapy* (2nd ed.). New York: Plenum Press.

Freeman, A., Schrodt, G. R., Gilson, M., & Ludgate, J. W. (1993). Group cognitive therapy with inpatients. In J. H. Wright, A. T. Beck, M. E. Thase, & J. W. Ludgate (Eds.), *Cognitive therapy with inpatients: Developing a cognitive milieu* (pp. 123–153). New York: Guilford Press.

Freeston, M. H., & Ladouceur, R. (1997). What do patients do with their obsessive thoughts? *Behaviour Research and Therapy, 35*, 335–348.

Frommer, M. S., Ames, J. R., Gibson, J. W., & Davis, W. N. (1987). Patterns of symptom change in the short-term group treatment of bulimia. *International Journal of Eating Disorders, 6*, 469–476.

Frost, R. O., & Steketee, G. (2002). *Cognitive approaches to obsessions and compulsions: Theory, assessment, and treatment*. Oxford, UK: Elsevier.

Furer, P., Walker, J. R., Chartier, M. J., & Stein, M. B. (1997). Hypochondriacal concerns and somatization in panic disorder. *Depression and Anxiety, 6*, 78–85.

Fydrich, T., Chambless, D. L., Perry, K. J., Buergener, F., & Beazley, M. B. (1998). Behavioral assessment of social performance: A rating system for social phobia. *Behaviour Research and Therapy, 36*, 995–1010.

Garety, P., Dunn, G., Fowler, D., & Kuipers, E. (1998). The evaluation of cognitive behavioural therapy for psychosis. In T. Wykes, N. Tarrier, & S. Lewis (Eds.), *Outcome and innovation in psychological treatment of schizophrenia* (pp. 101–118). Chichester, UK: Wiley.

Garety, P. A., Everitt, B. S., & Hemsley, D. R. (1988). The characteristics of delusions: A cluster analysis of deluded subjects. *European Archives of Psychiatry and Neurological Sciences, 237*, 112–114.

Garety, P. A., Fowler, D., & Kuipers, E. (2000). Cognitive-behavioral therapy for medication-resistant symptoms. *Schizophrenia Bulletin, 26*, 73–86.

Garety, P. A., & Freeman, D. (1999). Cognitive approaches to delusions: A critical review of theories and evidence. *British Journal of Clinical Psychology, 38*, 113–154.

Garety, P. A., Hemsley, D. R., & Wessely, S. (1991). Reasoning in deluded schizophrenic and paranoid patients. *Journal of Nervous and Mental Disease, 179*, 194–201.

Garner, D. M. (1991). *Eating Disorder Inventory–2 manual*. Odessa, FL: Psychological Assessment Resources.

Garner, D. M. (1997). Psychoeducational principles in treatment. In P. E. Garfinkel & D. M. Garner (Eds.), *Handbook of treatment for eating disorders* (2nd ed., pp. 145–177). New York: Guilford Press.

Garner, D. M. (2005). *Eating Disorder Inventory–3 manual*. Odessa, FL: Psychological Assessment Resources.

Garner, D. M., & Bemis, K. M. (1982). A cognitive-behavioral approach to anorexia nervosa. *Cognitive Therapy and Research, 6,* 123–150.

Garner, D. M., & Bemis, K. M. (1985). Cognitive therapy for anorexia nervosa. In *Handbook of treatment for eating disorders* (pp. 94–144). New York: Guilford Press.

Garner, D. M., Fairburn, C. G., & Davis, R. (1987). Cognitive-behavioral treatment of bulimia nervosa. *Behavior Modification, 11,* 398–431.

Garner, D. M., & Garfinkel, P. E. (1979). The Eating Attitudes Test: An index of the symptoms of anorexia nervosa. *Psychological Medicine, 9,* 273–279.

Garner, D. M., Olmsted, M. P., & Polivy, J. (1983). Development and validation of a multidimensional Eating Disorder Inventory for anorexia nervosa and bulimia. *International Journal of Eating Disorders, 2,* 15–34.

Garner, D. M., Vitousek, K. M., & Pike, K. M. (1997). Cognitive-behavioral therapy for anorexia nervosa. In D. M. Garner & P. E. Garfinkel (Eds.), *Handbook of treatment for eating disorders* (2nd ed., pp. 94–144). New York: Guilford Press.

Gelernter, C. S., Uhde, T. W., Cimbolic, P., Arnkoff, D. B., Vittone, B. J., & Tancer, M. E. (1991). Cognitive-behavioral and pharmacological treatments of social phobia: A controlled study. *Archives of General Psychiatry, 48,* 938–945.

Glass, C. R., & Arnkoff, D. B. (2000). Consumers' perspectives on helpful and hindering factors in mental health treatment. *Journal of Clinical Psychology, 56,* 1467–1480.

Gledhill, A., Lobban, F., & Sellwood, W. (1998). Group CBT for people with schizophrenia: A preliminary evaluation. *Behavioural and Cognitive Psychotherapy, 26,* 63–75.

Goodman, W. K., Price, L. H., Rasmussen, S. A., Mazure, C., Delgado, P., Heninger, G. R., et al. (1989a). The Yale–Brown Obsessive Compulsive Scale: II. Validity. *Archives of General Psychiatry, 46,* 1012–1016.

Goodman, W. K., Price, L. H., Rasmussen, S. A., Mazure, C., Fleischmann, R. L., Hill, C. L., et al. (1989b). The Yale–Brown Obsessive Compulsive Scale: I. Development, use, and reliability. *Archives of General Psychiatry, 46,* 1006–1011.

Goodwin, F. K., & Jamison, K. R. (1990). *Manic–depressive illness.* New York: Oxford University Press.

Gorin, A. A., Le Grange, D., & Stone, A. A. (2003). Effectiveness of spouse involvement in cognitive behavioral treatment for binge eating disorder. *International Journal of Eating Disorders, 33,* 421–433.

Gottesman, I. (1991). *Schizophrenia genesis: The origins of madness.* New York: Freeman.

Gould, R. A., Buckminster, S., Pollack, M. H., Otto, M. W., & Yap, L. (1997). Cognitive-behavioral and pharmacological treatment for social phobia: A meta-analysis. *Clinical Psychology: Science and Practice, 4,* 291–306.

Gould, R. A., Mueser, K. T., Bolton, E., Mays, V., & Goff, D. (2001). Cognitive therapy for psychosis in schizophrenia: An effect size analysis. *Schizophrenia Research, 48,* 335–342.

Gould, R. A., Otto, M. W., & Pollack, M. H. (1995). A meta-analysis of treatment outcome for panic disorder. *Clinical Psychology Review, 15,* 819–844.

Grant, D. A., Bieling, P. J., Antony, M. M., & McCabe, R. E. (2006). *Group versus individual cognitive therapy for depression: A meta-analytic and qualitative review.* Manuscript submitted for publication.

Greenberger, D., & Padesky, C. A. (1995). *Mind over mood: Change how you feel by changing the way you think.* New York: Guilford Press.

Greene, L. R. (2000). Process analysis of group interaction in therapeutic groups. In A. P. Beck & C. M. Lewis (Eds.), *The process of group psychotherapy systems for analyzing change* (pp. 23–48). Washington, DC: American Psychological Association.

Gumley, A., O'Grady, M., McNay, L., Reilly, J., Power, K., & Norrie, J. (2003). Early intervention for relapse in schizophrenia: Results of a 12-month randomized controlled trial of cognitive behavioural therapy. *Psychological Medicine, 33,* 419–431.

Gunther, L. M., Denniston, J. C., & Miller, R. R. (1998). Conducting exposure treatment in multiple contexts can prevent relapse. *Behaviour Research and Therapy, 36,* 75–91.

Gwilliam, P., Wells, A., & Cartwright-Hatton, S. (2004). Does meta-cognition or responsibility predict obsessive–compulsive symptoms: A test of the metacognitive model. *Clinical Psychology and Psychotherapy, 11,* 137–144.

Hackmann, A., Surawy, C., & Clark, D. M. (1998). Seeing yourself through others' eyes: A study of spontaneously occurring images in social phobia. *Behavioural and Cognitive Psychotherapy, 26,* 3–12.

Haddock, G., McCarron, J., Tarrier, N., & Faragher, E. B. (1999). Scales to measure dimensions of hallucinations and delusions: The psychotic symptom rating scales (PSYRATS). *Psychological Medicine, 29,* 879–889.

Haddock, G., Tarrier, N., Morrison, A. P., Hopkins, R., Drake, R., & Lewis, S. A. (1999). A pilot study evaluating the effectiveness of individual inpatient cognitive-behavioral therapy in early psychosis. *Social Psychiatry and Psychiatric Epidemiology, 34,* 254–258.

Haddock, G., Tarrier, N., Spaulding, W., Yusupoff, L., Kinney, C., & McCarthy, E. (1998). Individual cognitive-behavioral therapy in the treatment of hallucinations and delusions: A review. *Clinical Psychology Review, 18,* 821–838.

Hafner, H., Nowotny, B., Loffler, W., van der Heiden, W., & Maurer, K. (1995). When and how does schizophrenia produce social deficits? *European Archives of Psychiatry and Clinical Neuroscience, 246,* 17–28.

Hahlweg, K., Fiegenbaum, W., Frank, M., Schroeder, B., & von Witzleben, I. (2001). Short- and long term effectiveness of an empirically supported treatment for agoraphobia. *Journal of Consulting and Clinical Psychology, 69,* 375–382.

Halford, W. K., & Hayes, R. L. (1995). Social skills in schizophrenia: Assessing the relationship between social skills, psychopathology, and community functioning. *Social Psychiatry and Psychiatric Epidemiology, 30,* 14–19.

Hall, A. (1985). Group psychotherapy for anorexia nervosa. In D. M. Garner & P. E. Garfinkel (Eds.), *Handbook of psychotherapy for anorexia nervosa and bulimia* (pp. 213–239). New York: Guilford Press.

Halperin, S., Nathan, P., Drummond, P., & Castle, D. (2000). A cognitive-behavioral, group-based intervention for social anxiety in schizophrenia. *Australian and New Zealand Journal of Psychiatry, 34,* 809–813.

Hardy, G. E., Barkham, M., Shapiro, D. A., Stiles, W. B., Rees, A., & Reynolds, S. (1995). Impact of cluster C personality disorders on outcomes of contrasting brief psychotherapies for depression. *Journal of Consulting and Clinical Psychology, 63,* 997–1004.

Harrow, M., Goldberg, J. F., Grossman, L. S., & Meltzer, H. Y. (1990). Outcome in manic disorders: A naturalistic follow-up study. *Archives of General Psychiatry, 47,* 665–671.

Hartmann, A., Herzog, T., & Drinkmann, A. (1992). Psychotherapy of bulimia nervosa: What is effective?: A meta-analysis. *Journal of Psychosomatic Research, 36,* 159–167.

Haug, T. T., Blomhoff, S., Hellström, K., Holme, I., Humble, M., Madsbu, H. P., et al. (2003). Exposure therapy and sertraline in social phobia: 1-year follow-up of a randomized controlled trial. *British Journal of Psychiatry, 182,* 312–318.

Hawkins, R. C., II, & Clement, P. F. (1980). Development and construct validation of a self-report measure of binge eating tendencies. *Addictive Behaviors, 5,* 219–226.

Hawton, K., & Kirk, J. (1989). Problem solving. In K. S. Hawton, P. M. Salkovskis, J. Kirk, & D. M. Clark (Eds.), *Cognitive behaviour therapy for psychiatric problems: A practical guide* (pp. 406–426). Oxford, UK: Oxford University Press.

Hayes, S. C., Follette, V. M., & Linehan, M. M. (2004). *Mindfulness and acceptance: Expanding the cognitive-behavioral tradition.* New York: Guilford Press.

Heimberg, R. G. (2003, March). Cognitive-behavioral and psychotherapeutic strategies for social anxiety disorder. In M. R. Liebowitz (Chair), *Beyond shyness: Recognition, diagnosis, and treatment of social anxiety disorder.* Symposium presented at the meeting of the Anxiety Disorders Association of America, Toronto, Ontario, Canada.

Heimberg, R. G., & Becker, R. E. (2002). *Cognitive-behavioral group therapy for social phobia: Basic mechanisms and clinical strategies.* New York: Guilford Press.

Heimberg, R. G., Dodge, C. S., Hope, D. A., Kennedy, C. R., Zollo, L. J., & Becker, R. E. (1990). Cognitive behavioral group treatment for social phobia: Comparison with a credible placebo control. *Cognitive Therapy and Research, 14,* 1–23.

Heimberg, R. G., Liebowitz, M. R., Hope, D. A., Schneier, F. R., Holt, C. S., Welkowitz, L. A., et al. (1998). Cognitive-behavioral group treatment versus phenelzine in social phobia: 12-week outcome. *Archives of General Psychiatry, 55,* 1113–1141.

Heimberg, R. G., Salzman, D. G., Holt, C. S., & Blendell, K. A. (1993). Cognitive-behavioral group treatment for social phobia: Effectiveness at five-year follow-up. *Cognitive Therapy and Research, 17,* 325–339.

Heinrichs, N., Spiegel, D. A., & Hofmann, S. G. (2002). Panic disorder with agoraphobia. In F. W. Bond & W. Dryden (Eds.), *Handbook of brief cognitive behaviour therapy* (pp. 55–76). Chichester, UK: Wiley.

Herbert, J. D., Rheingold, A. A., Gaudiano, B. A., & Myers, V. H. (2004). Standard versus extended cognitive behavior therapy for social anxiety disorder: A randomized-controlled trial. *Behavioural and Cognitive Psychotherapy, 32,* 131–147.

Higgitt, A., & Fonagy, P. (1992). Psychotherapy in borderline and narcissistic personality disorder. *British Journal of Psychiatry, 161,* 23–43.

Himle, J. A., Rassi, S., Haghighatgou, H., Krone, K. P., Nesse, R. M., & Abelson, J.

(2001). Group behavioral therapy of obsessive–compulsive disorder: Seven vs. twelve-week outcomes. *Depression and Anxiety, 13,* 161–165.

Hirsch, C. R., & Clark, D. M. (2004). Information-processing bias in social phobia. *Clinical Psychology Review, 24,* 799–825.

Hoek, H. W., & van Hoeken, D. (2003). Review of the prevalence and incidence of eating disorders. *International Journal of Eating Disorders, 34,* 383–396.

Hoffman, L. (2002). *Psychotherapy for personality disorders* (Book review). *American Journal of Psychiatry, 159,* 504–507.

Hoffman, R. E. (1986). Verbal hallucinations and language production processes in schizophrenia. *Behavioral and Brain Sciences, 9,* 503–548.

Hofmann, S. G., & Barlow, D. H. (1999). The costs of anxiety disorders: Implications for psychosocial interventions. In N. E. Miller & K. M. Magruder (Eds.), *Cost-effectiveness of psychotherapy* (pp. 224–234). New York: Oxford University Press.

Hofmann, S. G., Newman, M. G., Becker, E., Taylor, C. B., & Roth, W. T. (1995). Social phobia with and without avoidant personality disorder: Preliminary behavior therapy outcome findings. *Journal of Anxiety Disorders, 9,* 427–438.

Hoge, S. K., Appelbaum, P. S., Lawlor, T., Beck, J. C., Litman, R., & Greer, A. (1990). Prospective multi-centre study of patients' refusal of anti-psychotic medication. *Archives of General Psychiatry, 47,* 949–956.

Hohagen, F., Winkelmann, G., Rasche-Räuchle, H., Hand, I., König, A., Münchau, N., et al. (1998). Combination of behaviour therapy with fluvoxamine in comparison with behaviour therapy and placebo: Results of a multicentre study. *British Journal of Psychiatry, 173*(Suppl. 35), 71–78.

Hollon, S. D., & Shaw, B. F. (1979). Group cognitive therapy for depressed patients. In A. T. Beck, A. J. Rush, B. F. Shaw, & G. Emery (Eds.), *Cognitive therapy of depression* (pp. 328–353). New York: Guilford Press.

Hope, D. A., Heimberg, R. G., Juster, H. R., & Turk, C. L. (2000). *Managing social anxiety.* New York: Oxford University Press.

Hope, D. A., Herbert, J. D., & White, C. (1995). Diagnostic subtype, avoidant personality disorder, and efficacy of cognitive-behavioral group therapy for social phobia. *Cognitive Therapy and Research, 19,* 399–417.

Houck, P. R., Spiegel, D. A., Shear, M. K., & Rucci, P. (2002). Reliability of the self-report version of the Panic Disorder Severity Scale. *Depression and Anxiety, 15,* 183–185.

Hsu, L. K. G. (1990). *Eating disorders.* New York: Guilford Press.

Humphreys, K., & Klaw, E. (2001). Can targeting nondependent problem drinkers and providing internet-based services expand access to assistance for alcohol problems?: A study of the moderation management self-help/mutual aid organization. *Journal of Studies on Alcohol, 62,* 528–532.

Huppert, J. D., & Baker-Morissette, S. L. (2003). Beyond the manual: The insider's guide to panic control treatment. *Cognitive and Behavioral Practice, 10,* 2–13.

Huppert, J. D., Bufka, L. F, Barlow, D. H., Gorman, J. M., Shear, M. K., & Woods, S. W. (2001). Therapists, therapist variables and cognitive-behavioral therapy outcome in a multicenter trial for panic disorder. *Journal of Consulting and Clinical Psychology, 69,* 747–755.

Huppert, J. D., Schultz, L. T., Foa, E. B., Barlow, D. H., Davidson, J. R. T., Gorman, J. M., et al. (2004). Differential response to placebo among patients with social phobia, panic disorder, and obsessive–compulsive disorder. *American Journal of Psychiatry, 161,* 1485–1487.

Huq, S. F., Garety, P. A., & Hemsley, D. R. (1988). Probabilistic judgments in deluded and nondeluded subjects. *Quarterly Journal of Experimental Psychology, 40A,* 801–812.

Hyman, B. M., & Pedrick, C. (1999). *The OCD workbook: Your guide to breaking free from obsessive–compulsive disorder.* Oakland, CA: New Harbinger.

Inbody, D. R., & Ellis, J. J. (1985). Group therapy with anorexic and bulimic patients: Implications for therapeutic intervention. *American Journal of Psychotherapy, 39,* 411–420.

Ingersoll, K., Wagner, C., & Gharib, S. (1997). *Motivational groups in community substance abuse programs.* Richmond, VA: Mid-Atlantic Addiction Technology Transfer Center.

Isohanni, I., Jones, P. B., Jarvelin, M. -R., Nieminen, P., Rantakallio, P., Jokelainen, J., et al. (2001). Educational consequences of mental disorders treated in hospital: A 31-year follow-up of the Northern Finland 1966 Birth Cohort. *Psychological Medicine, 31,* 339–349.

Jacobi, C., Dahme, B., & Dittmann, R. (2002). Cognitive-behavioural, fluoxetine and combined treatment for bulimia nervosa: Short- and long-term results. *European Eating Disorders Review, 10,* 179–198.

Jarrett, R. B., Kraft, D., Doyle, J., Foster, B. M., Eaves, G. G., & Silver, P. C. (2001). Preventing recurrent depression using cognitive therapy with and without a continuation phase: A randomized clinical trial. *Archives of General Psychiatry, 58,* 381–388.

Jenike, M. A. (1998). Neurosurgical treatment of obsessive–compulsive disorder. *British Journal of Psychiatry, 173*(Suppl. 35), 79–90.

Johns, L. C., Sellwood, W., McGovern, J., & Haddock, G. (2002). Battling boredom: Group cognitive behavioural therapy for negative symptoms of schizophrenia. *Behavioural and Cognitive Psychotherapy, 30,* 341–346.

Jones, C., Cormac, I., Mota, J., & Campbell, C. (2000). Cognitive behaviour therapy for schizophrenia. *Cochrane Database of Systematic Reviews* [computer file], 2, CD000524.

Jones, M. K., & Menzies, R. G. (1998). The relevance of associative learning pathways in the development of obsessive–compulsive washing. *Behaviour Research and Therapy, 36,* 273–283.

Kadden, R. M., Cooney, N. L., Getter, H., & Litt, M. D. (1989). Matching alcoholics to coping skills or interactional therapies: Posttreatment results. *Journal of Consulting and Clinical Psychology, 57,* 698–704.

Kampman, M., Keijsers, G. P., Hoogduin, C. A., & Hendriks, G. J. (2002). A randomized, double-blind, placebo-controlled study of the effects of adjunctive paroxetine in panic disorder patients unsuccessfully treated with cognitive-behavioral therapy alone. *Journal of Clinical Psychiatry, 63,* 772–777.

Kampman, M., Keijsers, G. P. J., Hoogduin, C. A. L., & Verbraak, M. J. P. M. (2002). Addition of cognitive-behaviour therapy for obsessive–compulsive disorder patients non-responding to fluoxetine. *Acta Psychiatrica Scandinavica, 106,* 314–319.

Kandel, D. B. (Ed.). (2002). *Stages and pathways of drug involvement: Examining the gateway hypothesis.* New York: Cambridge University Press.

Kane, J. M., & Marder, S. R. (1993). Psychopharmacologic treatment of schizophrenia. *Schizophrenia Bulletin, 19,* 287–302.

Kaney, S., & Bentall, R. P. (1989). Persecutory delusions and attributional style. *British Journal of Medical Psychology, 62,* 191–198.

Karterud, S., Vaglum, S., Friis, S., Irion, T., Johns, S., & Vaglum, P. (1992). Day hospital therapeutic community treatment for patients with personality disorders. *Journal of Mental Disorders, 180,* 238–243.

Kay, S. R., Fiszbein, A., & Opler, L. A. (1987). The Positive and Negative Syndrome Scale (PANSS) for schizophrenia. *Schizophrenia Bulletin, 13,* 261–276.

Keel, P. K., Mitchell, J. E., Davis, T. L., & Crow, S. L. (2002). Long-term impact of treatment in women diagnosed with bulimia nervosa. *International Journal of Eating Disorders, 31,* 151–158.

Keesey, R. E. (1993). Physiological regulation of body energy: Implications for obesity. In A. J. Stunkard & T. A. Wadden (Eds.), *Obesity: theory and therapy* (2nd ed., pp. 77–96). New York: Raven Press.

Keijsers, G. P., Hoogduin, C. A., & Schnaap, C. P. D. R. (1994). Prognostic factors in the behavioral treatment of panic disorder with and without agoraphobia. *Behavior Therapy, 25,* 689–708.

Keller, M. B., Harrison, W., Fawcett, J. A., Gelenberg, A., Hirschfeld, R. M., Klein, D., et al. (1995). Treatment of chronic depression with sertralineor imipramine: Preliminary blinded response rates and high rates of undertreatment in the communicy. *Psychopharmacology Bulletin, 31,* 205–212.

Keller, M. B., Yonkers, K. A., Warshaw, M. G., Pratt, L. A., Golan, J., Mathews, A. O., et al. (1994). Remission and relapse in subjects with panic disorder and panic with agoraphobia: A prospective short-interval naturalistic follow-up. *Journal of Nervous and Mental Disease, 182,* 290–296.

Kessler, R. C., Barber, C., Birnbaum, H. G., Frank, R. G., Greenberg, P. E., Rose, R. M., et al. (1999). Depression in the workplace: Effects on short-term disability. *Health Affairs (Millwood), 18,* 163–171.

Khantzian, E. J. (1985). The self-medication hypothesis of addictive disorders: Focus on heroin and cocaine dependence. *American Journal of Psychiatry, 142,* 1259–1264.

Khawaja, N. G., & Oei, T. P. S. (1998). Catastrophic cognitions in panic disorder with and without agoraphobia. *Clinical Psychology Review, 18,* 341–365.

Khawaja, N. G., Oei, T. P. S., & Baglioni, A. J. (1994). Modification of the Catastrophic Cognition Questionnaire (CCQ-M) for normals and patients: Exploratory and LISREL analyses. *Journal of Psychopathology and Behavioral Assessment, 16,* 325–342.

Kim, C. -H., Chang, J. W., Koo, M. -S., Kim, J. W., Suh, H. S., Park, I. H., et al. (2003). Anterior cingulotomy for refractory obsessive–compulsive disorder. *Acta Psychiatrica Scandinavica, 107,* 283–290.

Kinderman, P., & Bentall, R. P. (1997). Causal attributions in paranoia: Internal, personal and situational attributions for negative events. *Journal of Abnormal Psychology, 106,* 341–345.

Kingsep, P., Nathan, P., & Castle, D. (2003). Cognitive behavioural group treatment for social anxiety in schizophrenia. *Schizophrenia Research, 63,* 121–129.

Klerman, G. L., Weissman, M. M., Ouellette, R., Johnson, J., & Greenwald, S. (1991). Panic attacks in the community: Social morbidity and health care utilization. *Journal of the American Medical Association, 265,* 742–746.

Kobak, K. A., Greist, J. H., Jefferson, J. W., & Katzelnick, D. J. (2002). Fluoxetine in social phobia: A double-blind, placebo-controlled pilot trial. *Journal of Clinical Psychopharmacology, 22,* 257–262.

Kobak, K. A., Taylor, L. V., Warner, G., & Futterer, R. (2005). St. John's wort versus placebo in social phobia: Results from a placebo-controlled pilot study. *Journal of Clinical Psychopharmacology, 25,* 51–58.

Kretschmer, E. (1936). *Physique and character.* London: Routledge & Kegan Paul.

Krochmalik, A., & Menzies, R. G. (2003). The classification and diagnosis of obsessive compulsive disorder. In R. G. Menzies, & P. de Silva (Eds.), *Obsessive compulsive disorder: Theory, research and treatment* (pp. 3–20). Chichester, UK: Wiley.

Kuipers, E., Fowler, D., Garety, P., Chisholm, D., Freeman, D., Dunn, G., et al. (1998). The London–East Anglia randomised controlled trial of cognitive behavioral therapy for psychosis: III. Follow-up and economic evaluation at 18 months. *British Journal of Psychiatry, 173,* 61–68.

Kuipers, E., Garety, P., Fowler, D., Dunn, G., Bebbington, P., Freeman, D., et al. (1997). London–East Anglia randomized controlled trial of cognitive-behavioural therapy for psychosis: I. Effects of the treatment phase. *British Journal of Psychiatry, 171,* 319–327.

Lacey, H. (1983). Bulimia nervosa, binge eating, and psychogenic vomiting: A controlled treatment study and long term outcome. *British Medical Journal, 286,* 1609–1613.

Lader, M., Stender, K., Bürger, V., & Nil, R. (2004). Efficacy and tolerability of escitalopram in 12- and 24-week treatment of social anxiety disorder: Randomized, double-blind, placebo-controlled, fixed-dose study. *Depression and Anxiety, 19,* 241–248.

Ladouceur, R., Blais, F., Freeston, M. H., & Dugas, M. J. (1998). Problem solving and problem orientation in generalized anxiety disorder. *Journal of Anxiety Disorders, 12,* 139–152.

Laliberté, M., & McKenzie, J. (2003). *Making changes: A manual for group-based cognitive behavior therapy for eating disorders.* Hamilton, ON: Crieff Hollow Press.

Lam, D. H., Watkins, E. R., Hayward, P., Bright, J., Wright, K., Kerr, N., et al. (2003). A randomized controlled study of cognitive therapy for relapse prevention for bipolar affective disorder: Outcome of the first year. *Archives of General Psychiatry, 60,* 145–152.

Lang, A. J., & Craske, M. G. (2000). Manipulations of exposure-based therapy to reduce return of fear: A replication. *Behaviour Research and Therapy, 38,* 1–12.

LaSalle, V. H., Cromer, K. R., Nelson, K. N., Kazuba, D., Justement, L., & Murphy, D. L. (2004). Diagnostic interview assessed neuropsychiatric disorder comorbidity in 334 individuals with obsessive–compulsive disorder. *Depression and Anxiety, 19,* 163–173.

Leahy, R. L. (2001). *Overcoming resistance in cognitive therapy.* New York: Guilford Press.

Leahy, R. L. (2003). *Cognitive therapy techniques: A practitioner's guide.* New York: Guilford Press.

Lecomte, T., Cyr, M., Lesage, A. D., Wilde, J., Leclerc, C., & Richard, N. (1999). Efficacy of a self-esteem module in the empowerment of individuals with schizophrenia. *Journal of Nervous and Mental Disease, 187,* 406–413.

Lecomte, T., Leclerc, C., Wykes, T., & Lecomte, J. (2003). Group CBT for clients with a first episode of schizophrenia. *Journal of Cognitive Psychotherapy: An International Quarterly, 17,* 375–383.

Leichsenring, F., & Leibing, E. (2003). The effectiveness of psychodynamic therapy and cognitive behavior therapy in the treatment of personality disorders: A meta-analysis. *American Journal of Psychiatry, 160,* 1223–1232.

Leigh, B. C., & Stacy, A. W. (2004). Alcohol expectancies and drinking in different age groups. *Addiction, 99,* 215–227.

Lenze, E. J., Dew, M. A., Mazumdar, S., Begley, A. E., Cornes, C., Miller, M. D., et al. (2002). Combined pharmacotherapy and psychotherapy as maintenance treatment for late-life depression: Effects on social adjustment. *American Journal of Psychiatry, 159,* 466–468.

Leon, A. C., Portera, L., & Weissman, M. M. (1995). The social costs of anxiety disorders. *British Journal of Psychiatry, 166,* 19–22.

Leung, N., Waller, G., & Thomas, G. (1999). Group cognitive-behavioural therapy for anorexia nervosa: A case for treatment? *European Eating Disorders Review, 7,* 351–361.

Leung, N., Waller, G., & Thomas, G. (2000). Outcome of group cognitive-behavior therapy for bulimia nervosa: The role of cores beliefs. *Behaviour Research and Therapy, 38,* 145–156.

Lewinsohn, P. M., Striegel-Moore, R. H., & Seeley, J. R. (2000). Epidemiology and natural course of eating disorders in young women from adolescence to young adulthood. *Journal of the American Academy of Child and Adolescent Psychiatry, 39,* 1284–1292.

Lewis, S., Tarrier, N., Haddock, G., Bentall, R., Kinderman, P., Kingdon, D., et al. (2002a). Cognitive therapy improves 18-month outcomes but not time to relapse in first episode schizophrenia. *Schizophrenia Research, 53*(Suppl. 1), 14.

Lewis, S., Tarrier, N., Haddock, G., Bentall, R., Kinderman, P., Kingdon, D., et al. (2002b). Randomised controlled trial of cognitive-behavioural therapy in early schizophrenia: Acute-phase outcomes. *British Journal of Psychiatry, 181*(Suppl. 43), s91–s97.

Libermann, R. P., Eckman, T. (1981). Behavior therapy vs. insight oriented therapy for repeated suicide attempters. *Archives of General Psychiatry, 38,* 1126–1130.

Lidren, D. M., Watkins, P. L., Gould, R. A., Clum, G. A., Asterino, M., & Tulloch, H. L. (1994). A comparison of bibliotherapy and group therapy in the treatment of panic disorder. *Journal of Consulting and Clinical Psychology, 62,* 865–869.

Liebowitz, M. R. (1987). Social phobia. *Modern Problems in Pharmacopsychiatry, 22,* 141–173.

Linehan, M. M. (1993). *Cognitive behavioral treatment of borderline personality disorder.* New York: Guilford Press.

Linehan, M. M., Armstrong, H. E., Suarez, A., Allmon, D., & Heard, H. L. (1991). Cognitive-behavioral treatment of chronically parasuicidal borderline patients. *Archives of General Psychiatry, 48,* 1060–1064.

Linehan, M. M., Heard, H. L., & Armstrong, H. E. (1993). Naturalistic follow-up of a behavioral treatment of chronically parasuicidal borderline patients. *Archives of General Psychiatry, 50,* 971–974.

Linehan, M. M., Tutek, D. A., Heard, H. L., & Armstrong, H. E. (1994). Interpersonal outcome of cognitive behavioral treatment for chronically suicidal borderline patients. *American Journal of Psychiatry, 151,* 1771–1776.

Lock, J. (2002). Treating adolescents with eating disorders in the family context: Empirical and theoretical considerations. *Child and Adolescent Psychiatric Clinics of North America, 11,* 331–342.

Logan, A. M., & Tonigan, J. S. (2003). Religiosity, psychopathology, twelve-step therapy, and AA attendance. *Alcoholism: Clinical and Experimental Research, 26*(Suppl. 5), 632A. (Abstract)

Lopatka, C. L. (1989). *The role of unexpected events in avoidance.* Unpublished Master's thesis, State University of New York, Albany.

Lovibond, P. F., & Lovibond, S. H. (1995a). The structure of negative emotional states: Comparison of the Depression Anxiety Stress Scales (DASS) with the Beck Depression and Anxiety Inventories. *Behaviour Research and Therapy, 33,* 335–342.

Lovibond, S. H., & Lovibond, P. F. (1995b). *Manual for the Depression Anxiety Stress Scales* (2nd ed.). Sydney, Australia: Psychology Foundation of Australia.

Lucas, R. A., & Telch, M. J. (1993, November). *Group versus individual treatment of social phobia.* Paper presented at the meeting of the Association for Advancement of Behavior Therapy, Atlanta, GA.

Lundh, L. G., & Öst, L. G. (1996). Recognition bias for critical faces in social phobics. *Behaviour Research and Therapy, 34,* 787–794.

Lydiard, R. B., Greenwald, S., Weissman, M. M., Johnson, J., Drossman, D. A., & Ballenger, J. C. (1994). Panic disorder and gastrointestinal symptoms: Findings from the NIMH Epidemiologic Catchment Area project. *American Journal of Psychiatry, 151,* 64–70.

Lyon, H. M., Kaney, S., & Bentall, R. P. (1994). The defensive function of persecutory delusions: Evidence from attribution tasks. *British Journal of Psychiatry, 164,* 637–646.

Macdonald, E. M., Jackson, H. J., Hayes, R. L., Baglioni, A. J., & Madden, C. (1998). Social skill as a determinant of social networks and perceived social support in schizophrenia. *Schizophrenia Research, 29,* 275–286.

MacDonald, P., Antony, M. M., MacLeod, C., & Richter, M. A. (1997). Memory and confidence in memory judgments among individuals with obsessive compulsive disorder and non-clinical controls. *Behaviour Research and Therapy, 35,* 497–505.

MacKenzie, K. R., & Harper-Guiffre, H. (1992). Developing a health relationship with your body. *Group psychotherapy for eating disorders* (pp. 329–333). Washington, DC: American Psychiatric Press.

MacPhillamy, D. J., & Lewinsohn, P. M. (1982). The pleasant events schedule: Studies on reliability, validity, and scale intercorrelation. *Journal of Consulting and Clinical Psychology, 50,* 363–380.

Maher, B. A. (1988). Anomolous experience and delusional thinking: The logic of explanation. In T. F. Oltmanns & B. A. Maher (Eds.), *Delusional beliefs* (pp. 15–33). New York: Wiley.

Maidenberg, E., Chen, E., Craske, M., Bohn, P., & Bystritsky, A. (1996). Specificity of attentional bias in panic disorder and social phobia. *Journal of Anxiety Disorders, 10,* 529–541.

Maj, M., Sartorius, N., Okasha, A., & Zohar, J. (Eds.). (2002). *Obsessive–compulsive disorder* (2nd ed.). Chichester, UK: Wiley.

Manassis, K., Mendlowitz, S. L., Scapillato, D., Avery, D., Fiksenbaum, L., Freire, M., et al. (2002). Group and individual cognitive-behavioral therapy for childhood anxiety disorders: A randomized trial. *Journal of the American Academy of Child and Adolescent Psychiatry, 41*, 1423–1430.

Marcaurelle, R., Bélanger, C., & Marchand, A. (2003). Marital relationship and the treatment of panic disorder with agoraphobia: A critical review. *Clinical Psychology Review, 23*, 247–276.

Margraf, J., Barlow, D. H., Clark, D. M., & Telch, M. J. (1993). Psychological treatment of panic: Work in progress on outcome, active ingredients, and follow-up. *Behaviour Research and Therapy, 31*, 1–8.

Margraf, J., & Ehlers, A. (1988). Etiological models of panic—psychophysiological and cognitive aspects. In R. Baker (Ed.), *Panic disorder: Theory, research and therapy* (pp. 205–231). Chichester, UK: Wiley.

Marlatt, G. A., & Gordon, J. R. (1985). *Relapse prevention: Maintenance strategies in the treatment of addictive behaviors.* New York: Guilford Press.

Mattick, R. P., & Clarke, J. C. (1998). Development and validation of measures of social phobia scrutiny fear and social interaction anxiety. *Behaviour Research and Therapy, 36*, 455–470.

Maude-Griffin, P. M., Hohenstein, J. M., Humfleet, G. L., Reilly, P. M., Tusel, D. J., & Hall, S. M. (1998). Superior efficacy of cognitive-behavioral therapy for urban crack cocaine abusers: Main and matching effects. *Journal of Consulting and Clinical Psychology, 66*, 832–837.

McCabe, R. E. (2001). Overview and assessment of panic disorder and agoraphobia. In M. M. Antony, S. Orsillo, & L. Roemer (Eds.), *Practitioner's guide to empirically-based measures of anxiety* (pp. 87–94). New York: Kluwer Academic/Plenum Press.

McCabe, R. E., & Antony, M. M. (2002). Specific and social phobias. In M. M. Antony & D. H. Barlow (Eds.), *Handbook of assessment and treatment planning psychological disorders* (pp. 113–146). New York: Guilford Press.

McCabe, R. E., & Antony, M. M. (2005). Panic disorder with and without agoraphobia. In M. Antony, D. Roth & R. Heimberg (Eds.), *Improving outcomes and preventing relapse following cognitive behavior therapy* (pp. 1–37). New York: Guilford Press.

McCabe, R. E., Chudzik, S., Antony, M. M., Summerfeldt, L. J., & Swinson, R. P. (2004, November). In S. G. Hofmann & D. A. Moscovitch (Chairs), *Comorbidity in anxiety disorders: Psychopathology and treatment.* Paper presented at the meeting of the Association for Advancement of Behavior Therapy, New Orleans, LA.

McCabe, R. E., McFarlane, T. L., & Olmsted, M. P. (2003). *The overcoming bulimia workbook.* Oakland, CA: New Harbinger.

McCabe, R. E., Rowa, K., Antony, M. M., Swinson, R. P., & Ladak, Y. (2001, July). *The exposure hierarchy as a measure of cognitive and behavioral change, treatment progress and efficacy.* Paper presented at the World Congress of Behavioural and Cognitive Therapies, Vancouver, British Columbia.

McCrady, B. S., Horvath, A. T. & Delaney, S. (2002). Self-help groups. In R. K. Hester & W. R. Miller, (Eds.), *Handbook of alcoholism treatment approaches: Effective alternatives* (3rd ed., pp. 165–187). Boston: Allyn & Bacon.

McDonough, M. (2003). Pharmacological and neurosurgical treatment for obsessive-compulsive disorder. In R. G. Menzies & P. de Silva (Eds.), *Obsessive-compulsive disorder: Theory, research and treatment* (pp. 291–310). Chichester, UK: Wiley.

McDougle, C. J., Epperson, C. N., Pelton, G. H., Wasylink, S., & Price, L. H. (2000). A double-blind, placebo-controlled study of risperidone addition in serotonin reuptake inhibitor-refractory obsessive–compulsive disorder. *Archives of General Psychiatry, 57,* 794–801.

McElroy, S. L., Altshuler, L. L., Suppes, T., Keck, P. E., Frye, M. A., Denicoff, K. D., et al. (2001). Axis I psychiatric co-morbidity and its relationship to historical illness variables in 288 patients with bipolar disorder. *American Journal of Psychiatry, 158,* 420–426.

McKay, M., Davis, M., & Fanning, P. (1995). *Messages: The communications skills book, second edition.* Oakland, CA: New Harbinger.

McKellar, J. D., Stewart, E., & Humphreys, K. (2003). AA involvement and positive alcohol-related outcomes: Cause, consequence, or just a correlate? *Journal of Consulting and Clinical Psychology, 71,* 302–308.

McKisack, C., & Waller, G. (1996). Why is attendance variable at groups for women with bulimia nervosa?: The role of eating psychopathology and other characteristics. *International Journal of Eating Disorders, 20,* 205–209.

McLean, P. D., Whittal, M. L., Sochting, I., Koch, W. J., Paterson, R., Thordarson, D. S., et al. (2001). Cognitive versus behavior therapy in the group treatment of obsessive–compulsive disorder. *Journal of Consulting and Clinical Psychology, 69,* 205–214.

McMahon, J., & Jones, B. T. (1993a). Negative expectancy and motivation. *Addiction Research, 1,* 145–155.

McMahon, J., & Jones, B. T. (1993b). The Negative Alcohol Expectancy Questionnaire. *Journal of the Association of Nurses on Substance Abuse, 12,* 17.

McMullin, R. E. (2000). *The new handbook of cognitive therapy techniques.* New York: Norton.

Meichenbaum, D. S., & Jaremko, M. E. (Eds.). (1983). *Stress reduction and prevention.* New York: Plenum Press.

Mennin, D. S., & Heimberg, R. G. (2000). The impact of comorbid mood and personality disorders in the cognitive-behavioral treatment of panic disorder. *Clinical Psychology Review, 20,* 339–357.

Mennin, D. S., Heimberg, R. G., & MacAndrew, J. S. (2000). Comorbid generalized anxiety disorder in primary social phobia: Symptom severity, functional impairment, and treatment response. *Journal of Anxiety Disorders, 14,* 325–343.

Menzies, R. G., & Clarke, J. C. (1993). A comparison of *in vivo* and vicarious exposure in the treatment of childhood water phobia. *Behaviour Research and Therapy, 31,* 9–15.

Menzies, R. G., & de Silva, P. (Eds.). (2003). *Obsessive–compulsive disorder: Theory, research, and treatment.* Chichester, UK: Wiley.

Meyer, V. (1966). Modifications of expectations in cases with obsessional rituals. *Behaviour Research and Therapy, 4,* 273–280.

Middelboe, T., Mackeprang, T., Hansson, L., Werdelin, G., Karlsson, H., Bjarnason, O., et al. (2001). The Nordic study on schizophrenic patients living in the community: Subjective needs and perceived help. *European Psychiatry, 16,* 207–214.

Miller, W. R. (2000). Rediscovering fire: Small interventions, large effects. *Psychology of Addictive Behaviors, 14,* 6–18.

Miller, W. R. & Rollnick, S. (2002). *Motivational interviewing: Preparing people to change* (2nd ed.). New York: Guilford Press.

Miller, W. R., & Tonigan, J. S. (1996). Assessing drinkers' motivation for change: The Stages of Change Readiness and Treatment Eagerness Scale (SOCRATES). *Psychology of Addictive Behaviors, 10,* 81–89.

Miller, W. R., Willbourne, P. L., & Hettema, J. E. (2003). What works?: A summary of alcohol treatment outcome research. In R. K. Hester & W. R. Miller (Eds.), *Handbook of alcoholism treatment approaches: Effective alternatives* (3rd ed., pp. 13–63). Boston: Allyn & Bacon.

Millon, T. (1981). *Disorders of personality.* New York: Wiley.

Mineka, S., Davidson, M., Cook, M., & Keir, R. (1984). Observational conditioning of fear in rhesus monkeys. *Journal of Abnormal Psychology, 93,* 355–372.

Mitchell, J. E., Agras, W. S., Wilson, G. T., Halmi, K., Kraemer, H., & Crow, S. (2004). A trial of a relapse prevention strategy in women with bulimia nervosa who respond to cognitive-behavior therapy. *International Journal of Eating Disorders, 35,* 549–555.

Mitchell, J. E., Halmi, K., Wilson, G. T., Agras, W. S., Kraemer, H., & Crow, S. (2002). A randomized secondary treatment study of women with bulimia nervosa who fail to respond to CBT. *International Journal of Eating Disorders, 32,* 271–281.

Monti, P. M., Kadden, R., Rohsenow, D. J., Cooney, N., & Abrams, D. (2002). *Treating alcohol dependence: A coping skills training guide* (2nd ed.). New York: Guilford Press.

Morgan, H., & Raffle, C. (1999). Does reducing safety behaviours improve treatment response in patients with social phobia? *Australia and New Zealand Journal of Psychiatry, 33,* 503–510.

Morgenstern, J. M., Frey, R., McCrady, B. S., Labouvie, E., & Neighbors, C. (1996). Mediators of change in traditional chemical dependency treatment. *Journal of Studies on Alcohol, 57,* 53–64.

Moritz, S., Jacobsen, D., Kloss, M., Fricke, S., Rufer, M., & Hand, I. (2004). Examination of emotional Stroop interference in obsessive–compulsive disorder. *Behaviour Research and Therapy, 42,* 671–682.

Morrison, A. P. (2001). The interpretation of intrusions in psychosis: An integrative cognitive approach to hallucinations and delusions. *Behavioural and Cognitive Psychotherapy, 29,* 257–276.

Morrison, A. P., Haddock, G., & Tarrier, N. (1995). Intrusive thoughts and auditory hallucinations: A cognitive approach. *Behavioural and Cognitive Psychotherapy, 23,* 265–280.

Morrison, N. (2001). Group cognitive therapy: Treatment of choice or sub-optimal option? *Behavioural and Cognitive Psychotherapy, 29,* 311–332.

Motherwell, L., & Shay, J. J. (Eds.). (2004). *Complex dilemmas in group psychotherapy.* New York: Brunner-Routledge.

Mowrer, O. H. (1960). *Learning theory and behavior.* New York: Wiley.

Mueser, K. (1993). Schizophrenia. In A. S. Bellack & M. Hersen (Eds.), *Handbook of behavior therapy in the psychiatric setting: Critical issues in psychiatry* (pp. 269–291). New York: Plenum Press.

Mueser, K. T. (1998). Social skills training and problem solving. In A. S. Bellack & M. Hersen (Eds.), *Comprehensive clinical psychology* (Vol. 6, pp. 183–201). New York: Elsevier.

Mueser, K. T., & Bellack, A. S. (1998). Social skills and social functioning in schizophrenia. In K. T. Mueser & N. Tarrier (Eds.), *Handbook of social functioning in schizophrenia* (pp. 74–96). Needham Heights, MA: Allyn & Bacon.

Murray, C. J., & Lopez, A. D. (1997a). Global mortality, disability, and the contribution of risk factors: Global burden of disease study. *Lancet, 349,* 1436–1442.

Murray, C. J., & Lopez, A. D. (1997b). Alternative projections of mortality and disability by cause, 1990–2020: Global burden of disease study. *Lancet, 349,* 1498–1504.

Nadiga, D. N., Hensley, P. L., & Uhlenhuth, E. H. (2003). Review of the long-term effectiveness of cognitive behavioral therapy compared to medications in panic disorder. *Depression and Anxiety, 17,* 58–64.

Néron, S., Lacroix, D., & Chaput, Y. (1995). Group vs individual cognitive behaviour therapy in panic disorder: An open clinical trial with a six month follow up. *Canadian Journal of Behavioural Science, 27,* 379–392.

Newman, C. F., Leahy, R. L., Beck, A. T., Reilly-Harrington, N. A., & Gyulai, L. (2002). *Bipolar disorder: A cognitive therapy approach.* Washington, DC: American Psychological Association.

Newman, D. L., Moffitt, T. E., Caspi, A., & Silva, P. A. (1998). Comorbid mental disorders: Implications for treatment and sample selection. *Journal of Abnormal Psychology, 107,* 305–311.

Newton, E., Landau, S., Smith, P., Monks, P., Shergill, S., & Wykes, T. (2005). Early psychological intervention for auditory hallucinations: An exploratory study of young people's voices groups. *Journal of Nervous and Mental Disease, 193,* 58–61.

Nezu, A. M., Ronan, G. F., Meadows, E. A., & McClure, K. (2000). *Practitioner's guide to empirically based measures of depression.* New York: Kluwer Academic/Plenum Press.

Noyes, R., Garve, M. J., & Cook, B. (1991). Controlled discontinuation of benzodiazepine treatment for patients with panic disorder. *American Journal of Psychiatry, 148,* 517–523.

Obsessive Compulsive Cognitions Working Group. (1997). Cognitive assessment of obsessive compulsive disorder. *Behaviour Research and Therapy, 35,* 667–681.

O'Connor, K., Freeston, M. H., Gareau, D., Careau, Y., Dufour, M. J., Aardema, F., et al. (2005). Group versus individual treatment in obsessions without compulsions. *Clinical Psychology and Psychotherapy, 12,* 87–96.

O'Connor, K., Todorov, C., Robillard, S., Borgeat, F., & Brault, M. (1999). Cognitive-behaviour therapy and medication in the treatment of obsessive–compulsive disorder: A controlled study. *Canadian Journal of Psychiatry, 44,* 64–71.

Ojehagen, A., & Berglund, M. (1989). Changes of drinking goals in a two-year outpatient alcoholic treatment program. *Addictive Behaviors, 14,* 1–9.

Okasha, A. (2002). Diagnosis of obsessive–compulsive disorder. In M. Maj, N. Sartorius, A. Okasha, & J. Zohar (Eds.), *Obsessive–compulsive disorder* (2nd ed., pp. 1–41). Chichester, UK: Wiley.

Oliver, J. M., & Baumgart, E. P. (1985). The Dysfunctional Attitude Scale: Psychometric properties and relation to depression in an unselected adult population. *Cognitive Therapy and Research, 9,* 161–167.

Olmsted, M. P., Davis, R., Garner, D. M., Rockert, W., Irvine, M. J., & Eagle, M. (1991). Efficacy of a brief group psychoeducational intervention for bulimia nervosa. *Behaviour Research and Therapy, 28,* 71–83.

Olmsted, M. P., Kaplan, A. S., & Rockert, W. (1994). Rate and prediction of relapse in bulimia nervosa. *American Journal of Psychiatry, 151,* 738–743.

Orsillo, M. M. (2001). Measures for social phobia. In M. M. Antony, S. M. Orsillo, & L. Roemer (Eds.), *Practitioner's guide to empirically-based measures of anxiety* (pp. 165–187). New York: Kluwer Academic/Plenum Press.

Öst, L., Sedvall, H., Breitholz, E., Hellström, K., & Lindwall, R. (1995, July). *Cognitive-behavioral treatment for social phobia: Individual, group, and self-administered treatment.* Paper presented at the meeting of the World Congress of Behavioural and Cognitive Therapies, Copenhagen, Denmark.

Otto, M. W., Pollack, M. H., Gould, R. A., Worthington J. J., III, McArdle, E. T., Rosenbaum, J. F., et al. (2000). A comparison of the efficacy of clonazepam and cognitive-behavioral group therapy for the treatment of social phobia. *Journal of Anxiety Disorders, 14,* 345–358.

Otto, M. W., Pollack, M. H., & Maki, K. M. (2000). Empirically supported treatments for panic disorder: Costs, benefits and stepped care. *Journal of Consulting and Clinical Psychology, 68,* 556–563.

Otto, M. W., Pollack, M. H., Penava, S. J., & Zucker, B. G. (1999). Group cognitive-behavior therapy for patients failing to respond to pharmacotherapy for panic disorder: A clinical case series. *Behaviour Research and Therapy, 37,* 763–770.

Otto, M. W., Pollack, M. H., Sachs, G. S., Reiter, S. R., Meltzer-Brody, S., & Rosenbaum, J. F. (1993). Discontinuation of benzodiazepine treatment: Efficacy of cognitive behavioral therapy for patients with panic disorder. *American Journal of Psychiatry, 150,* 1485–1490.

Palmer, A. G., Williams, H., Gorsefield, D., & Adams, M. (1995). CBT in a group format for bipolar affective disorder. *Behavioral and Cognitive Psychotherapy, 23,* 153–168.

Pantelis, C., & Barnes, T. R. (1996). Drug strategies and treatment resistant schizophrenia. *Australia and New Zealand Journal of Psychiatry, 30,* 20–37.

Parikh, S. V., Wasylenki, D., Goering, P., & Wong, J. (1996). Mood disorders: Rural/urban differences in prevalence, health care utilization, and disability in Ontario. *Journal of Affective Disorders, 38,* 57–65.

Patelis-Siotis, I., Young, L. T., Robb, J. C., Marriott, M., Bieling, P. J., Cox, L. C., et al. (2001). Group cognitive behavioral therapy for bipolar disorder: A feasibility and effectiveness study. *Journal of Affective Disorders, 65,* 145–153.

Patterson, G. A., & Forgatch, M. S. (1985). Therapist behavior as a determinant for client noncompliance: A paradox for the behavior modifier. *Journal of Consulting and Clinical Psychology, 53,* 846–851.

Paul, G., & Lentz, R. (1977). *Psychosocial treatment of the chronic mental patient.* Cambridge, MA: Harvard University Press.

Paul, G. L. (1969). Behavior modification research. In C. M. Franks (Ed.), *Behavior therapy: Appraisal and status* (pp. 29–62). New York: McGraw-Hill.

Penn, D., Mueser, K. T., Tarrier, N., Gloege, A., Cather, C., Serrano, D., et al. (2004). Supportive therapy for schizophrenia: Possible mechanisms and implications for adjunctive psychosocial treatments. *Schizophrenia Bulletin, 30,* 101–112.

Pérez-López, J. R., & Woody, S. R. (2001). Memory for facial expressions in social phobia. *Behaviour Research and Therapy, 39,* 967–975.

Perlman, L. M., & Hubbard, B. A. (2000). A self-control skills group for persistent auditory hallucinations. *Cognitive and Behavioral Practice, 7,* 17–21.

Perry, A., Tarrier, N., Morriss, R., McCarthy, E., & Limb, K. (1999). Randomised controlled trial of efficacy of teaching patients with bipolar disorder to identify early symptoms of relapse and obtain treatment. *British Medical Journal, 318,* 149–153.

Perry, J. C., Banon, E., & Lanni, F. (1999). Effectiveness of psychotherapy for personality disorders. *American Journal of Psychiatry, 156*, 1312–1321.

Persons, J. B. (1989). *Cognitive therapy in practice: A case formulation approach*. New York: Norton.

Perugi, G., & Akiskal, H. S. (2002). The soft bipolar spectrum redefined: Focus on the cyclothymic, anxious-sensitive, impulse-dyscontrol, and binge-eating connection of bipolar II and related conditions. *Psychiatric Clinics of North America, 25*, 713–737.

Peterson, C., Semmel, A., von Baeyer, C., Abramson, L. Y., Metalsky, G. I., & Seligman, M. E. P. (1982). The Attributional Style Questionnaire. *Cognitive Therapy and Research, 6*, 287–300.

Peterson, C. B., & Miller, K. B. (2005). Assessment of eating disorders. In S. Wonderlich, J. Mitchell, M. de Zwann, & H. Steiger (Eds.), *Eating disorders review, Part I* (pp. 105–126). Oxon, UK: Radcliffe.

Peterson, R. A., & Reiss, S. (1993). *Anxiety Sensitivity Index—Revised test manual*. Worthington, OH: IDS Publishing Corporation.

Pilling, S., Bebbington, P., Kuipers, E., Garety, P., Geddes, J., Orback, G., et al. (2002). Psychological treatments in schizophrenia: I. Meta-analysis of family intervention and cognitive behaviour therapy. *Psychological Medicine, 32*, 763–782.

Pini, S., Cassano, G. G., Simonini, E., Savino, M., Russo, A., & Montgomery, S. A. (1997). Prevalence of anxiety disorders co-morbidity in bipolar depression, unipolar depression and dysthymia. *Journal of Affective Disorders, 42*, 145–153.

Pinkham, A. E., Gloege, A. T., Flanagan, S., & Penn, D. L. (2004). Group cognitive-behavioral therapy for auditory hallucinations: A pilot study. *Cognitive and Behavioral Practice, 11*, 93–98.

Pinto, A., La Pia, S., Mennella, R., Giorgio, D., & DeSimone, L. (1999). Cognitive behavioral therapy and clozapine for clients with treatment-refractory schizophrenia. *Psychiatric Services, 50*, 901–904.

Piper, W. E. (1994). Client variables. In A. Fuhriman & G. M. Burlingame (Eds.), *Handbook of group psychotherapy: An empirical and clinical synthesis* (pp. 83–113). New York: Wiley.

Polivy, J., & Federoff, I. (1997). Group psychotherapy. In P. E. Garfinkel & D. M. Garner (Eds.), *Handbook of treatment for eating disorders* (2nd ed., pp. 462–475). New York: Guilford Press.

Polivy, J., & Garfinkel, P. E. (1984). Group treatments for specific medical disorders: Anorexia nervosa. In H. B. Roback (Ed.), *Helping patients and their families cope with medical problems* (pp. 60–78). San Francisco: Jossey-Bass.

Pollack, M. H., Otto, M. W., Kaspi, S. P., Hammerness, P. G., & Rosenbaum, J. F. (1994). Cognitive behavior therapy for treatment-refractor panic disorder. *Journal of Clinical Psychiatry, 55*, 200–205.

Prochaska, J. O., & DiClemente, C. C. (1983). Stages and processes of self-change of smoking: Toward an integrative model of change. *Journal of Consulting and Clinical Psychology, 51*, 390–395.

Prochaska, J. O., Velicer, W. F., Rossi, J. S., Goldstein, M. G., Marchus, B., Rakowski, W., Fiore, C., Harlow, L. L. Redding, C. A., Rosenbloom, D. & Rossi, S. R. (1994). Stages of change and decisional balance for 12 problem behaviors. *Health Psychology, 13*, 39–46.

Purdon, C. (1999). Thought suppression and psychopathology. *Behaviour Research and Therapy, 37*, 1029–1054.

Purdon, C., Rowa, K., & Antony, M. M. (in press). Diary records of thought suppression attempts by individuals with obsessive–compulsive disorder. *Behavioral and Cognitive Psychotherapy*.

Rabkin, J., Wagner, G., & Griffin, K. W. (2000). Quality of life measures. In American Psychiatric Association, *Handbook of psychiatric measures*. Washington, DC: American Psychiatric Association.

Rachman, S. (1978). The anatomy of obsessions. *Behavioural Analysis and Modification, 2*, 253–278.

Rachman, S. (1997). A cognitive theory of obsessions. *Behaviour Research and Therapy, 35*, 793–802.

Rachman, S. (1998). A cognitive theory of obsessions: Elaborations. *Behaviour Research and Therapy, 36*, 385–401.

Rachman, S. (2002). A cognitive theory of compulsive checking. *Behaviour Research and Therapy, 40*, 625–639.

Rachman, S., Craske, M. G., Tallman, K., & Solyom, C. (1984). Does escape behaviour strengthen agoraphobic avoidance? A replication. *Behavior Therapy, 17*, 366–384.

Rachman, S., & Shafran, R. (1999). Cognitive distortions: Thought-action fusion. *Clinical Psychology and Psychotherapy, 6*, 80–85.

Radomsky, A. S., Gilchrist, P. T., & Dussault, D. (2003, November). *Repeated checking really does cause memory distrust*. Paper presented at the meeting of the Association for Advancement of Behavior Therapy, Boston, MA.

Radomsky, A. S. & Rachman, S. (1999). Memory bias in obsessive-compulsive disorder (OCD). *Behaviour Research and Therapy, 37*, 605–618.

Ramacciotti, C. E., Coli, E., Paoli, R., Gabriellini, G., Schulte, F., Castrogiovanni, S., Dell'Osso, L., Garfinkel, P. E. (2005). The relationship between binge eating disorder and non-purging bulimia nervosa. *Eating and Weight Disorders, 10*, 8–12.

Rapee, R. M. (1999). *I think they think...Overcoming social phobia (video tape)*. New York: Guilford.

Rapee, R. M., & Heimberg, R. G. (1997). A cognitive-behavioral model of social anxiety in social phobia. *Behaviour Research and Therapy, 35*, 741–756.

Rapee, R. M., & Lim, L. (1992). Discrepancy between self- and observer ratings of performance in social phobics. *Journal of Abnormal Psychology, 101*, 728–731.

Rapee, R. M., & Spence, S. H. (2004). The etiology of social phobia: Empirical evidence and an initial model. *Clinical Psychology Review, 24*, 737–767.

Rector, N. A., & Beck, A. T. (2001). Cognitive Behavioral Therapy for Schizophrenia: An empirical review. *The Journal of Nervous and Mental Disease, 189*, 278–287.

Rector, N. A., Seeman, M. V., & Segal, Z. V. (2003). Cognitive therapy for schizophrenia: A preliminary randomized controlled trial. *Schizophrenia Research, 63*, 1–12.

Regier, D. A., Farmer, M. E., Rae, D. S., Locke, B. Z., Keith, S. J., Judd, L. L., & Goodwin, F. K. (1990). Comorbidity of mental disorder with alcohol and other drug abuse: Results from the Epidemiologic Catchment Area (ECA) Study. *Journal of the American Medical Association, 264*, 2511–2518.

Reiss, S., & McNally, R. J. (1985). The expectancy model of fear. In S. Reiss & R. R. Bootzin (Eds.), *Theoretical issues in behavior therapy* (pp. 107–121). New York: Academic Press.

Reiss, S., Peterson, R. A., Gursky, M., & McNally, R. J. (1986). Anxiety sensitivity, anxiety frequency, and the prediction of fearfulness. *Behaviour Research and Therapy, 24,* 1–8.

Rickels, K., Mangano, R., & Khan, A. (2004). A double-blind, placebo-controlled study of a flexible dose of venlafaxine ER in adult outpatients with generalized social anxiety disorder. *Journal of Clinical Psychopharmacology, 24,* 488–496.

Robb, J. C., Cooke, R. G., Devins, G. M., Young, L. T., & Joffe, R. T. (1997). Quality of life and lifestyle disruption in bipolar disorder—euthymic phase. *Journal of Psychiatric Research, 31,* 509–517.

Robert Wood Johnson Foundation (2001). *Substance abuse: The nation's number one health problem. Key Indicators for Policy Update, 2001.* Princeton: Author.

Robinson, L. A., Berman, J. S., & Neimeyer, R. A. (1990). Psychotherapy for the treatment of depression: A comprehensive review of controlled outcome research. *Psychological Bulletin, 108,* 30–49.

Rodebaugh, T. L., Holaway, R. M., & Heimberg, R. G. (2004). The treatment of social anxiety disorder. *Clinical Psychology Review, 24,* 883–908.

Rollnick, S., Heather, N., Gold, R., & Hall, W. (1992). Development of a short "readiness to change" questionnaire for use in brief, opportunistic interventions among excessive drinkers. *British Journal of Addiction, 87,* 743–754.

Rollnick, S., Mason, P., & Butler, C. (1999). *Health behavior change: A guide for practitioners.* New York: Churchill Livingstone.

Rose, D. T., Abramson, L. Y., Hodulik, C. J., Halberstadt, L., & Leff, G. (1994). Heterogeneity of cognitive style among depressed inpatients. *Journal of Abnormal Psychology, 103,* 419–429.

Rose, S. D., Tolman, R., & Tallant, S. (1985). Group process in cognitive-behavioral therapy. *Behavior Therapist, 8,* 71–75.

Rosenthal, R. N., & Westreich, L. (1999). Treatment of persons with dual diagnosis of substance use disorder and other psychological problems. In B. S. McCrady & E. E. Epstein (Eds.), *Addictions: A comprehensive guidebook* (pp. 439–476). New York: Oxford University Press.

Rosqvist, J. (2005). *Exposure treatments for anxiety disorders: A practitioner's guide to concepts, methods, and evidence-based practice.* New York: Routledge.

Rotgers, F. (2003). Cognitive behavioral theories of substance abuse. In F. Rotgers, J. Morgenstern, & S. T. Walters (Eds.), *Treating substance abuse: Theory and technique* (2nd ed., pp. 166–189). New York: Guilford Press.

Rotgers, F., & Graves, G. (2004). *Motivational enhancement treatment manual, version 3.0.* Available from authors.

Rotgers, F., Kern, M. F., & Hoeltzel, R. (2002). *Responsible drinking: A Moderation Management approach for problem drinkers.* Oakland, CA: New Harbinger.

Rotgers, F., & Kishline, A. (1999). Moderation Management®: A support group for persons who want to reduce their drinking, but not necessarily abstain. *International Journal of Self-Help and Self-Care, 1,* 145–158.

Rowa, K., Antony, M. M., & Swinson, R. P. (in press). Exposure and ritual prevention. In M. M. Antony, C. Purdon, & L. J. Summerfeldt (Eds.), *Psychological treatment of OCD: Fundamentals and beyond.* Washington, DC: American Psychological Association.

Rowa, K., Bieling, P. J., & Segal, Z. V. (2005). Improving outcomes in cognitive-behavioral treatment of depression. In M. M. Antony, D. R. Ledley, & R. G. Heimberg (Eds.), *Improving outcomes and preventing relapse in cognitive-*

behavioral therapy: A clinical handbook (pp. 204–245). New York: Guilford Press.

Rowe, M. K., & Craske, M. G. (1998). Effects of varied-stimulus exposure training on fear reduction and return of fear. *Behaviour Research and Therapy, 36,* 719–734.

Roy-Byrne, P., Lee-Benner, K., & Yager, J. (1984). Group therapy for bulimia. *International Journal of Eating Disorders, 3,* 97–116.

Roy-Byrne, P. P., Stein, M. B., Russo, J., Mercier, E., Thomas, R., McQuaid, J., et al. (1999). Panic disorder in the primary care setting: Comorbidity, disability, service utilization, and treatment. *Journal of Clinical Psychiatry, 60,* 492–499.

Safran, J. D., & Segal, Z. V. (1990). *Interpersonal process in cognitive therapy.* New York: Basic Books.

Salkovskis, P. M. (1985). Obsessional–compulsive problems: A cognitive-behavioural analysis. *Behaviour Research and Therapy, 23,* 571–583.

Salkovskis, P. M. (1998). Psychological approaches to the understanding of obsessional problems. In R. P. Swinson, M. M. Antony, S. Rachman, & M. A. Richter (Eds.), *Obsessive–compulsive disorder: Theory, research, and treatment* (pp. 33–50). New York: Guilford Press.

Salkovskis, P. M., Clark, D. M., Hackmann, A., Wells, A., & Geldner, M. G. (1999). An experimental investigation of the role of safety-seeking behaviors in the maintenance of panic disorder with agoraphobia. *Behaviour Research and Therapy, 37,* 559–574.

Salkovskis, P. M., & Forrester, E. (2002). Responsibility. In R. O. Frost & G. Steketee (Eds.), *Cognitive approaches to obsessions and compulsions: Theory, assessment, and treatment* (pp. 45–61). Oxford, UK: Elsevier.

Sanchez-Craig, M., & Lei, H. (1986). Disadvantages of imposing the goal of abstinence on problem drinkers: An empirical study. *British Journal of Addiction, 81,* 505–512.

Satterfield, J. M. (1994). Integrating group dynamics and cognitive-behavioral groups: A hybrid model. *Clinical Psychology: Science and Practice, 1,* 185–196.

Schmidt, N. B. (1999). Prospective evaluations of anxiety sensitivity. In S. Taylor (Ed.), *Anxiety sensitivity: Theory, research, and treatment of the fear of anxiety* (pp. 217–235). Mahwah, NJ: Erlbaum.

Schmidt, N. B., & Bates, M. J. (2003). Evaluation of a pathoplastic relationship between anxiety sensitivity and panic disorder. *Anxiety, Stress and Coping: An International Journal, 16,* 17–30.

Schmidt, N. B., Lerew, D. R., & Jackson, R. J. (1997). The role of anxiety sensitivity in the pathogenesis of panic: Prospective evaluation of spontaneous panic attacks during acute stress. *Journal of Abnormal Psychology, 106,* 355–364.

Schmidt, N. B., McCreary, B. T., Trakowski, J., Santiago, H., Woolaway-Bickel, K., & Ialongo, N. (2003). Effects of cognitive-behavioral treatment on physical health status in patients with panic disorder. *Behavior Therapy, 34,* 49–63.

Schmidt, N. B., & Woolaway-Bickel, K. (2000). The effects of treatment compliance on outcome in cognitive-behavioral therapy for panic disorder: Quality versus quantity. *Journal of Consulting and Clinical Psychology, 68,* 13–18.

Schmidt, N. B., Woolaway-Bickel, K., Trakowski, J., Santiago, H., Storey, J., Koselka, M., et al. (2000). Dismantling cognitive-behavioral treatment for panic disorder: Questioning the utility of breathing retraining. *Journal of Consulting and Clinical Psychology, 68,* 417–424.

Schmidt, N. B., Woolaway-Bickel, K., Trakowski, J. H., Santiago, H. T., & Vasey, M. (2002). Antidepressant discontinuation in the context of cognitive behavioral treatment for panic disorder. *Behaviour Research and Therapy, 40,* 67–73.

Scholing, A., & Emmelkamp, P. M. (1993). Exposure with and without cognitive therapy for generalized social phobia: Effects of individual and group treatment. *Behaviour Research and Therapy, 31,* 667–681.

Schuckit, M. A., Smith, T. L., Tipp, J. E. (1997). The Self-Rating of the Effects of Alcohol (SRE) form as a retrospective measure of the risk for alcoholism. *Addiction, 92,* 979–988.

Schwannauer, M. (2004). Cognitive behavioural therapy for bipolar affective disorder. In M. Power (Ed.), *Mood disorders: A handbook of science and practice* (pp. 259–273). Chichester, UK: Wiley.

Scott, J. (2001). Cognitive therapy as an adjunct to medication in bipolar disorder. *British Journal of Psychiatry Suppl., 41,* s164–s168.

Scott, J., Garland, A., & Moorhead, S. (2001). A pilot study of cognitive therapy in bipolar disorders. *Psychological Medicine, 31,* 459–467.

Scott, J., Stanton, B., Garland, A., & Ferrier, I. N. (2000). Cognitive vulnerability in patients with bipolar disorder. *Psychological Medicine, 30,* 467–472.

Scott, M. J., & Stradling, S. G. (1990). Group cognitive therapy for depression produces clinically significant reliable change in community-based settings. *Behavioural Psychotherapy, 18,* 1–19.

Segal, Z. V., Williams, J. M. G., & Teasdale, J. D. (2002). *Mindfulness-based cognitive therapy for depression: A new approach to preventing relapse.* New York: Guilford Press.

Sensky, R., Turkington, D., Kingdon, D., Scott, J. L., Scott, J., Siddle, R., et al. (2000). A randomized controlled trial of cognitive-behavioral therapy for persistent symptoms in schizophrenia resistant to medication. *Archives of General Psychiatry, 57,* 165–172.

Serfaty, M. A., Turkington, D., Heap, M., Ledsham, L., & Jolley, E. (1999). Cognitive therapy versus dietary counseling in the outpatient treatment of anorexia nervosa: Effects of the treatment phase. *European Eating Disorders Review, 7,* 334–350.

Shafran, R., & de Silva, P. (2003). Cognitive-behavioral models. In J. T. Treasure, U. Schmidt, & E. van Furth (Eds.), *Handbook of eating disorders* (2nd ed., pp. 121–138). West Sussex, UK: Wiley.

Shafran, R., Thordarson, D. S., & Rachman, S. (1996). Thought–action fusion in obsessive–compulsive disorder. *Journal of Anxiety Disorders, 10,* 379–391.

Shapira, N. A., Ward, H. E., Mandoki, M., Murphy, T. K., Yang, M. C. K., Blier, P., et al. (2004). A double-blind, placebo-controlled trial of olanzapine addition in fluoxetine-refractory obsessive–compulsive disorder. *Biological Psychiatry, 550,* 553–555.

Sharp, D. M., & Power, K. G. (1999). Predicting treatment outcome for panic disorder and agoraphobia in primary care. *Clinical Psychology and Psychotherapy, 6,* 336–348.

Sharp, D. M., Power, K. G., & Swanson, V. (2004). A comparison of the efficacy and acceptability of group versus individual cognitive behaviour therapy in the treatment of panic disorder and agoraphobia in primary care. *Clinical Psychology and Psychotherapy, 11,* 73–82.

Shear, M. K., Brown, T. A., Barlow, D. H., Money, R., Sholomskas, D. E., Woods, S.

W., et al. (1997). Multicenter collaborative panic disorder severity scale. *American Journal of Psychiatry, 154,* 1571–1575.

Sheehan, D. V. (1983). *The anxiety disease.* New York: Scribner.

Sheehan, D. V., Lecrubier, Y., Sheehan, K. H., Amorim, P., Janavs, J., Weiller, E., et al. (1998). The Mini-International Neuropsychiatric Interview (M. I. N. I.): The development and validation of a structured diagnostic psychiatric interview for DSM-IV and ICD-10. *Journal of Clinical Psychiatry, 59*(Suppl. 20), 22–23, 34–57.

Sheikh, J. I., Leskin, G. A., & Klein, D. F. (2002). Gender differences in panic disorder: Findings from the National Comorbidity Survey. *American Journal of Psychiatry, 159,* 55–58.

Siris, S. G. (2000). Depression in schizophrenia: Perspective on the era of atypical antipsychotic agents. *American Journal of Psychiatry, 157,* 1379–1389.

Slade, M., Phelan, M., Thornicroft, G., & Parkman, S. (1996). The Camberwell Assessment of Need (CAN): Comparison of assessments by staff and patients of the needs of the severely mentally ill. *Social Psychiatry and Psychiatric Epidemiology, 31,* 109–113.

Slade, P. D. (1982). Towards a functional analysis of anorexia nervosa and bulimia nervosa. *British Journal of Clinical Psychology, 21,* 167–179.

Slade, P. D., & Bentall, R. P. (1988). *Sensory deception: A scientific analysis of hallucination.* Baltimore: Johns Hopkins University Press.

Smith, T. E., & Docherty, J. P. (1998). Standards of care and clinical algorithms for treating schizophrenia. *Psychiatric Clinics of North America, 21,* 203–220.

Spiegel, D. A., Bruce, . J., Gregg, S. F., & Nuzzarello, A. (1994). Does cognitive behavior therapy assist slow-taper alprazolam discontinuation in panic disorder? *American Journal of Psychiatry, 151,* 876–881.

Spitzer, R. L., Williams, J. B., Kroenke, K., Linzer, M., deGruy, F. V., III, Hahn, S. R., et al. (1994). Utility of a new procedure for diagnosing mental disorders in primary care: The PRIME-MD 1000 study. *Journal of the American Medical Association, 272,* 1749–1756.

Stangier, U., Heidenreich, T., Peitz, M., Lauterbach, W., & Clark, D. M. (2003). Cognitive therapy for social phobia: Individual versus group treatment. *Behaviour Research and Therapy, 41,* 991–1007.

Stanley, M. A., & Averill, P. M. (1998). Psychosocial treatments for obsessive-compulsive disorder: Clinical applications. In R. P. Swinson, M. M. Antony, S. Rachman, & M. A. Richter (Eds.), *Obsessive–compulsive disorder: Theory, research and treatment* (pp. 277–297). New York: Guilford Press.

Steketee, G., Frost, R. O., Wincze, J., Greene, K. A. I., & Douglass, H. (2000). Group and individual treatment of compulsive hoarding: A pilot study. *Behavioural and Cognitive Psychotherapy, 28,* 259–268.

Steketee, G., & Pruyn, N. A. (1998). Families of individuals with obsessive–compulsive disorder. In R. P. Swinson, M. M. Antony, S. Rachman, & M. A. Richter (Eds.), *Obsessive–compulsive disorder: Theory, research, and treatment* (pp. 120–140). New York: Guilford Press.

Steketee, G., Quay, S., & White, K. (1991). Religion and guilt in OCD patients. *Journal of Anxiety Disorders, 5,* 359–367.

Steketee, G. S. (1993). *Treatment of obsessive compulsive disorder.* New York: Guilford Press.

Stern, R., & Marks, I. (1973). Brief and prolonged flooding: A comparison in agoraphobic patients. *Archives of General Psychiatry, 28,* 270–276.

Stompe, T., Friedman, A., Ortwein, G., Strobl, R., Chaudhry, H. R., Najam, N., et al. (1999). Comparison of delusions among schizophrenics in Austria and in Pakistan. *Psychopathology, 32,* 225–234.

Stone, M. (1983). Psychotherapy with schizotypal borderline patients. *Journal of the American Academy of Psychoanalysis, 11,* 87–111.

Stopa, L., & Clark, D. M. (1993). Cognitive processes in social phobia. *Behaviour Research and Therapy, 31,* 255–267.

Stopa, L., & Clark, D. M. (2000). Social phobia and interpretation of social events. *Behaviour Research and Therapy, 38,* 273–283.

Stravynski, A., Bond, S., & Amado, D. (2004). Cognitive causes of social phobia: A critical appraisal. *Clinical Psychology Review, 24,* 421–440.

Striegel-Moore, R. H., & Franko, D. L. (2003). The epidemiology of binge eating disorder. *International Journal of Eating Disorders, 34*(Suppl.), S19–S29.

Striegel-Moore, R. H., Silberstein, L. R., & Rodin, J. (1986). Toward an understanding of risk factors for bulimia. *American Psychologist, 41,* 146–163.

Summerfeldt, L. J. (2001). Obsessive–compulsive disorder: A brief overview and guide to assessment. In M. M. Antony, S. M. Orsillo, & L. Roemer (Eds.), *Practitioner's guide to empirically-based measures of anxiety* (pp. 211–218). New York: Kluwer Academic/Plenum Press.

Summerfeldt, L. J., & Antony, M. M. (2002). Structured and semistructured interviews. In M. M. Antony & D. M. Barlow (Eds.), *Handbook of assessment and treatment planning for psychological disorders* (pp. 3–37). Toronto: Guilford Press.

Summerfeldt, L. J., & Endler, N. S. (1998). Examining the evidence for anxiety-related cognitive biases in obsessive–compulsive disorder. *Journal of Anxiety Disorders, 12,* 579–598.

Swales, M., Heard, H. L., & Williams, J. M. G. (2000). Linehan's dialectical behavior therapy (DBT) for borderline personality disorder: Overview and adaptation. *Journal of Mental Health, 9,* 7–23.

Tarrier, N. (1987). An investigation of residual psychotic symptoms in discharged schizophrenic patients. *British Journal of Clinical Psychology, 26,* 141–143.

Tarrier, N., Beckett, R., Harwood, S., Baker, A., Yusupoff, L., & Ugarteburu, I. (1993). A trial of two cognitive-behavioural methods of treating drug resistant residual psychotic symptoms in schizophrenic patients: I. Outcome. *British Journal of Psychiatry, 162,* 524–532.

Tarrier, N., Harwood, S., Yusupoff, L., Beckett, R., & Baker, A. (1990). Coping strategy enhancement (CSE): A method of treating residual schizophrenic symptoms. *Behavioural Psychotherapy, 18,* 283–293.

Tarrier, N., Kinney, C., McCarthy, E., Humphreys, L., Wittkowski, A., & Morris, J. (2000). Two year follow-up of cognitive-behaviour therapy and supportive counseling in the treatment of persistent positive symptoms in chronic schizophrenia. *Journal of Consulting and Clinical Psychology, 68,* 917–922.

Tarrier, N., Kinney, C., McCarthy, E., Wittkowski, A., Yusupoff, L.,Gledhill, A., et al. (2001). Are some types of psychotic symptoms more responsive to cognitive-behavior therapy? *Behavioural and Cognitive Psychotherapy, 29,* 45–55.

Tarrier, N., Wittkowski, A., Kinney, C., McCarthy, E., Morris, J., & Humphreys, L.

(1999). Durability of the effects of cognitive-behavioral therapy in the treatment of chronic schizophrenia: 12-month follow-up. *British Journal of Psychiatry, 174,* 500–504.

Tarrier, N., & Wykes, T. (2004). Cognitive-behavioural treatments of psychosis: Clinical trials and methodological issues in clinical psychology. In S. Day, S. Green, & D. Machin (Eds.), *Textbook of clinical trials* (pp. 273–296). Chichester, UK: Wiley.

Tarrier, N., Yusupoff, L., Kinney, C., McCarthy, E., Gledhill, A., & Haddock, G. (1998). Randomised controlled trial of intensive cognitive behavior therapy for patients with chronic schizophrenia. *British Medical Journal, 317,* 303–307.

Tasca, G., Flynn, C., & Bissada, H. (2002). Comparison of group climate in an eating disorders partial hospital group and a psychiatric partial hospital group. *International Journal of Group Psychotherapy, 52,* 409–417.

Tata, P. R., Leibowitz, J. A., Prunty, M. J., Cameron, M., & Pickering, A. D. (1996). Attentional bias in obsessional compulsive disorder. *Behaviour Research and Therapy, 34,* 53–60.

Taylor, S. (1996). Meta-analysis of cognitive behavioral treatment for social phobia. *Journal of Behavior Therapy and Experimental Psychiatry, 27,* 1–9.

Taylor, S. (2000). *Understanding and treating panic disorder: Cognitive behavioural approaches.* New York: Wiley.

Taylor, S., Thordarson, D. S., & Söchting, I. (2002). Obsessive–compulsive disorder. In M. M. Antony & D. H. Barlow (Eds.), *Handbook of assessment and treatment planning for psychological disorders* (pp. 182–214). New York: Guilford Press.

Telch, C. F., & Agras, W. S. (1992). *Cognitive behavioral therapy for binge eating disorder therapist manual.* Stanford, CA: Stanford University Press.

Telch, M. J., Lucas, J. A., Schmidt, N. B., Hanna, H. H., Jaimez, T. L., & Lucas, R. A. (1993). Group cognitive-behavioral treatment of panic disorder. *Behaviour Research and Therapy, 31,* 279–287.

Telch, M. J., Schmidt, N. B., LaNae Jaimez, T., Jacquin, K. M., & Harrington, P. J. (1995). Impact of cognitive-behavioral treatment on quality of life in panic disorder patients. *Journal of Consulting and Clinical Psychology, 63,* 823–830.

Thelen, M. H., Farmer, J., Wonderlich, S., & Smith, M. (1991). A revision of the Bulimia Test: The BULIT-R. *Psychological Assessment, 3,* 119–124.

Thompson, L. W., Powers, D. V., Coon, D. W., Takagi, K., McKibbin, C., & Gallagher-Thompson, D. (2000). Older adults. In J. R. White & A. S. Freeman (Eds.), *Cognitive-behavioral group therapy: For specific problems and populations* (pp. 235–261). Washington, DC: American Psychological Association.

Tien, A. Y. (1991). Distributions of hallucinations in the population. *Social Psychiatry and Psychiatric Epidemiology, 26,* 287–292.

Tiffany, S. T. (1990). A cognitive model of drug urges and drug-use behavior: Role of automatic and non-automatic processes. *Psychological Review, 97,* 147–168.

Tolin, D. F., Abramowitz, J. S., Brigidi, B. D., & Foa, E. B. (2003). Intolerance of uncertainty in obsessive–compulsive disorder. *Journal of Anxiety Disorders, 17,* 233–242.

Tolin, D. F., Woods, C. M., & Abramowitz, J. S. (2003). Relationship between obsessive beliefs and obsessive–compulsive symptoms. *Cognitive Therapy and Research, 27,* 657–669.

Tollefson, G. D., & Sanger, T. M. (1999). Anxious-depressive symptoms in schizophrenia: A new treatment target for pharmacotherapy? *Schizophrenia Research, 35*, S13–S21.

Toni, C., Perugi, G., Frare, F., Mata, B., Voitale, B., Mengali, F., et al. (2000). A prospective naturalistic study of 326 panic-agoraphobic patients treated with antidepressants. *Pharamacopsychiatry, 33*, 121–131.

Tsao, J. C. I., & Craske, M. G. (2000). Timing of treatment and return of fear: Effects of massed, uniform-, and expanding-spaced exposure schedules. *Behavior Therapy, 31*, 479–497.

Tsao, J. C. I., Mystkowski, J. L., Zucker, B., & Craske, M. G. (2002). Effects of cognitive-behavioral therapy for panic disorder on comorbid conditions: Replication and extension. *Behavior Therapy, 33*, 493–509.

Turgeon, L., Marchand, A., & Dupuis, G. (1998). Clinical features in panic disorder with agoraphobia: A comparison of men and women. *Journal of Anxiety Disorders, 12*, 539–553.

Turk, C. L., Coles, M., & Heimberg, R. G. (2002). Psychotherapy for social phobia. In D. J. Stein & E. Hollander (Eds.), *Textbook of anxiety disorders* (pp. 323–339). Washington, DC: American Psychiatric Press.

Turkington, D., Kingdon, D., & Turner, T. (2002). Effectiveness of a brief cognitive-behavioural therapy intervention in the treatment of schizophrenia. *British Journal of Psychiatry, 180*, 523–527.

Turner, S. M., Beidel, D. C., Cooley, M. R., & Woody, S. R. (1994). A multicomponent behavioral treatment for social phobia: Social effectiveness therapy. *Behaviour Research and Therapy, 32*, 381–390.

Turner, S. M., Beidel, D. C., Wolff, P. L., Spaulding, S., & Jacob, R. G. (1996). Clinical features affecting treatment outcome in social phobia. *Behaviour Research and Therapy, 34*, 795–804.

Turner, S. M., Johnson, M. R., Beidel, D. C., Heiser, N. A., & Lydiard, R. B. (2003). The Social Thoughts and Beliefs Scale: A new inventory for assessing cognitions in social phobia. *Psychological Assessment, 15*, 384–391.

Uren, T. H., Szabó, M., & Lovibond P. F. (2004). Probability and cost estimates for social and physical outcomes in social phobia and panic disorder. *Journal of Anxiety Disorders, 18*, 481–498.

van Balkom, A. J. L. M., & van Dyck, R. (1998). Combination treatments for OCD. In R. P. Swinson, M. M. Antony, S. Rachman, & M. A. Richter (Eds.), *Obsessive–compulsive disorder: Theory, research, and treatment* (pp. 349–366). Guilford Press.

van Balkom, A. J., van Oppen, P., Vermeulen, A. W., & van Dyck, R. (1994). A meta-analysis on the treatment of obsessive–compulsive disorder: A comparison of antidepressants, behavior, and cognitive therapy. *Clinical Psychology Review, 14*, 359–381.

van Dam-Baggen, R., & Kraaimaat, F. (2000). Group social skills training or cognitive group therapy as the clinical treatment of choice for generalized social phobia? *Journal of Anxiety Disorders, 14*, 437–451.

van Hout, W. J. P. J., & Emmelkamp, P. M. G. (1994). Overprediction of fear in panic disorder patients with agoraphobia: Does the (mis)match model generalize to exposure *in vivo* therapy? *Behaviour Research and Therapy, 32*, 723–734.

Van Noppen, B., Steketee, G., McCorkle, B. H., & Pato, M. (1997). Group and multifamily behavioral treatment for obsessive compulsive disorder: A pilot study. *Journal of Anxiety Disorders, 11*, 431–446.

van Oppen, P., de Haan, E., van Balkom, A. J. L. M., Spinhoven, P., Hoogduin, K., & van Dyck, R. (1995). Cognitive therapy and exposure *in vivo* in the treatment of obsessive compulsive disorder. *Behaviour Research and Therapy, 33*, 379–390.

van Os, J., Hanssen, M., & Vollebergh, W. (2001). Prevalence of psychotic disorder and community level psychotic symptoms. *Archives of General Psychiatry, 58*, 663–668.

van Velzen, C. J. M., Emmelkamp, P. M. G., & Scholing, A. (1997). The impact of personality disorders on behavioral treatment outcome for social phobia. *Behaviour Research and Therapy, 35*, 889–900.

Velasquez, M. M., Maurer, G. G., Crouch, C., & DiClemente, C. C. (2001). *Group treatment for substance abuse: A stages-of-change therapy manual.* New York: Guilford Press.

Ventura, J., Green, M., Shaner, A., & Liberman, R. P. (1993). Training and quality assurance with the Brief Psychiatric Rating Scale. *International Journal of Methods in Psychiatric Research, 3*, 221–244.

Vitousek, K. B., & Ewald, L. S. (1993). Self-representation in eating disorders: A cognitive perspective. In Z. V. Segal & S. J. Blatt (Eds.), *The self in emotional distress: Cognitive and psychodynamic perspectives* (p. 221–266). New York: Guilford Press.

Vitousek, K. B., & Hollon, S. D. (1990). The investigation of schematic content and processing eating disorders. *Cognitive Therapy and Research, 14*, 191–214.

Wade, W. A., Treat, T. A., & Stuart, G. L. (1998). Transporting an empirically supported treatment for panic disorder to a service clinic setting: A benchmarking strategy. *Journal of Consulting and Clinical Psychology, 66*, 231–239.

Weissman, A. N., & Beck, A. T. (1978, November). *Development and validation of the Dysfunctional Attitude Scale.* Paper presented at the annual meeting of the Association for the Advancement of Behavior Therapy, Chicago, IL.

Weissman, M. M. (1991). Panic disorder: Impact on quality of life. *Journal of Clinical Psychiatry, 52*, 6–9.

Weissman, M. M. (2000). Social Adjustment Scale (SAS). In American Psychiatric Association (Ed.), *Handbook of psychiatric measures* (pp. 109–113). Washington, DC: American Psychiatric Association.

Weissman, M. M., & Bothwell, S. (1976). Assessment of social adjustment by patient self-report. *Archives of General Psychiatry, 33*, 1111–1115.

Wells, A. (1995). Meta-cognition and worry: A cognitive model of generalized anxiety disorder. *Behavioural and Cognitive Psychotherapy, 23*, 301–320.

Wells, A., Clark, D. M., Salkovskis, P., Ludgate, J., Hackman, A., & Gelder, M. (1995). Social phobia: The role of in-situation safety behaviors in maintaining anxiety and negative beliefs. *Behavior Therapy, 26*, 153–161.

Wells, A., & Papageorgiou, C. (1999). The observer perspective: Biased imagery in social phobia, agoraphobia, and blood/injury phobia. *Behaviour Research and Therapy, 37*, 653–658.

Wenzel, A., & Holt, C. S. (2002). Memory bias against threat in social phobia. *British Journal of Clinical Psychology, 41*, 73–79.

White, J. R. (2000). Depression. In J. R. White & A. S. Freeman (Eds.), *Cognitive-behavioral group therapy: For specific problems and populations* (pp. 29–61). Washington, DC: American Psychological Association.

White J. R., & Freeman A. S. (Eds.). (2000). *Cognitive-behavioral group therapy: For specific problems and populations.* Washington, DC: American Psychological Association.

Whittal, M. L., & McLean, P. D. (2002). Group cognitive behavioral therapy for obsessive compulsive disorder. In R. O. Frost & G. Steketee (Eds.), *Cognitive approaches to obsessions and compulsions: Theory, assessment, and treatment* (pp. 417–433). Oxford, UK: Elsevier.

Whittal, M. L., Otto, M. W., & Hong, J. J. (2001). Cognitive-behavior therapy for discontinuation of SSRI treatment of panic disorder: A case series. *Behaviour Research and Therapy, 39,* 939–945.

Whittal, M. L., Thordarson, D. S., & McLean, P. D. (2005). Treatment of obsessive–compulsive disorder: Cognitive behavior therapy vs. exposure and response prevention. *Behaviour Research and Therapy, 43,* 1559–1576.

Wiersma, D., Nienhuis, F. J., & Slooff, C. J. (1998). Natural course of schizophrenic disorders: A 15 year follow-up of a Dutch incidence cohort. *Schizophrenia Bulletin, 24,* 75–85.

Wilfley, D. E., Friedman, M. A., Dounchis, J. Z., Stein, R. I., Welch, R., & Ball, S. A. (2000). Comorbid psychopathology in binge eating disorder: Relation to eating disorder severity at baseline and following treatment. *Journal of Consulting and Clinical Psychology, 68,* 296–305.

Wilfley, D. E., Schwartz, M., Spurrell, E. B., & Fairburn, C. G. (2000). Using the Eating Disorder Examination to identify the specific psychopathology of binge eating disorder. *International Journal of Eating Disorders, 27,* 259–269.

Wilfley, D. E., Welch, R. R., Stein, R. I., Spurrell, E. B., Cohen, L. R., Saelens, B. E., et al. (2002). A randomized comparison of group cognitive-behavioral therapy and group interpersonal psychotherapy for the treatment of overweight individuals with binge-eating disorder. *Archives of General Psychiatry, 59,* 713–721.

Wilhelm, S., McNally, R. J., Baer, L., & Florin, I. (1996). Directed forgetting in obsessive–compulsive disorder. *Behaviour Research and Therapy, 34,* 633–641.

Williams, J. B. W. (2000). Mental health status, functioning, and disabilities measures. In American Psychiatric Association (Eds.), *Handbook of psychiatric measures* (pp. 93–100). Washington, DC: American Psychiatric Association.

Williams, K. E., & Chambless, D. L. (1990). The relationship between therapist characteristics and outcome of *in vivo* exposure treatment for agoraphobia. *Behavior Therapy, 21,* 111–116.

Wilson, G. T. (1999). Cognitive behavior therapy for eating disorders: Progress and problems. *Behaviour Research and Therapy, 37*(Suppl. 1), S79–S97.

Wilson, G. T., & Fairburn, C. G. (2002). Treatments for eating disorders. In P. E. Nathan & J. M. Gorman (Eds.), *A guide to treatments that work* (2nd ed., pp. 559–592). New York: Oxford University Press.

Wilson, G. T., Fairburn, C. G., & Agras, W. S. (1997). Cognitive-behavioral therapy for bulimia nervosa. In D. M. Garner & P. E. Garfinkel (Eds.), *Handbook of treatment for eating disorders* (2nd ed., pp. 67–93). New York: Guilford Press.

Wiseman, C. V., Sunday, S. R., Klapper, F., Klein, M., & Halmi, K. A. (2002). Short-term group CBT versus psycho-education on an inpatient eating disorder unit. *Eating Disorders: The Journal of Treatment and Prevention, 10,* 313–320.

Wlazlo, Z., Schroeder-Hartwig, K., Hand, I., Kaiser, G., & Münchau, N. (1990). Exposure in vivo vs. social skills training for social phobia: Long term outcome and differential effects. *Behaviour Research and Therapy, 28,* 181–193.

Wolpe, J. (1958). *Psychotherapy by reciprocal inhibition.* Stanford, CA: Stanford University Press.

Woods, C. M., Chambless, D. L., & Steketee, G. (2002). Homework compliance and behavior therapy outcome for panic with agoraphobia and obsessive compulsive disorder. *Cognitive Behaviour Therapy, 31,* 88–95.

Woods, C. M., Vevea, J. L., Chambless, D. L. ., & Bayen, U. J. (2002). Are compulsive checkers impaired in memory?: A meta-analytic review. *Clinical Psychology: Science and Practice, 9,* 353–366.

Woody, S. R., Detweiler-Bedell, J., Teachman, B. A., & O'Hearn, T. (2003). *Treatment planning in psychotherapy: Taking the guesswork out of clinical care.* New York: Guilford Press.

Woody, S. R., Taylor, S., McLean, P. D., & Koch, W. J. (1998). Cognitive specificity in panic and depression: Implications for comorbidity. *Cognitive Therapy and Research, 22,* 427–443.

World Health Organization. (1993). *International classification of diseases* (10th ed.). Geneva: Author.

Wykes, T., Parr, A., & Landau, S. (1999). Group treatment of auditory hallucinations: Exploratory study of effectiveness. *British Journal of Psychiatry, 175,* 180–185.

Yalom, I. D. (1970). *The theory and practice of group psychotherapy.* New York: Basic Books.

Yalom, I. D. (1985). *The theory and practice of group psychotherapy* (3rd ed.). New York: Basic Books.

Yalom, I. D. (1995). *The theory and practice of group psychotherapy* (4th ed.). New York: Basic Books.

Yonkers, K. A., & Samson, J. (2000). Mood disorders measures. In American Psychiatric Association (Ed.), *Handbook of psychiatric measures* (pp. 515–548). Washington, DC: American Psychiatric Association.

Yonkers, K. A., Zlotnick, C., Allsworth, J., Warshaw, M., Shea, T., & Keller, M. B. (1998). Is the course of panic disorder the same in women and men? *American Journal of Psychiatry, 155,* 596–602.

Young, J. E. (1990). *Cognitive therapy for personality disorders: A schema-focused approach* (3rd ed.). Sarasota, FL: Professional Resource Press.

Young, R. C., Biggs, J. T., Ziegler, V. E., & Meyer, D. A. (1978). A rating scale for mania: Reliability, validity, and sensitivity. *British Journal of Psychiatry, 133,* 429–435.

Zaretsky, A. E., Segal, Z. V., & Gemar, M. (1999). Cognitive therapy for bipolar depression: A pilot study. *Canadian Journal of Psychiatry, 44,* 491–494.

Zucker, B. G., Craske, M. G., Barrios, V., & Holguin, M. (2002). Thought–action fusion: Can it be corrected? *Behaviour Research and Therapy, 40,* 653–664.

Zung, W. W. K. (1965). A self-rating depression scale. *Archives of General Psychiatry, 12,* 63–70.

Index